T0331123

Spider Behaviour

Flexibility and Versatility

Spiders are often underestimated as suitable behavioural models because it is generally believed that, due to their small brains, their behaviour is innate and mostly invariable. Challenging this assumption, this fascinating book shows that spiders display surprising cognitive abilities, changing their behaviour to suit their situational needs. The team of authors unravels the considerable intra-specific as well as intra-individual variability and plasticity in different behaviours, ranging from foraging and web building to communication and courtship. An introductory chapter on spider biology, systematics and evolution provides the reader with the necessary background information to understand the behaviours discussed, and helps to place them into an evolutionary context.

Highlighting an underexplored area of behaviour, this book will provide new ideas for behavioural researchers and students unfamiliar with spiders, as well as a valuable resource for those already working in this intriguing field.

MARIE ELISABETH HERBERSTEIN is an Associate Professor in the Department of Biological Sciences at Macquarie University, Sydney. Her research investigates a range of behaviours in spiders such as web building, learning, mating (including sexual cannibalism) and the use of deceptive signals.

Spider Behaviour

Flexibility and Versatility

Edited by
MARIE ELISABETH HERBERSTEIN
Macquarie University, Sydney, Australia

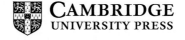

CAMBRIDGE
UNIVERSITY PRESS

CAMBRIDGE
UNIVERSITY PRESS

University Printing House, Cambridge CB2 8BS, United Kingdom

One Liberty Plaza, 20th Floor, New York, NY 10006, USA

477 Williamstown Road, Port Melbourne, VIC 3207, Australia

4843/24, 2nd Floor, Ansari Road, Daryaganj, Delhi - 110002, India

79 Anson Road, #06-04/06, Singapore 079906

Cambridge University Press is part of the University of Cambridge.

It furthers the University's mission by disseminating knowledge in the pursuit of education, learning and research at the highest international levels of excellence.

www.cambridge.org
Information on this title: www.cambridge.org/9780521765299

© Cambridge University Press 2011

First published 2011
Reprinted 2012

A catalogue record for this publication is available from the British Library

ISBN 978-0-521-76529-9 Hardback

Contents

The colour plates are situated between pages 116 and 117.

Contributors

Maydianne Andrade

Integrative Behaviour and Neuroscience Group, Department of Biological Sciences, University of Toronto Scarborough, 1265 Military Trail, Scarborough, Ontario, Canada, M1C 1A4

Trine Bilde

Department of Biological Sciences, Aarhus University, Ny Munkegade 1540, 8000 Aarhus C, Denmark

Damian O. Elias

Department of Environmental Science, Policy and Management, University of California, Berkeley, 137 Mulford Hall, Berkeley, CA 94720-3114, USA

Marie E. Herberstein

Department of Biological Sciences, Macquarie University, North Ryde, NSW 2109, Australia

Robert R. Jackson

School of Biological Sciences, University of Canterbury, Private Bag 4800, Christchurch, New Zealand, and International Centre of Insect Physiology and Ecology, Thomas Odhiambo Campus, P.O. Box 30, Mbita Point, Kenya

Elizabeth Jakob

Department of Psychology, Tobin Hall, University of Massachusetts, Amherst, MA 01003, USA

Skye Long

Organismic and Evolutionary Biology Graduate Program, Morrill Hall, University of Massachusetts Amherst, Amherst, MA 01003, USA

Yael Lubin
Mitrani Department of Desert Ecology, Blaustein Institutes for Desert Research, Ben-Gurion University of the Negev, Sede Boqer Campus 84990, Israel

Ximena J. Nelson
School of Biological Sciences, University of Canterbury, Private Bag 4800, Christchurch, New Zealand

Jutta Schneider
Department of Ethology, Biozentrum Grindel, University of Hamburg, Martin Luther King Platz 3, 20146 Hamburg, Germany

Christa Skow
Department of Biological Sciences, 106 Central Street, Wellesley College, MA 02481, USA

I-Min Tso
Department of Life Science, Tunghai University, Taichung 40704, Taiwan

Gabriele Uhl
Department of General and Systematic Zoology, Ernst-Mortiz-Arndt University of Greifswald, Anklame Strasse 20, 17487 Greifswald, Germany

Mary Whitehouse
CSIRO Ecosystem Sciences – Myall Vale, Australian Cotton Research Unit, Wee Waa Road, Myall Vale (via Narrabri), NSW 2390, Australia

Anne Wignall
Department of Biological Sciences, Macquarie University, North Ryde, NSW 2109, Australia

How this book came about

This book is a community effort! We are a community of researchers who are fascinated by the behaviour of animals. We endeavour to describe behaviour and understand the proximate and ultimate mechanisms of behaviour. In this pursuit we are only few among the many other researchers in animal behaviour and behavioural ecology. What sets us apart is our choice of model: spiders. If you, valued reader, assume we have chosen to work on spiders because we have been ensnared by their curious biology you may be partly right. The main reason, however, why we address theoretical questions about behaviour in spiders is because we recognise their scientific value, versatility and often superiority over other animal models. We believe that the utility of spiders in behavioural research is grossly underestimated. The motivation behind this book is to showcase spider behaviour to the broader research community. The ten chapters of the book describe most aspects of spider behaviour, from foraging to communication to mating and deception. Some behaviour crosses these, often arbitrary, classifications, and hence it is not surprising to find a discussion of the same species and behaviour in more than one chapter. Some chapters are more extensive than others, not because that particular topic is more important than other topics, but primarily because we decided not to subdivide certain chapters into two or more smaller chapters.

Our efforts in putting this book together have been generously supported by our colleagues who provided helpful feedback and suggestions throughout as well as photographs. In particular we would like to thank Ingi Agnarsson, Suresh Benjamin, Jonathan Coddington, Fiona Cross, Sharon Downes, Bill Eberhard, Rainer Foelix, Matthias Foellmer, Volker Framenau, Lutz Fromhage, Felipe Gawryszewski, Rosie Gillespie, Madeline Girard, Charles Griswold, Aaron Harmer, Astrid Heiling, Karen Hollis, Rudy Jocqué, Michael

Kasumovic, Sara Kross, Christine Lambkin, Daiqin Li, Emily MacLeod, Paul McDonald, Tadashi Miyashita, Maria Modanu, Ron Oldfield, Dan Papaj, David Penney, Adam Porter, John Prenter, Helma Roggenbuck, Nicole Ruppel, Stefan Schulz, Paul Selden, Jeff Stoltz, Nicholas Strausfeld, Janice Ting, Klaas Welke, Hannah Wood, Steffi Zimmer, Samuel Zschokke and Daniel Zurek.

1

Introduction: spider biology

MARIE E. HERBERSTEIN AND ANNE WIGNALL

The introductory chapter has been written especially for readers unfamiliar with the finer details of spider systematics, terminology and biology. The introduction is by no means intended to be a complete account of spider biology, which can be found in the excellent *Biology of Spiders* by Rainer Foelix (1996). Instead, here we concentrate on those aspects of spider biology that prepare the reader for the behavioural chapters to follow. The sections on systematics, fossil record and evolutionary milestones will help place the various behaviours discussed into an evolutionary context. The biology section will familiarise the reader with the spider-specific terminology and reveal some of the peculiarities of spiders: did you know that in modern spiders females have two separate copulatory openings and that spiders can produce up to seven different types of silk? For readers already familiar with spiders, the introduction offers a succinct and up-to-date summary of spider biology.

1.1   Scope of this book

The aim of this book is to illustrate the incredible diversity and often bewildering complexity of spider behaviour. Researchers that regularly work with spiders are well aware of their behavioural potential, and yet spiders still surprise us constantly with behaviours and phenomena that are intriguing, often bizarre and uncommon in other animals. Here we aim to enthuse readers that may have not considered spiders as models for behavioural studies, perhaps assuming that they are limited in their behavioural repertoires. Behavioural variation can be found in all aspects of spider biology, including foraging,

Spider Behaviour: Flexibility and Versatility, ed. Marie Elisabeth Herberstein. Published by Cambridge University Press. © Cambridge University Press 2011.

building webs, courtship and mating. While variation is high between different species, it is surprisingly high between individuals of the same species, and also within the same individual. This book highlights that spiders are not simple robots with a limited behavioural repertoire. Rather, they show great cognitive abilities, changing their behaviour to suit their situational needs. We hope that this book will serve two functions: first, encourage behavioural and evolutionary biologists to consider spiders as potential study models and, second, become a resource for researchers already working on spider behaviour. Most of all, we hope you enjoy the book!

1.2   Spider biology

1.2.1   *Systematics of the main spider groups*

Spiders (Order Araneae) belong to the Class Arachnida along with several other Orders including mites and ticks (Acari), scorpions (Scorpiones), harvestmen (Opiliones), whiptailed scorpions and vinegaroons (Thelyphonida), whipspiders (or tailless whipscorpions (Amblypygi)), micro whipscorpions (Palpigradi), false scorpions (Pseudoscorpiones), sun spiders (Solifugae) and windscorpions (Ricinulei) (Wheeler and Hayashi, 1998). There is strong evidence that the spiders form a monophyletic group based on the presence of chelicerae (mouthparts) with venom glands, modified legs for sperm transfer (pedipalps) and abdominal silk glands and spinnerets (Coddington, 2005, Coddington and Levi, 1991). In terms of arachnid diversity, spiders only trail the ticks and mites in the number of described species. Currently, there are 41 719 taxonomically recognised spider species from 3802 genera (Platnick, 2010).

The two main suborders of spiders are the basal Mesothelae and the more derived Opisthothelae (Figure 1.1). The Mesothelae, unlike the Opisthothelae, still exhibit external and internal segmentation of the opisthosoma. This group only occurs in South-East Asia and is represented by a single family (Liphistiidae) with five genera and 89 species (Coddington, 2005, 2010). The opisthothele spiders include the Mygalomorphae and the Araneomorphae. The former comprise the tarantulas, funnel-web and trapdoor spiders represented by 15 families with around 2600 species in 321 genera (Hedin and Bond, 2006, Platnick, 2010). Most mygalomorphs are relatively large, ground-dwelling spiders that live in permanent burrows. Their dispersal is limited as the spiderlings of most species do not balloon (Coddington, 2005, Hedin and Bond, 2006). Mygalomorph systematics is still somewhat problematic. Molecular data support the split of the mygalomorphs into two main groups: the atypoids (including the Atypidae, Antrodiaetidae and Mecicobothriidae) and the non-atypoids (the remaining 12 families). However, the remaining relationships between

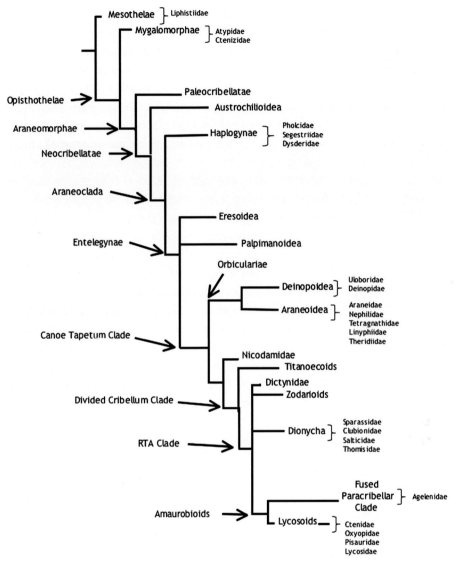

Figure 1.1 Phylogeny of the Araneae, simplified from Coddington (2005). The listed families are not exhaustive but predominantly include those that are also frequently referred to throughout the book.

families and the monophyly of some families remain contentious (Ayoub *et al.*, 2007, Hedin and Bond, 2006).

By far the most diverse suborder of spiders is the Araneomorphae, the sister group to the Mygalomorphae. It contains more than 38 000 described species in 3407 genera and 90 families (Platnick, 2010). There are several synapomorphic characters common to all araneomorphs, including the cribellum – a sclerotised plate bearing thousands of silk extruding spigots (secondarily lost in many araneomorph families). Other synapomorphies are the major ampullate glands, the piriform glands and diaxial chelicerae (Coddington, 2005).

On the basis of the presence of two rather than one pair of book lungs, the Paleocribellatae (with only one family, the Hypochilidae) are sister to the Neocribellatae, which include all other araneomorphs. The large Neocribellatae group is split into the Haplogynae and Entelegynae clades (Figure 1.1). Entelegyne females have fertilisation ducts that are separate from the copulation ducts, which are lacking in haplogynes (Figures 1.2, 1.5). In most entelegynes (but also some haplogynes), a sclerotised plate, the epigynum, covers the genital opening (Coddington, 2005, Coddington and Levi, 1991). The monophyly of the Entelegynae is supported by morphological and genetic evidence, but the monophyly of the Haplogynae is contentious (Ayoub et al., 2007, Coddington, 2005).

Among the Entelegynae two major clades are responsible for most of the current spider diversity: the RTA clade (with over 21 000 species in 39 families) and the Orbiculariae (over 11 000 species in 15 families; Blackledge et al., 2009, Coddington, 2005). The retrolateral tibial apophysis (RTA) located on the tibia of the male pedipalp is the synapomorphy that defines the RTA clade. The function of this structure is to anchor the male pedipalp to the female genital opening during copulation (Coddington, 2005, Coddington and Levi, 1991). Many families within this clade have mostly lost the ability to build webs, such as the wolf spiders (Lycosidae), crab spiders (Thomisidae) or the jumping spiders (Salticidae), although some wolf and jumping spider species still build webs (Coddington, 2005, Coddington and Levi, 1991).

The Orbiculariae, the orb-web spiders, consist of two main groups distinguished by the type of silk they produce. The Deinopoidea produce dry cribellate silk while the Araneoidea spin ecribellate, sticky silk. Despite this fundamental difference in silk type, the monophyly of the Orbiculariae and the single origin of the orb-web spiders have recently received molecular support (Blackledge et al., 2009, Garb et al., 2006). Within the Araneoidea, the orb web has subsequently been lost in favour of three-dimensional space webs such as the sheet webs of the Linyphiidae or the tanglefoot/cob webs of the Theridiidae (Blackledge et al., 2003, Coddington, 2005).

1.2.2   External morphology

Spiders have two major body regions, the prosoma and the opisthosoma (also called the cephalothorax and abdomen respectively) joined by a pedicel (Figure 1.2). The prosoma carries six pairs of appendages: the chelicerae, the pedipalps and four pairs of walking legs. The main podomeres (articles) of the

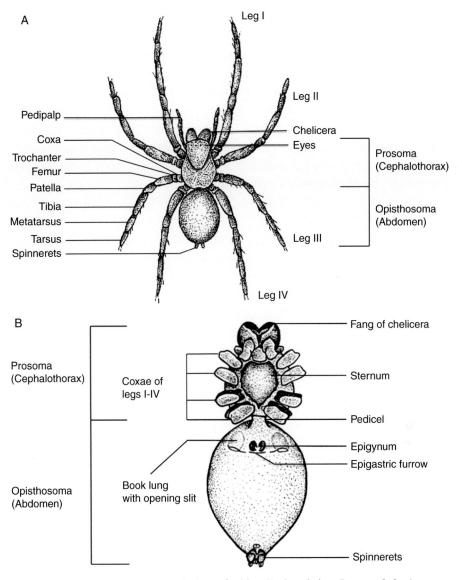

A

Leg I

Pedipalp

Leg II

Coxa

Chelicera

Trochanter

Eyes

Femur

Prosoma
(Cephalothorax)

Patella

Tibia

Opisthosoma
(Abdomen)

Metatarsus

Tarsus

Leg III

Spinnerets

Leg IV

B

Fang of chelicera

Prosoma
(Cephalothorax)

Coxae of
legs I-IV

Sternum

Pedicel

Epigynum
Epigastric furrow

Opisthosoma
(Abdomen)

Book lung
with opening slit

Spinnerets

Figure 1.2 External morphology of spiders (A, dorsal view; B, ventral view).
(Redrawn from Jocqué and Dippenaar-Schoeman, 2007, by Monika Hänel with kind
permission from Rudy Jocqué and Ansi Dippenaar-Schoeman.)

walking legs are the coxa, trochanter, femur, patella, tibia, metatarsus and
tarsus (from proximal to distal end of the legs). The pedipalps contain similar
podomeres to the walking legs, but are missing the metatarsus and have at their
base a maxilla that surrounds the mouth and connects to the coxa (McGregor
et al., 2008). The chelicerae, however, consist of only two segments, with a

movable distal fang that sits inside a groove in the basal segment when not being used (Yigit et al., 2009). The distal segment of the male pedipalp, the palpal bulb, is modified for sperm transfer and appears to be derived embryologically from the tarsal claw (see Eberhard and Huber, 2010, for a review). Also located on the prosoma are four pairs of eyes (in some groups the number of eyes may be reduced or even lacking).

The opisthosoma also has remnants of four pairs of appendages: two pairs develop into breathing organs called the book lungs while the other two pairs develop into spinnerets. The male and female genital openings are situated on the ventral opisthosoma in the epigastric furrow.

1.2.3   Locomotion

Spiders use their eight legs and their silk as a means of locomotion. The lifestyle (i.e. cursorial or sedentary web building) can usually be deduced from the morphology of the spider, particularly the structure of the tarsal claws (Vollrath and Selden, 2007).

Locomotion on silk

Web-building spiders tend to remain motionless for long periods of time at a hidden or central location in the web. Movement is initiated by stimuli (usually vibratory) indicating the presence of prey, a potential mate or a predator (Harwood, 1974, Venner et al., 2000, Zschokke, 1996). Spiders that build webs have morphological adaptations for walking on silk, such as modifications of the median tarsal claws that grip the silk thread, absent in cursorial spiders (Schütt, 1995). The median tarsal claw hooks onto the silk thread while serrated bristles on either side hold the thread in place (Foelix, 1970b, 1996). Orb-web spiders tend to grip the radial threads when traversing their webs rather than the sticky spirals (Yoshida, 1987).

Spiders leave behind dragline silk (extruded from the anterior spinnerets) as they move about. This acts as a safety line, or a means of communication between individuals such as to locate mates and competitors (e.g. Clark and Jackson, 1994, Leonard and Morse, 2006). The strength of the dragline is altered depending on whether the spider is moving across a vertical or horizontal surface (Garrido et al., 2002). Draglines are also used for dispersal via ballooning. Ballooning spiders release a line of silk into the airstream, release the substrate and are lifted into the air (Suter, 1999a). Ballooning spiders can move distances from a few metres to kilometres (Reynolds et al., 2006). Ballooning is a common method of spiderling dispersal in most spider groups, although rarer in mygalomorphs (Coddington, 2005, Coyle et al., 1985, Hedin and Bond, 2006).

Locomotion on land

Many cursorial spiders use scopulae on the leg tips (claw tufts) to help them walk and climb smooth, steep surfaces. These claw tufts comprise many setae covered with small extensions that end in spatula-shaped tips (Foelix and Chu-Wang, 1975, Niederegger and Gorb, 2006, Roscoe and Walker, 1991).

Jumping spiders have, as indicated by their name, the ability to jump great distances, up to several times their own body lengths. The thrust for the jump is almost entirely generated from the sudden hydraulic straightening of the fourth pair of legs (Parry and Brown, 1959). Jumping is not only an efficient means to bridge gaps but also an effective tool for prey capture (e.g. Bartos, 2002).

Locomotion on water

Spider species that are found in regular association with water may rely on water for foraging (Shultz, 1987a), predator evasion (Johnson and Sih, 2007) and mate location (Arnqvist, 1992). Water is a denser medium than air, and hence requires particular adaptations for locomotion. Spiders that traverse the surface of the water have hydrophobic exoskeletons and cuticular hairs that prevent the animal breaking the surface tension (Suter *et al.*, 1997). The main forms of aquatic locomotion by spiders are rowing, walking, galloping, sailing and diving under the water surface (Barnes and Barth, 1991, Shultz, 1987b, Suter *et al.*, 2003). Sailing is probably one of the least energetically expensive forms of aquatic locomotion, although direction cannot be controlled. It involves the spider using wind currents close to the surface of the water to propel it across the water surface by extending and elevating either the first pair of legs or the entire body from the surface (Suter, 1999b).

Spiders that associate consistently with water are cursorial spiders, particularly the wolf spiders (Lycosidae), while only two species of jumping spiders have been observed to move on water (Stratton *et al.*, 2004). Some spiders, such as the semi-aquatic *Dolomedes* fishing spiders (Lycosidae), are very good at walking, running or rowing on water (Stratton *et al.*, 2004). *Dolomedes* has even been observed jumping vertically on the water surface, a behaviour that has only recently been discounted as an anti-predator behaviour (Suter and Gruenwald, 2000). Only one species of spider, *Argyroneta aquatica* (Cybaeidae), spends its whole life in water (Schütz and Taborsky, 2003). Occasionally, web-building spiders will walk on water, most notably tetragnathids (Suter *et al.*, 2003).

1.2.4   *Silk production*

Silk plays a central role in the life of spiders. Its function in foraging through webs is obviously best known, but silk is also used to build egg sacs and

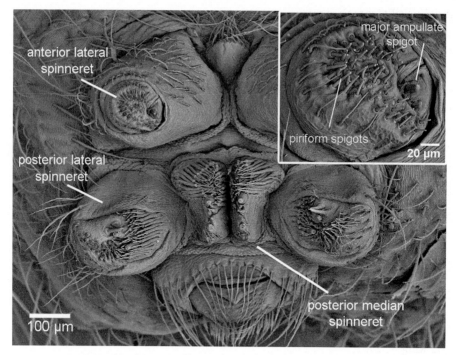

Figure 1.3 Ventral view of orb-web spider spinnerets (Araneidae: *Telaprocera maudae*). Inset: anterior lateral spinneret. Dragline silk is produced from the major ampullate spigot. (Photo credit: Aaron Harmer.)

to line burrows; it facilitates communication between the sexes, and aids in the dispersal of spiderlings (see Craig, 1997, 2003, for review). The silk-spinning apparatus consists of one or more types of silk glands within the opisthosoma that lead via a duct to the numerous spigots located on the external spinnerets (up to four pairs; Craig, 1997, 2003; Figure 1.3).

Silks are semi-crystalline biopolymers, characterised by repeated sequences of amino acids, such as alanine, glycine and serine (Craig, 1997, Kishore *et al.*, 2002). Silk consists of crystalline regions that are dominated by alanine, forming structured β-sheets, and non-crystalline regions. It is thought that β-sheets are responsible for the renowned strength of spider silk. The non-crystalline region is rich in glycine, somewhat less structured and thought to provide the elastic properties of spider silk (see Craig, 1997, Vollrath and Knight, 2001, for review). However, recent models suggest that spider silk may contain various conformations challenging the perhaps simplistic crystalline–amorphous silk concept (Vollrath and Knight, 2001).

The production of a solid silk strand from a liquid protein solution is very complex and generally not very well understood but is best studied in the dragline silk from the major ampullate gland (see Vollrath and Knight, 2001, for a review). Dragline silk is produced as a liquid in the major ampullate glands and collects in the central lumen (Vollrath, 1999). The liquid is then drawn into a looped duct where water is successively removed. At the distal end of this duct, cells pump hydrogen ions into the duct, thereby increasing the pH within the lumen. The acidic conditions in the distal duct may assist the formation of the silk's β-sheets. An internal valve grips the thread when it passes to the outside via the elastic lips of the spigots, which remove the final coating of water from the silk. The spigots are also important for putting the emerging silk thread under pressure during the air-drawn phase that finalises the transformation from liquid to the solid silk thread (see Vollrath, 1999, Vollrath and Knight, 2001, Vollrath *et al.*, 1998, for a summary).

What distinguishes spider silk from other arthropod silk is the sheer diversity of silk glands and the silk types they produce. For example, orb-web spiders (Araneidae) maintain up to seven different gland types (aciniform, tubuliform, piriform, major ampullate, minor ampullate, flagelliform and aggregate glands; Craig, 1997, Vollrath and Knight, 2001). Silk types are characterised by different fibre compositions and chemical profiles as well as physical properties (Vollrath and Knight, 2001; Figure 1.4).

Even more remarkable is the intraspecific and even intra-individual variation in structure, composition and properties of spider silk. Amino acid composition can vary with diet (Craig *et al.*, 2000, Tso *et al.*, 2005) and the mechanical properties of silk vary with environmental conditions such as climate (Craig *et al.*, 2000, Vollrath, 1999), prey availability (Tso *et al.*, 2007), diet (Zax *et al.*, 2004), spider condition (Crews and Opell, 2006, Madsen *et al.*, 1999) and the speed at which the silk is reeled from the spinneret (Madsen and Vollrath, 2000). The muscular and nervous control over spigots and spinnerets allows the spider to further adjust the diameter of the thread as well as the rate at which it is drawn, affecting the mechanical properties of the finished silk (Craig, 1997). This incredible variation in silk structure and mechanics between and within species

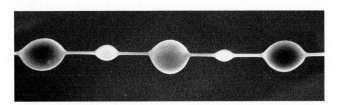

Figure 1.4 SEM of a sticky capture thread in an orb web. Sticky droplets are arranged along an axial fibre. (Reprinted with kind permission from Rainer Foelix.)

and especially within an individual is a fascinating but not well understood phenomenon.

1.2.5   *Genitalia, mating and reproduction*

Spider internal and external genitalia are extremely variable across taxa but several elements are common to most spiders. The male internal system consists of paired testes in the abdomen that fuse and open through the ventral genital pore in the epigastric furrow (Figure 1.2B). A variety of associated glandular structures may nourish the sperm but may also produce substances that are transferred to the female during mating (e.g. Michalik and Uhl, 2005; see also Chapter 7).

Males do not possess copulatory organs that are directly connected with the testes. Instead the sperm is transferred indirectly via modified appendages, the pedipalps. The male ejaculates sperm through the genital pore onto a specially constructed sperm web. He then dips his pedipalps into the sperm droplet and takes the sperm up into a reservoir in the distal pedipalps. This process is called sperm induction. With the pedipalps charged, males search for females, although in some sheet-web spiders (Linyphiidae) males only fill their pedipalps once they have located a female (Eberhard and Huber, 2010, Foelix, 1996, Weygoldt, 1996).

Spider sperm itself shows very interesting characteristics and variation in morphology across taxa (Alberti, 1990). Unlike most animal sperm, spider sperm is inactive, with a rolled-up tail, when transferred into the female. After a period of storage, the female apparently activates the sperm, which then swim actively to fertilise the eggs. The process responsible for sperm activation is currently unknown. In the more basal spider groups (Mesothelae and Mygalomorphae) sperm is transferred in large aggregates of more than 20 individual sperm encapsulated by a common secretion sheath (coenospermia). Cleistospermia, where each sperm is enclosed and transferred individually, occurs in the more derived araneomorphs, such as the entelegynes and haplogynes. Some haplogynes also transfer completely fused sperm cells (synspermia) that are no longer separated by cell membranes but are surrounded by a common sheath (Michalik *et al.*, 2004). The adaptive value of the different sperm morphologies is intriguing but not well understood.

The female internal reproductive system consists of paired ovaries that fuse to form the uterus externus, which opens in the epigastric furrow. In the Mygalomorphae and Haplogynae (Araneomorphae) the female external genitalia consist of a single opening located near the anterior book lungs leading to a genital cavity (Figure 1.5). A single duct connects the genital cavity with single or multiple sperm storage organs, the spermatheca. Eggs travel from the ovary via

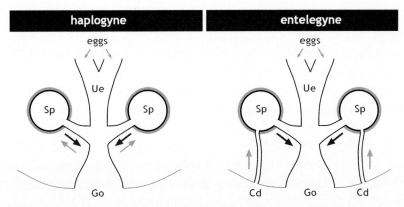

Figure 1.5 Schematic of female haplogyne and entelegyne genitalia. Cd, copulatory duct; Go, genital opening; Sp, spermathecae; Ue, uterus externus. (Reprinted from Uhl *et al.*, 2010, with kind permission from Springer Science+Business Media.)

the oviduct to the genital cavity where they are fertilised by sperm from the spermatheca. The fertilised eggs are extruded via the genital opening. Thus the copulatory duct also functions as the fertilisation duct (Figure 1.5).

In most entelegyne araneomorphs, a sclerotised plate, the epigyne, covers the primary genital opening. There are two copulatory openings, each leading to separate spermathecae (Figure 1.5). The spermathecae connect with the uterus externus, where fertilisation occurs via the fertilisation duct, thus copulation and fertilisation occur in separate ducts (Austad, 1984, Foelix, 1996, Uhl, 2000, Uhl and Vollrath, 1998). The morphological arrangement of fertilisation and copulatory ducts can have implications for patterns of fertilisation and paternity (Austad, 1984), which are discussed in greater detail in Chapter 7.

Mate location and courtship behaviour is facilitated by airborne or contact pheromones, usually emitted by the female (Gaskett, 2007; see Chapter 5 for discussion). Copulation is generally preceded by some form of courtship that may include vibratory or visual signals. Copulation occurs when the male inserts his pedipalp into the female genital opening. As the distal pedipalp of most spiders lacks musculature, hydraulics inflate the soft membranes deep into the female reproductive system and extrude the sperm (Huber, 2004a). Mesothele and mygalomorph males may insert both pedipalps at the same time, while araneomorph spiders tend to insert their pedipalps sequentially (Foelix, 1996). Sexual cannibalism and genital damage occur in some groups of spiders and will be discussed in greater detail in Chapter 7.

Female spiders provide a range of parental care. Some, like many orb-web spiders (Araneidae) only wrap the eggs in a protective silk cocoon, which is subsequently attached to the substrate. Others, such as hunting spiders (Pisauridae), carry the egg sac with them either attached to the mouthparts or the spinnerets.

These spiders may also assist in opening the cocoon and carrying the newly hatched spiderlings on their backs until they are ready to disperse. More extreme forms of maternal care involve feeding the spiderlings with regurgitated food or even matriphagy where the spiderlings eventually ingest the mother (Evans *et al.*, 1995, Kullmann, 1972, Schneider, 2002; see Chapter 8 for more detail). Male spiders are not known to provide any parental care.

1.2.6   Mouthparts and feeding

Spiders have two pairs of appendages surrounding the mouth, the chelicerae and pedipalps. The mouth opening itself (which leads into the pharynx) is bordered by the maxillae (modified coxae of the pedipalps), labium and rostrum (Butt and Taylor, 1986, Foelix, 1996). The chelicerae are used to manipulate items as well as during prey capture (Cohen, 1995). The cheliceral fang connects via a duct to a poison gland that is located inside the chelicerae in mygalomorph spiders, or the cephalothorax in araneomorph spiders (Foelix, 1996). The methods of prey capture correlate strongly with the structure of the chelicerae. For example, spitting spiders that spit venom on their prey from a distance have much larger poison glands and smaller chelicerae than wolf spiders that envenomate their prey directly by biting it (Suter and Stratton, 2005). The venom itself is delivered through a small pore in the tip of the fang (Moon and Yu, 2007, Yigit *et al.*, 2009). Spider venom may kill or just paralyse prey (Rash and Hodgson, 2002). Many spiders use the chelicerae to crush and chew their prey (Cohen, 1995, Lang and Klarenberg, 1997).

Most spiders feed by releasing digestive fluid from the midgut into or onto their prey that digests the internal tissues of the prey (Cohen, 1995, Weng *et al.*, 2006). Once the digestive fluid has digested the prey, the spider uses muscles in its pharynx and sucking stomach to ingest the contents of the prey (Butt and Taylor, 1986, Rash and Hodgson, 2002, Weng *et al.*, 2006). The maxillae, while also used for chewing in some spiders, filter prey fluids to prevent large particles entering the narrow oesophagus (Butt and Taylor, 1986, Cohen, 1995, Foelix, 1996). The pharynx has an elaborate back wall (palate plate) that also filters food particles (Foelix, 1996).

1.2.7   Sense organs

The major sense organs of spiders are eyes, lyriform organs, trichobothria and chemosensory organs. The size, sensitivity, frequency, distribution of and reliance on these sense organs are related to the spider's lifestyle. For example, cursorial spiders tend to have much more highly developed eyes due to their reliance on visual stimuli to guide them around their environment. Web-building spiders, however, tend to rely more on their vibratory senses.

Eyes

There has been considerable research effort into the structure and abilities of cursorial spider eyes, particularly salticid eyes. This is probably due to the fact that the visual abilities of cursorial spiders are much better than in web-building spiders.

Most spiders have eight eyes, although some may have a reduced number of eyes or have lost their eyes all together (Barth *et al.*, 1993a, Dacke *et al.*, 2001, Platnick, 1994). In jumping spiders (Salticidae), the eyes are arranged in four pairs, with the frontmost pair called the anterior median eyes (AME), or principal eyes. The other three pairs of eyes are often called secondary eyes and are important for motion detection. They include the anterior lateral eyes (ALE) used for range finding and to control prey pursuit. The posterior median eyes (PME) are very small in jumping spiders but are large motion detectors in some jumping spider families (Spartaeinae, Lyssomaninae). The posterior lateral eyes (PLE) contain the widest field of view. Together, these four pairs of eyes cover almost the full 360° range of vision (Figure 1.6).

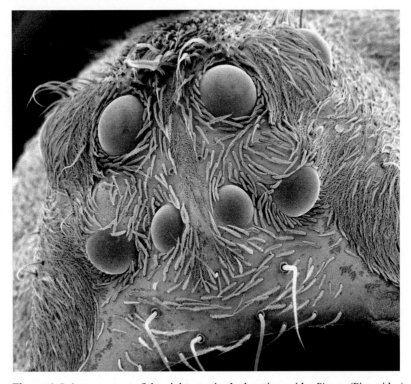

Figure 1.6 Arrangement of the eight eyes in the hunting spider *Pisaura* (Pisauridae). (Reprinted with kind permission from Rainer Foelix.)

While there is considerable diversity between spider species in the fine structure of eyes, all have a cornea that refracts light entering the eye, a lens underneath the cornea, a vitreous layer and a retina with photoreceptor cells (Land, 1969, Land and Nilsson, 2006). Differences in the fine structure of the eyes can be attributed to the ecology and behaviour of the spiders. Web-building spiders, such as *Argiope amoena*, tend to have a simple structure in the anterior median eyes, consisting of 400–500 receptor cells (Uehara *et al.*, 1977). This is in contrast to some species of jumping spiders that have many more receptors in the anterior median eyes (e.g. 1184 in *Phidippus johnsoni*; Land 1969). There is some suggestion that *A. amoena* and *A. bruennichii* have receptors sensitive to ultraviolet, blue and green light, but as yet there is no behavioural evidence (Yamashita and Tateda, 1978). The relative simplicity in the structure of *A. amoena* eyes probably relates to their reliance on vibrations in the spider web to inform them about their world, rather than visual input.

Salticid spiders also have a more complicated structure inside the anterior median eyes, including a movable retina and four layers of receptor cells, providing high visual acuity (Land, 1969, Land and Nilsson, 2006). Salticids and other cursorial spiders tend to use their anterior median eyes as their principal, 'image-forming' eyes, and the other three pairs of eyes as motion-detection eyes. These accessory eyes tend to be smaller, incapable of movement and have a simpler retina (Land, 1969). In non-cursorial spiders, there does not seem to be this structural differentiation between principal and accessory eyes (e.g. *Argiope amoena* (Uehara *et al.*, 1977). Generally, cursorial spiders such as the salticids tend to detect movement with their accessory eyes, then orientate towards the item of interest with their anterior median eyes to obtain fine image resolution.

The incredible visual ability of cursorial spiders is best illustrated by observations of their behaviour. Jumping spiders display to their own image in a mirror and respond to (motionless) mates, rivals and prey (Harland *et al.*, 1999, Jackson and Pollard, 1996) while wolf spiders can discriminate between images of prey and conspecifics on a television screen (Jackson and Pollard, 1996, Uetz and Roberts, 2002). Colour vision in spiders is less well understood, but there is direct and indirect evidence that some spiders can discriminate different colours ranging from ultraviolet to light red (for more detail see Chapter 6). Some insects (bees) are well known for their ability to detect polarised light. There is good evidence that some cursorial spiders are also able to do so, which they can use for navigation (Dacke *et al.*, 1999, 2001).

Slit sensilla and lyriform organs

Vibrations can provide information about the presence of prey, mates and enemies for both web-building and cursorial spiders. Spiders detect

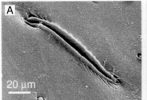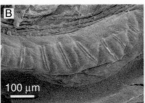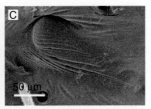

Figure 1.7 Slit sense organs (SEM) of the wandering spider *Cupiennius salei*. (A) Single slit on the sternum. (B) Grouping on the petiolus. (C) Lyriform organ on the trochanter. (Reprinted from Hößl *et al.*, 2006, with kind permission from Elsevier.)

vibrations through slits in the exoskeleton (slit sensilla) or specialised sensory hairs (trichobothria). Slit sensilla are distributed over most of the body, but are more common on the legs (Barth, 1982, Patil *et al.*, 2006; Figure 1.7). Lyriform organs comprise two or more slits in the exoskeleton, often parallel to each other (Patil *et al.*, 2006). Lyriform organs on the legs of spiders lie close to joints and can measure the particular position of a leg joint.

In the wandering spider *Cupiennius salei*, a model species for studies of vibration reception, slits in the metatarsal lyriform organ are relatively insensitive to very low frequencies (*c.* 10–40 Hz) below the range of biologically relevant vibrations (Barth, 2002). Frequencies above this range are detected much better. The central nervous system of the spider then discriminates vibrations that are within the frequency ranges of biologically interesting stimuli (i.e. prey, predators and conspecifics, see Section 1.2.8; Barth, 1997, Speck-Hergenröder and Barth, 1987).

While lyriform organs can be vibration receptors, there is some evidence that they are involved in kinaesthetic orientation as well. Spiders use information from previous movement sequences to return to an original position. However, when certain lyriform organs on the legs are damaged, spiders can no longer return to their previous position (Seyfarth and Barth, 1972).

Trichobothria

Trichobothria are vibration-sensitive hairs that detect air movements and are found on the legs and pedipalps of spiders (Barth, 2000). Like the slits of lyriform organs, trichobothria are tuned to frequency ranges between 40 Hz and 600 Hz (Barth *et al.*, 1993b). The length of the hair determines the hair's sensitivity, with the shorter hairs tuned to higher frequency ranges than longer hairs (Barth *et al.*, 1993b). The sensitivities of trichobothria receptors tend to coincide with the frequencies of vibrations generated by prey and courting males (Barth and Höller, 1999, Speck-Hergenröder and Barth, 1988). Further, spiders can determine the location and direction of air movements from the stimulation of trichobothria, as well as the strength of the stimulus by the number of trichobothria that are stimulated (Friedel and Barth, 1997, Speck-Hergenröder and Barth, 1988). While trichobothria are important for cursorial spiders, in particular for prey detection, web-building spiders also use trichobothria for the detection of predators and parasites, as well as prey, through air movements as they approach the web (Henderson and Elgar, 1999, Reißland and Görner, 1978).

Chemosensory organs

Some hairs are taste receptors and are located on the legs and pedipalps of spiders (Foelix, 1970a, Foelix and Chu-Wang, 1973). The hairs are curved, with blunt tips that are open to the outside. These chemoreceptive hairs are important for both prey and conspecific recognition, and in particular the recognition of potential mates (Vallet et al., 1998). Male wandering spiders (Cupiennius salei) have chemosensory hairs (also called tip pore sensillae) to detect female sex pheromones (Tichy et al., 2001). Spiders also possess a tarsal organ, a pore that can be exposed or encapsulated, located on the dorsal side of each tarsus (Anton and Tichy, 1994, Foelix and Chu-Wang, 1973). These were shown to serve as humidity and temperature sensors (Anton and Tichy, 1994, Ehn and Tichy, 1994).

1.2.8   Neurobiology

Most of our current knowledge of the neurobiology of spiders comes from studies of wandering spiders (specifically Cupiennius salei, Ctenidae), jumping spiders (Salticidae) and wolf spiders (Lycosidae). These studies mostly focused on how vibrational and visual information is processed by these cursorial spiders.

Central nervous system

The morphology of the spider central nervous system (CNS) has been described in several species, most notably in cursorial spiders such as the wandering spider Cupiennius salei (Ctenidae), jumping spiders (Salticidae) and wolf spiders (Lycosidae) (Babu and Barth, 1984, 1989, Kovoor et al., 2005, Meyer and Idel, 1977). The spider CNS comprises two ganglia – the dorsal supraoesophageal ganglion ('brain') and the suboesophageal ganglion, which is separated from the former by the oesophagus. Within the supraoesophageal ganglion is the arcuate body ('central body') and the mushroom body. The supraoesophageal ganglion is particularly important for processing visual information and learning (Weltzien and Barth, 1991), while the suboesophageal ganglion controls motor and body functions (Hwang and Moon, 2003, Meyer and Idel, 1977, Seyfarth et al., 1993).

Hormones

Control of moulting in spiders is via the hormone ecdysone (Bonaric and De Reggi, 1977). Ecdysone and its titers also play a role in oocyte maturation in spiders (Pourié and Trabalon, 2003, Trabalon *et al.*, 1992), inhibiting cannibalism during sexual activity and changing the production of sex pheromones in *Tegenaria atrica* (Trabalon *et al.*, 2005). In some species, such as *Amaurobius ferox* and the colonial spider *Parawixia bistriata*, synchronised moulting may be controlled by a moulting hormone in the cuticles of other individuals (Fowler and Diehl, 1978, Kim, 2001). Very little is known, however, about other spider hormones, clearly an area with great potential for further research.

Sensory integration

Spiders begin processing stimuli even before the information reaches the central nervous system. For example, the slit sensilla of spiders show reduced sensitivity to vibrations that are below the frequency thresholds of biologically important stimuli (Barth, 2002). Fine-scale discrimination of stimuli occurs inside the central nervous system, with different types of neurons in the suboesophageal ganglion in *Cupiennius salei* sensitive to frequencies within the range of different stimuli such as courtship and prey vibrations (Barth, 1997, Speck-Hergenröder and Barth, 1987). The supraoesophageal ganglion processes visual information from the primary eyes in the arcuate body ('central body') and information from the lateral eyes in the mushroom body (Kovoor *et al.*, 2005, Strausfeld *et al.*, 1993). Integration of sensory information from other sensory modalities also appears to be coordinated in the arcuate body (Strausfeld *et al.*, 2006).

1.3   The evolutionary history of spiders

1.3.1   *The spider fossil record*

Spider fossils are relatively rare compared with insect and other arthropod fossils as spiders usually do not preserve well outside amber inclusions (see Selden and Penney, 2010, for a discussion). Nevertheless, there are now over 1000 recognised fossil spider species (Dunlop *et al.*, 2009, Selden and Penney, 2010). Spiders were already present in some of the earliest terrestrial habitats (Penney, 2004). The Late Carboniferous is the earliest period for which we have evidence for the presence of spiders. The oldest spider fossil, *Palaeothele*, is around 300 million years old and represents the extant Mesothelae (Penney, 2004, Selden *et al.*, 2008). There are few spider fossils from the Permian (300–250 MYA) despite an abundance of insect fossils from this period. Only two specimens from the Permian are known: *Permarachne* and *Arthrolycosa*, both

Mesothelae (Selden and Penney, 2010). The end of the Permian is characterised by one of the greatest extinction events on Earth, although the effect of this event on spider diversity is difficult to assess due to the paucity of spider fossils from this period (Vollrath and Selden, 2007).

The fossil record from the Triassic period (250–205 MYA) not only contains mesothele spiders but also the first evidence for opisthothele spiders (Penney, 2004, Selden *et al.*, 1999). Considerable radiation in spiders must have occurred already before the Late Triassic (Penney, 2004, Selden *et al.*, 1991), possibly due to co-radiation with their insect prey (Penney, 2004). Fossils from the Jurassic (200–145 MYA) comprise spiders (mygalomorphs and araneomorphs) that are already modern-looking, including a considerable diversity of orb-web spiders (Orbiculariae; Vollrath and Selden, 2007).

Amber fossils from the Cretaceous (145–65 MYA) and the Tertiary (65–1.8 MYA) are particularly numerous. For example, more than 300 spider species have been identified from Tertiary Baltic amber alone including several extant genera (Penney *et al.*, 2003). An interesting aspect of amber fossils is that entire sections of webs, predatory and cannibalistic events are sometimes preserved, giving us a better understanding of the evolution of web silk and the behaviour of these spiders (Vollrath and Selden, 2007).

Overall, spiders seem to have been resistant to the various extinction events, including the best known, the Cretaceous–Tertiary (K/T) extinction event (65 MYA; Penney *et al.*, 2003). Unlike other groups, spiders did not suffer any reduction at the family level, but increased in number throughout the Cretaceous. It may be that as generalist predators, they may have shifted to new prey that were unaffected by the K/T extinction (Penney *et al.*, 2003). Indeed, throughout their evolutionary history, only a few spider families have become extinct and are known exclusively from fossils (Penney, 2004).

Whilst far from complete, the spider fossil record has contributed to interesting discussions such as the effects of extinctions, predator–prey coevolution through geological time or the comparison of fossil and recent faunas (Selden and Penney, 2010). Today, spiders are amongst the most diverse terrestrial arthropods and are considered the most important terrestrial predators (Wise, 1993). Their fossil record suggests that they have held this position for a very long time.

1.3.2   *The evolution of spider silk*

Silks are only produced by insects and arachnids. Among the insects, the ability to produce silk has evolved several times independently through different types of silk glands (Craig, 2003). The ability to produce silk from opisthosomal glands is ancestral in spiders and a defining feature for all spiders

(Order Araneae; Craig, 2003, Selden *et al.*, 2008). Almost all spiders, even those that have lost the ability to build webs, retain silk glands (Craig, 2003).

With the exception of the cheliceral glands of spitting spiders (family Scytodidae; Craig, 2003), silk glands appear to have evolved *de novo* from epidermal invaginations (Craig, 1997). The morphology of the spinning apparatus is linked to the phylogenetic status of the spider. Basal groups tend to have fewer and simple silk glands producing only one or two different silk types. Derived groups produce a greater diversity of silks from more silk glands, some of which are complex (Craig, 2003). The spinnerets are thought to derive from opisthosomal appendages and the spigots from setae (Selden *et al.*, 2008).

The most ancient spiders, the Mesothelae, have up to four different types of silk glands that produce up to three different types of protein fibres through four pairs of spinnerets (Craig, 2003, Haupt and Kovoor, 1993). The silk types are produced to line their burrows (Coddington and Levi, 1991, Craig, 2003). The Mygalomorphae have lost two pairs of spinnerets, the anterior median and the anterior lateral spinnerets. They only have one type of silk gland and a limited diversity in spigot type producing only two different types of proteins (Coddington and Levi, 1991, Craig, 2003, Palmer, 1985). Mygalomorphs use silk to line their burrows, build trip lines or even space webs and to wrap their eggs in a silk cocoon (Palmer, 1985).

The Araneomorphae are characterised by the presence of a cribellum – a homologue to the anterior median spinnerets found in the Mesothelae (Coddington and Levi, 1991). The cribellum is a sclerotised plate bearing thousands of tiny spigots. A comb-like structure on the spiders' fourth leg (the calamistrum) is used to brush the fine and very sticky, yet dry, silk threads from the cribellum (Kaston, 1964). The cribellum is a synapomorphy of the Araneomorphae, but has subsequently been lost several times independently (Coddington and Levi, 1991). The Araneomorphae produce up to seven different types of silk from several different silk glands. The fascinating aspect of this silk gland diversity is that even the more derived araneomorph spiders have retained the less complex ancestral gland types in addition to evolving more derived complex silk glands (Craig, 2003).

Spider silks are encoded by the spidroin gene family. Sequencing efforts have focused on araneomorph spiders, but the evolution of this gene family is not well understood. A recent phylogenetic analysis of spidroin sequences suggests that they are characterised by frequent gene duplications in both mygalomorph and araneomorph spiders. However, gene duplication in araneomorphs is far more frequent than in mygalomorphs, which may reflect the diversity in silk type and function of araneomorph spiders (Garb *et al.*, 2007).

1.3.3   The evolution of prey-capture methods

Extant spiders are almost exclusively carnivorous (Foelix, 1996, Vollrath and Selden, 2007) with the exception of a recently discovered spider whose diet predominantly consists of *Acacia* plant tissue and nectar (Meehan *et al.*, 2008). Spider morphology and physiology all point to a carnivorous ancestry. Early spiders were probably free-roaming hunters as silk may have initially been used as a protection from desiccation (Vollrath and Selden, 2007). Eventually, however, silk production was uncoupled from this protective function, resulting in increasingly efficient trapping devices. Early webs were likely to have been extensions of lined tubes trapping non-flying insect and other arthropod prey. This prey-capture method is still seen in segmented spiders (Liphistiidae), trapdoor spiders (Mygalomorphae) and funnel-web spiders (Araneomorphae), to name a few. As insects evolved the ability to fly (Late Carboniferous, 310 MYA) their spider predators followed them by shifting their ground webs higher into the vegetation; however, fossil evidence of webs from this period is lacking (Vollrath and Selden, 2007). This major evolutionary step was subsequently followed by the diversification of web and silk structure (see Chapter 3). Secondary loss of web building gave rise to free hunters that ambush prey (e.g. crab spiders: Thomisidae), actively hunt and pursue prey (e.g. wolf spiders: Lycosidae; jumping spiders: Salticidae; hunting spiders: Philodromidae, Oxyopidae, Pisauridae), stalk prey and even use aggressive mimicry (e.g. jumping spiders: Salticidae) (Foelix, 1996, Uetz, 1992). Chapter 2 discusses the foraging behaviour in spiders in greater detail.

1.3.4   The evolution of spider genitalia

The morphology of genitalia is extensively used in spider systematics and it represents one of the most important diagnostic characteristics to distinguish species (e.g. Huber, 2004b). Genital morphology in spiders also contains important phylogenetic information and genital character data have been incorporated into many cladistic analyses (Dimitrov *et al.*, 2007). Nevertheless, for most species detailed descriptions of external and internal reproductive structures are still lacking (Dimitrov *et al.*, 2007, Michalik *et al.*, 2005).

Female genitalia can be broadly classified into haplogyne and entelegyne types. The view that haplogyne genitalia are simple in structure while the entelegyne genitalia are more complex is probably oversimplified. Recent morphological investigations revealed surprising complexity in some haplogyne genitalia and low complexity in some entelegyne genitalia (Burger *et al.*, 2006a, 2006b, Dimitrov *et al.*, 2007, Michalik *et al.*, 2005, Uhl and Gunnarsson, 2001).

The haplogyne genital type is thought to be ancestral and found in the Mesothelae, Mygalomorphae and the Haplogynae (Araneopmorphae). In these groups the female external genitalia consist of a single opening and a single duct leading to the sperm storage organ. Thus the copulatory duct also functions as the fertilisation duct (Austad, 1984, Foelix, 1996, Uhl, 2000; for more detail see Section 1.2.5; Figure 1.5).

The more derived genitalia are found in the Entelegynae (Araneomorphae). Here the sclerotised epigyne covers the paired female genital openings each leading to two separate sperm storage organs and a separate copulatory and fertilisation duct. The entelegyne Tetragnathidae and some other species in the Entelegynae have reverted back to the haplogyne genital condition (Coddington and Levi, 1991). The reason behind the evolution of female entelegyne genitalia from the ancestral haplogyne genitalia is not yet resolved. It may be that entelegyne female genitalia allow for more female influence over fertilisation.

The evolutionary patterns in male genitalia are not quite as straightforward as for the females. The male genitalia of mygalomorphs and haplogyne araneomorphs consist of a pear-shaped bulb containing the male sperm, which is located on the tarsus of the pedipalp (Foelix, 1996). There are no further subdivisions to this structure (Eberhard and Huber, 2010). The male entelegyne pedipalps can comprise a quite complex bulb with sclerotised elements and protrusion connected by soft membranes (Foelix, 1996). Through hydraulic force, these soft membranes can be inflated (Eberhard and Huber, 2010). However, the pedipalps of most basal spiders, the Mesothelae, show a somewhat intermediate complexity, and it has been suggested that this may have been the ancestral state with the subsequent evolution to more complex (Entelegynae) and less complex (Mygalomorphae/Haplogynae) pedipalps (Eberhard and Huber, 2010).

1.4   Conclusion

There are numerous aspects of spider biology that set them apart from other invertebrates. These in turn strongly influence their behaviour. For example, the ability to produce silk is pivotal to their foraging strategies (e.g. web building), anti-predator behaviour (e.g. dropping on a dragline or throwing silk threads) as well as mating and communication systems (e.g. deposition of chemicals and vibratory courtship). The sensitivity of different sense organs is obviously related to their behaviour. Cursorial spiders tend to rely more on visual input to forage and court potential mates, while web-building spiders tend to rely more on vibratory input and respond to prey and courtship vibrations. The combination of a relatively conserved biology with considerable variation in the range and diversity of behaviour distinguishes spiders as superior models for many behavioural studies.

Acknowledgements

We thank Jonathan Coddington, Rainer Foelix, Volker Framenau and David Penney for helpful comments and suggestions and Aaron Harmer for permission to use his photograph.

References

Alberti, G. (1990). Comparative spermatology of Araneae. *Acta Zoologica Fennica*, **190**, 17–34.

Anton, S. and Tichy, H. (1994). Hygro- and thermoreceptors in tip-pore sensilla of the tarsal organ of the spider *Cupiennius salei*: innervation and central projection. *Cell and Tissue Research*, **278**, 399–407.

Arnqvist, G. (1992). Courtship behavior and sexual cannibalism in the semi-aquatic fishing spider, *Dolomedes fimbriatus* (Clerck) (Araneae: Pisauridae). *Journal of Arachnology*, **20**, 222–226.

Austad, S. N. (1984). Evolution of sperm priority patterns in spiders. In *Sperm Competition and the Evolution of Animal Mating Systems* (ed. R. L. Smith). New York: Academic Press.

Ayoub, N. A., Garb, J. E., Hedin, M. and Hayashi, C. Y. (2007). Utility of the nuclear protein-coding gene, elongation factor-1 gamma (EF-1 gamma), for spider systematics, emphasizing family level relationships of tarantulas and their kin (Araneae: Mygalomorphae). *Molecular Phylogenetics and Evolution*, **42**, 394–409.

Babu, K. S. and Barth, F. G. (1984). Neuroanatomy of the central nervous system of the wandering spider, *Cupiennius salei* (Arachnida, Araneida). *Zoomorphology*, **104**, 344–359.

Babu, K. S. and Barth, F. G. (1989). Central nervous projections of mechanoreceptors in the spider *Cupiennius salei* Keys. *Cell and Tissue Research*, **258**, 69–82.

Barnes, W. J. P. and Barth, F. G. (1991). Sensory control of locomotor mode in semi-aquatic spiders. In *Locomotor Neural Mechanisms in Arthropods and Vertebrates* (ed. D. M. Armstrong and B. M. H. Bush). Manchester, UK: Manchester Press.

Barth, F. G. (1982). Spiders and vibratory signals: sensory reception and behavioral significance. In *Spider Communication: Mechanisms and Ecological Significance* (ed. P. N. Witt and J. S. Rovner). Princeton, NJ: Princeton University Press.

Barth, F. G. (1997). Vibratory communication in spiders: adaptation and compromise at many levels. In *Orientation and Communication in Arthropods* (ed. M. Lehrer). Basel, Switzerland: Birkhäuser.

Barth, F. G. (2000). How to catch the wind: spider hairs specialized for sensing the movement of air. *Naturwissenschaften*, **87**, 51–58.

Barth, F. G. (2002). *A Spider's World: Senses and Behaviour*. Berlin: Springer.

Barth, F. G. and Höller, A. (1999). Dynamics of arthropod filiform hairs. V. The response of spider trichobothria to natural stimuli. *Philosophical Transactions of the Royal Society, B*, **354**, 183–192.

Barth, F. G., Nakagawa, T. and Eguchi, E. (1993a). Vision in the ctenid spider *Cupiennius salei*: spectral range and absolute sensitivity. *Journal of Experimental Biology*, **181**, 63–79.

Barth, F. G., Wastl, U., Humphrey, J. A. C. and Devarakonda, R. (1993b). Dynamics of arthropod filiform hairs. II. Mechanical properties of spider trichobothria (*Cupiennius salei* Keys.). *Philosophical Transactions of the Royal Society, B*, **340**, 445–461.

Bartos, M. (2002). Distance of approach to prey is adjusted to the prey's ability to escape in *Yllenus arenarius* Menge (Araneae, Salticidae). In *European Arachnology* (ed. S. Toft and N. Scharff). Aarhus, Denmark: Aarhus University Press.

Blackledge, T. A., Coddington, J. and Gillespie, R. G. (2003). Are three-dimensional spider webs defensive adaptations? *Ecology Letters*, **6**, 13–18.

Blackledge, T. A., Scharff, N., Coddington, J. A., *et al.* (2009). Reconstructing web evolution and spider diversification in the molecular era. *Proceedings of the National Academy of Sciences of the USA*, **106**, 5229–5234.

Bonaric, J. C. and De Reggi, M. (1977). Changes in ecdysone levels in the spider *Pisaura mirabilis* nymphs (Araneae: Pisauridae). *Experientia*, **33**, 1664–1665.

Burger, M., Graber, W., Michalik, P. and Kropf, C. (2006a). *Silhouettella loricatula* (Arachnida, Araneae, Oonopidae): a haplogyne spider with complex female genitalia. *Journal of Morphology*, **267**, 663–677.

Burger, M., Michalik, P., Graber, W., *et al.* (2006b). Complex genital system of a haplogyne spider (Arachnida, Araneae, Tetrablemmidae) indicates internal fertilization and full female control over transferred sperm. *Journal of Morphology*, **267**, 166–186.

Butt, A. G. and Taylor, H. H. (1986). Salt and water balance in the spider *Porrhothele antipodiana* (Mygalomorpha: Dipluridae): effects of feeding upon hydrated animals. *Journal of Experimental Biology*, **125**, 85–106.

Clark, R. J. and Jackson, R. R. (1994). Self recognition in a jumping spider: *Portia labiata* females discriminate between their own draglines and those of conspecifics. *Ethology, Ecology, and Evolution*, **6**, 371–375.

Coddington, J. A. (2005). Phylogeny and classification of spiders. In *Spiders of North America: An Identification Manual* (ed. D. Ubick, P. Paquin, P. E. Cushing and V. Roth). Poughkeepsie, NY: American Arachnological Society.

Coddington, J. A. and Levi, H. W. (1991). Systematics and evolution of spiders (Araneae). *Annual Review of Ecology and Systematics*, **22**, 565–592.

Cohen, A. C. (1995). Extra-oral digestion in predaceous terrestrial Arthropoda. *Annual Review of Entomology*, **40**, 85–103.

Coyle, F. A., Greenstone, M. H., Hultsch, A.-L. and Morgan, C. E. (1985). Ballooning mygalomorphs: estimates of the masses of *Sphodros* and *Ummidia* ballooners (Araneae: Atypidae, Ctenizidae). *Journal of Arachnology*, **13**, 291–296.

Craig, C. L. (1997). Evolution of arthropod silks. *Annual Review of Entomology*, **42**, 231–267.

Craig, C. L. (2003). *Spiderwebs and Silk*. Oxford, UK: Oxford University Press.

Craig, C. L., Reikel, C., Herberstein, M. E., *et al.* (2000). Evidence for diet effects on the composition of silk proteins produced by spiders. *Molecular Biology and Evolution*, **17**, 1904–1913.

Crews, S. C. and Opell, B. D. (2006). The features of capture threads and orb-webs produced by unfed *Cyclosa turbinata* (Araneae: Araneidae). *Journal of Arachnology*, **34**, 427–434.

Dacke, M., Doan, T. A. and O'Carroll, D. C. (2001). Polarized light detection in spiders. *Journal of Experimental Biology*, **204**, 2481–2490.

Dacke, M., Nilsson, D.-E., Warrant, E. J., *et al.* (1999). Built-in polarizers form part of a compass organ in spiders. *Nature*, **401**, 470–473.

Dimitrov, D., Alvarez-Padilla, F. and Hormiga, G. (2007). The female genital morphology of the orb weaving spider genus *Agriognatha* (Araneae, Tetragnathidae). *Journal of Morphology*, **268**, 758–770.

Dunlop, J. A., Penney, D. and Jekel, D. (2009) A summary list of fossil spiders. In *The World Spider Catalog*, Version 9.5 (ed. N. I. Platnick). American Museum of Natural History, online at http://research.amnh.org/entomology/spiders/catalog.

Eberhard, W. G. and Huber, B. A. (2010). Spider genitalia: precise maneuvers with a numb structure in a complex lock. In *Evolution of Primary Sexual Characters in Animals* (ed. J. Leonard and A. Córdoba-Aguilar). Oxford, UK: Oxford University Press.

Ehn, R. and Tichy, H. (1994). Hygro- and thermoreceptive tarsal organ in the spider *Cupiennius salei*. *Journal of Comparative Physiology, A*, **174**, 345–350.

Evans, T. A., Wallis, E. J. and Elgar, M. A. (1995). Making a meal of mother. *Nature*, **376**, 299.

Foelix, R. F. (1970a). Chemosensitive hairs in spiders. *Journal of Morphology*, **132**, 313–334.

Foelix, R. F. (1970b). Structure and function of tarsal sensilla in the spider *Araneus diadematus*. *Journal of Experimental Biology*, **175**, 99–124.

Foelix, R. F. (1996). *Biology of Spiders*, 2nd edn. Oxford, UK: Oxford University Press.

Foelix, R. F. and Chu-Wang, I.-W. (1973). The morphology of spider sensilla. II. Chemoreceptors. *Tissue and Cell*, **5**, 461–478.

Foelix, R. F. and Chu-Wang, I.-W. (1975). The structure of scopula hairs in spiders. In *Proceedings 6th International Arachnida Congress*. Amsterdam: Nederlandse Entomologische Vereniging, pp. 156–157.

Fowler, H. G. and Diehl, J. (1978). Biology of a Paraguayan colonial orb-weaver, *Eriophora bistriata* Rengger (Araneae, Araneidae). *Bulletin of the British Arachnological Society*, **4**, 241–250.

Friedel, T. and Barth, F. G. (1997). Wind-sensitive interneurons in the spider CNS (*Cupiennius salei*): directional information processing of sensory inputs from trichobothria on the walking legs. *Journal of Comparative Physiology, A*, **180**, 223–233.

Garb, J. E., Dimauro, T., Lewis, R. V. and Hayashi, C. Y. (2007). Expansion and intragenic homogenization of spider silk genes since the triassic: evidence from Mygalomorphae (tarantulas and their kin) spidroins. *Molecular Biology and Evolution*, **24**, 2454–2464.

Garb, J. E., Dimauro, T., Vo, V. and Hayashi, C. Y. (2006). Silk genes support the single origin of orb webs. *Science*, **312**, 1762.

Garrido, M. A., Viney, C. and Pérez-Rigueiro, J. (2002). Active control of spider silk strength: comparison of drag line spun on vertical and horizontal surfaces. *Polymer*, **43**, 1537–1540.

Gaskett, A. (2007). Spider sex pheromones: emission, reception, structures, and functions. *Biological Reviews*, **82**, 26–48.

Harland, D. P., Jackson, R. R. and Macnab, A. M. (1999). Distances at which jumping spiders (Araneae: Salticidae) distinguish between prey and conspecific rivals. *Journal of Zoology*, **247**, 357–364.

Harwood, R. H. (1974). Behavior of *Argiope aurantia* (Lucas). *American Midland Naturalist*, **91**, 130–139.

Haupt, J. and Kovoor, J. (1993). Silk-gland system and silk production in Mesothelae (Araneae). *Annales des Sciences Naturelles – Zoologie et Biologie Animale*, **14**, 35–48.

Hedin, M. and Bond, J. E. (2006). Molecular phylogenetics of the spider infraorder Mygalomorphae using nuclear rRNA genes (18S and 28S): conflict and agreement with the current system of classification. *Molecular Phylogenetics and Evolution*, **41**, 454–471.

Henderson, R. J. and Elgar, M. A. (1999). Foraging behaviour and the risk of predation in the black house spider, *Badumna insignis* (Desidae). *Australian Journal of Zoology*, **47**, 29–35.

Hößl, B., Böhm, H. J., Rammerstorfer, F. G., Müllan, R. and Barth, F. G. (2006). Studying the deformation of arachnid slit sensilla by a fracture mechanical approach. *Journal of Biomechanics*, **39**, 1761–1768.

Huber, B. A. (2004a). Evolutionary transformation from muscular to hydraulic movements in spider (Arachnida, Araneae) genitalia: a study based on histological serial sections. *Journal of Morphology*, **261**, 364–376.

Huber, B. A. (2004b). The significance of copulatory structures in spider systematics. In *Biosemiotik: Praktische Anwendung und Konsequenzen für die Einzelwissenschaften* (ed. J. Schult). Berlin: VWB Verlag.

Hwang, H.-J. and Moon, M.-J. (2003). Fine structural analysis of the central nervous system in the spider *Achaearanea tepidariorum* (Theridiidae: Araneae). *Korean Journal of Entomology*, **33**, 119–126.

Jackson, R. R. and Pollard, S. D. (1996). Predatory behavior of jumping spiders. *Annual Review of Entomology*, **41**, 287–308.

Jocqué, R. and Dippenaar-Schoeman, A. S. (2007). *Spider Families of the World*. Tervuren, Belgium: Royal Museum for Central Africa.

Johnson, J. C. and Sih, A. (2007). Fear, food, sex and parental care: a syndrome of boldness in the fishing spider, *Dolomedes triton*. *Animal Behaviour*, **74**, 1131–1138.

Kaston, B. J. (1964). The evolution of spider webs. *American Zoologist*, **4**, 191–207.

Kim, K. W. (2001). Social facilitation of synchronized molting behavior in the spider *Amaurobius ferox* (Araneaea, Amaurobiidae). *Journal of Insect Behavior*, **14**, 401–409.

Kishore, A. I., Herberstein, M. E., Craig, C. L. and Separovic, F. (2002). Solid-state NMR relaxation studies of Australian spider silks. *Biopolymers*, **61**, 287–297.

Kovoor, J., Muñoz-Cuevas, A. and Ortega-Escobar, J. (2005). The visual system of *Lycosa tarentula* (Araneae, Lycosidae): microscopic anatomy of the protocerebral optic centres. *Italian Journal of Zoology*, **72**, 205–216.

Kullmann, E. J. (1972). Evolution of social behavior in spiders (Araneae: Eresidae and Theridiidae). *American Zoologist*, **12**, 419–426.

Land, M. F. (1969). Structure of the retinae of the principal eyes of jumping spiders (Salticidae: Dendryphantinae) in relation to visual optics. *Journal of Experimental Biology*, **51**, 443–470.

Land, M. F. and Nilsson, D.-E. (2006). General-purpose and special-purpose visual systems. In *Invertebrate Vision* (ed. E. J. Warrant and D.-E. Nilsson). Cambridge, UK: Cambridge University Press.

Lang, A. and Klarenberg, A. J. (1997). Experiments on the foraging behaviour of the hunting spider *Pisaura mirabilis* (Araneae: Pisauridae): utilization of single prey items. *European Journal of Entomology*, **94**, 456–459.

Leonard, A. S. and Morse, D. H. (2006). Line-following preferences of male crab spiders, *Misumena vatia*. *Animal Behaviour*, **71**, 717–724.

Madsen, B., Shao, Z. Z. and Vollrath, F. (1999). Variability in the mechanical properties of spider silks on three levels: interspecific, intraspecific and intraindividual. *International Journal of Biological Macromolecules*, **24**, 301–306.

Madsen, B. and Vollrath, F. (2000). Mechanics and morphology of silk drawn from anesthetized spiders. *Naturwissenschaften*, **87**, 148–153.

McGregor, A. P., Hilbrant, M., Pechmann, M., *et al.* (2008). *Cupiennius salei* and *Achaearanea tepidariorum*: spider models for investigating evolution and development. *BioEssays*, **30**, 487–498.

Meehan, C. J., Olson, E. J. and Curry, R. L. (2008) Exploitation of the *Pseudomyrmex-Acacia* mutualism by a predominantly vegetarian jumping spider (*Bagheera kiplingi*). In *The 93rd ESA Annual Meeting*, held in Milwaukee, WI. Washington, DC: Ecological Society of America.

Meyer, W. and Idel, K. (1977). The distribution of acetylcholinesterase in the central nervous system of jumping spiders and wolf spiders (Arachnida, Araneida: Salticidae et Lycosidae). *Journal of Comparative Neurobiology*, **173**, 717–744.

Michalik, P. and Uhl, G. (2005). The male genital system of the cellar spider *Pholcus phalangioides* (Fuesslin, 1775) (Pholcidae, Araneae): development of spermatozoa and seminal secretion. *Frontiers in Zoology*, **2**, 12.

Michalik, P., Haupt, J. and Alberti, G. (2004). On the occurrence of coenospermia in mesothelid spiders (Araneae: Heptathelidae). *Arthropod Structure and Development*, **33**, 173–181.

Michalik, P., Reiher, W., Tintelnot-Suhm, M. and Coyle, F. A. (2005). Female genital system of the folding-trapdoor spider *Antrodiaetus unicolor* (Hentz, 1842) (Antrodiaetidae, Araneae): ultrastructural study of form and function with notes on reproductive biology of spiders. *Journal of Morphology*, **263**, 284–309.

Moon, M.-J. and Yu, M.-H. (2007). Fine structure of the chelicera in the spider *Nephila clavata*. *Entomological Research*, **37**, 167–172.

Niederegger, S. and Gorb, S. N. (2006). Friction and adhesion in the tarsal and metatarsal scopulae of spiders. *Journal of Comparative Physiology, A*, **192**, 1223–1232.

Palmer, J. M. (1985). The silk and silk production system of the funnel-web mygalomorph spider *Euagrus* (Araneae, Dipluridae) *Journal of Morphology*, **186**, 195–207.

Parry, D. A. and Brown, R. H. J. (1959). The hydraulic mechanism of the spider leg. *Journal of Experimental Biology*, **36**, 423–433.

Patil, B., Prabhu, S. and Rajashekhar, K. P. (2006). Lyriform slit sense organs on the pedipalps and spinnerets of spiders. *Journal of Biosciences*, **31**, 75–84.

Penney, D. (2004). Does the fossil record of spiders track that of their principal prey, the insects? *Transactions of the Royal Society of Edinburgh – Earth Sciences*, **94**, 275–281.

Penney, D., Wheater, C. P. and Selden, P. A. (2003). Resistance of spiders to Cretaceous-Tertiary extinction events. *Evolution*, **57**, 2599–2607.

Platnick, N. I. (1994). A review of the Chilean spiders of the family Caponiidae (Araneae, Haplogynae). *American Museum Novitates*, **3113**, 1–10.

Platnick, N. I. (2010) *The World Spider Catalog*, Version 11. American Museum of Natural History, online at http://research.amnh.org/iz/spiders/catalog.

Pourié, G. and Trabalon, M. (2003). The role of 20-hydroxyecdysone on the control of spider vitellogenesis. *General and Comparative Endocrinology*, **131**, 250–257.

Rash, L. D. and Hodgson, W. C. (2002). Pharmacology and biochemistry of spider venoms. *Toxicon*, **40**, 225–254.

Reißland, A. and Görner, P. (1978). Mechanics of trichobothria in orb-weaving spiders (Agelenidae, Araneae). *Journal of Comparative Physiology, A*, **123**, 59–69.

Reynolds, A. M., Bohan, D. A. and Bell, J. R. (2006). Ballooning dispersal in arthropod taxa with convergent behaviours: dynamic properties of ballooning silk in turbulent flows. *Biology Letters*, **2**, 371–373.

Roscoe, D. T. and Walker, G. (1991). The adhesion of spiders to smooth surfaces. *Bulletin of the British Arachnological Society*, **8**, 224–226.

Schneider, J. M. (2002). Reproductive state and care giving in *Stegodyphus* (Araneae: Eresidae) and the implications for the evolution of sociality. *Animal Behaviour*, **63**, 649–658.

Schütt, K. (1995). *Drapetisca socialis* (Araneae: Linyphiidae): web reduction – ethological and morphological adaptations. *European Journal of Entomology*, **92**, 553–563.

Schütz, D. and Taborsky, M. (2003). Adaptations to an aquatic life may be responsible for the reversed sexual size dimorphism in the water spider, *Argyroneta aquatica*. *Evolutionary Ecology Research*, **5**, 105–117.

Selden, P. A. and Penney, D. (2010). Fossil spiders. *Biological Reviews*, **85**, 171–206.

Selden, P. A., Anderson, J. M., Anderson, H. M. and Fraser, N. C. (1999). Fossil araneomorph spiders from the Triassic of South Africa and Virginia. *Journal of Arachnology*, **27**, 401–414.

Selden, P. A., Shear, W. A. and Bonamo, P. M. (1991). A spider and other arachnids from the Devonian of New York, and reinterpretations of Devonian Araneae. *Palaeontology*, **34**, 241–281.

Selden, P. A., Shear, W. A. and Sutton, M. D. (2008). Fossil evidence for the origin of spider spinnerets, and a proposed arachnid order. *Proceedings of the National Academy of Sciences of the USA*, **105**, 20 781–20 785.

Seyfarth, E.-A. and Barth, F. G. (1972). Compound slit sense organs on the spider leg: mechanoreceptors involved in kinesthetic orientation. *Journal of Comparative Physiology*, **78**, 176–191.

Seyfarth, E.-A., Hammer, K., Spörhase-Eichmann, U., Hörner, M. and Vullings, H. G. B. (1993). Octopamine immunoreactive neurons in the fused central nervous system of spiders. *Brain Research*, **611**, 197–206.

Shultz, J. W. (1987a). Walking and surface film locomotion in terrestrial and semi-aquatic spiders. *Journal of Experimental Biology*, **128**, 427–444.

Shultz, J. W. (1987b). The origin of the spinning apparatus in spiders. *Biological Reviews*, **62**, 89–113.

Speck-Hergenröder, J. and Barth, F. G. (1987). Tuning of vibration sensitive neurons in the central nervous system of a wandering spider, *Cupiennius salei* Keys. *Journal of Comparative Physiology, A*, **160**, 467–475.

Speck-Hergenröder, J. and Barth, F. G. (1988). Vibration sensitive hairs on the spider leg. *Experientia*, **44**, 13–14.

Stratton, G. E., Suter, R. B. and Miller, P. R. (2004). Locomotion on the water surface: propulsive mechanisms of the fisher spider *Dolomedes triton*. *Journal of Experimental Biology*, **200**, 2523–2538.

Strausfeld, N. J., Strausfeld, C. M., Stowe, S., Rowell, D. and Loesel, R. (2006). The organization and evolutionary implications of neuropils and their neurons in the brain of the onychophoran *Euperipatoides rowelli*. *Arthropod Structure and Development*, **35**, 169–196.

Strausfeld, N. J., Weltzien, P. and Barth, F. G. (1993). Two visual systems in one brain: neuropils serving the principal eyes of the spider *Cupiennius salei*. *Journal of Comparative Neurology*, **328**, 63–75.

Suter, R. B. (1999a). An aerial lottery: the physics of ballooning in a chaotic atmosphere. *Journal of Arachnology*, **27**, 287–293.

Suter, R. B. (1999b). Cheap transport for fishing spiders (Araneae, Pisauridae): the physics of sailing on the water surface. *Journal of Arachnology*, **27**, 489–496.

Suter, R. B. and Gruenwald, J. (2000). Predator avoidance on the water surface? Kinematics and efficacy of vertical jumping by *Dolomedes* (Araneae, Pisauridae). *Journal of Arachnology*, **28**, 201–210.

Suter, R. B. and Stratton, G. E. (2005). *Scytodes vs. Schizocosa*: predatory techniques and their morphological correlates. *Journal of Arachnology*, **33**, 7–15.

Suter, R. B., Rosenberg, O., Loeb, S., Wildman, H. and Long, Jr., J. H. (1997). Locomotion on the water surface: propulsive mechanisms of the fisher spider *Dolomedes triton*. *Journal of Experimental Biology*, **200**, 2523–2538.

Suter, R. B., Stratton, G. and Miller, P. R. (2003). Water surface locomotion by spiders: distinct gaits in diverse families. *Journal of Arachnology*, **31**, 428–432.

Tichy, H., Gingl, E., Ehn, R., Papke, M. and Schulz, S. (2001). Female sex pheromone of a wandering spider (*Cupiennius salei*): identification and sensory reception. *Journal of Comparative Physiology, A*, **187**, 75–78.

Trabalon, M., Bautz, A.-M., Moriniere, M. and Porcheron, P. (1992). Ovarian development and correlated changes in hemolymphatic ecdysteroid levels in two spiders, *Coelotes terrestris* and *Tegenaria domestica* (Araneae, Agelenidae). *General and Comparative Endocrinology*, **88**, 128–136.

Trabalon, M., Niogret, J. and Legrand-Frossi, C. (2005). Effect of 20-hydroxyecdysone on cannibalism, sexual behavior, and contact sex pheromone in the solitary female spider, *Tegenaria atrica*. *General and Comparative Endocrinology*, **144**, 60–66.

Tso, I. M., Chiang, S. Y. and Blackledge, T. A. (2007). Does the giant wood spider *Nephila pilipes* respond to prey variation by altering web or silk properties? *Ethology*, **113**, 324–333.

Tso, I. M., Wu, H. C. and Hwang, I. R. (2005). Giant wood spider *Nephila pilipes* alters silk protein in response to prey variation. *Journal of Experimental Biology*, **208**, 1053–1061.

Uehara, A., Toh, Y. and Tateda, H. (1977). Fine structure of the eyes of orb-weavers, *Argiope amoena* L. Koch (Araneae: Argiopidae). *Cell and Tissue Research*, **182**, 81–91.

Uetz, G. W. (1992). Foraging strategies in spiders. *Trends in Ecology and Evolution*, **7**, 155–159.

Uetz, G. W. and Roberts, J. A. (2002). Multisensory cues and multimodal communication in spiders: insights from video/audio playback studies. *Brain, Behavior and Evolution*, **59**, 222–230.

Uhl, G. (2000). Two distinctly different sperm storage organs in female *Dysdera erythrina* (Araneae: Dysderidae). *Arthropod Structure and Development*, **29**, 163–169.

Uhl, G. and Gunnarsson, B. C. (2001). Female genitalia in *Pityohyphantes phrygianus*, a spider with a skewed sex ratio. *Journal of Zoology*, **255**, 367–376.

Uhl, G. and Vollrath, F. (1998). Genital morphology of *Nephila edulis*: implications for sperm competition in spiders. *Canadian Journal of Zoology*, **76**, 39–47.

Uhl, G., Nessler, S. H. and Schneider, J. (2010). Securing paternity in spiders? A review on occurrence and effects of mating plugs and male genital mutilation. *Genetica*, **138**(1), 75–104.

Vallet, A. M., Marion-Poll, F. and Trabalon, M. (1998). Preliminary electrophysiological study of the contact chemoreceptors in a spider. *Comptes Rendus de l'Académie des Sciences, Series III, Sciences de la Vie*, **321**, 463–469.

Venner, S., Pasquet, A. and Leborgne, R. (2000). Web-building behaviour in the orb-weaving spider *Zygiella x-notata*: influence of experience. *Animal Behaviour*, **59**, 603–611.

Vollrath, F. (1999). Biology of spider silk. *International Journal of Biological Macromolecules*, **24**, 81–88.

Vollrath, F. and Knight, D. P. (2001). Liquid crystalline spinning of spider silk. *Nature*, **410**, 541–548.

Vollrath, F. and Selden, P. (2007). The role of behavior in the evolution of spiders, silks, and webs. *Annual Review of Ecology, Evolution, and Systematics*, **38**, 819–846.

Vollrath, F., Knight, D. P. and Hu, X. W. (1998). Silk production in a spider involves acid bath treatment. *Proceedings of the Royal Society of London, B*, **265**, 817–820.

Weltzien, P. and Barth, F. G. (1991). Volumetric measurements do not demonstrate that the spider brain 'central body' has a special role in web building. *Journal of Morphology*, **208**, 91–98.

Weng, J.-L., Barrantes, G. and Eberhard, W. G. (2006). Feeding by *Philoponella vicina* (Araneae, Uloboridae) and how uloborid spiders lost their venom glands. *Canadian Journal of Zoology*, **84**, 1752–1762.

Weygoldt, P. (1996). Chelicerata, Spinnentiere. In *Spezielle Zoologie* (ed. W. Westheide and R. Rieger). Stuttgart, Germany: Gustav Fisher Verlag.

Wheeler, W. C. and Hayashi, C. Y. (1998). The phylogeny of the extant chelicerate orders. *Cladistics – the International Journal of the Willi Hennig Society*, **14**, 173–192.

Wise, D. H. (1993). *Spiders in Ecological Webs*. Cambridge, UK: Cambridge University Press.

Yamashita, S. and Tateda, H. (1978). Spectral sensitivities of the anterior median eyes of the orb web spiders, *Argiope bruennichi* and *A. amoena*. *Journal of Experimental Biology*, **74**, 47–57.

Yigit, N., Bayram, A., Danisman, T., Sancak, Z. and Tel, M. G. (2009). Morphological characterization of the venom apparatus in the wolf spider *Lycosa singoriensis* (Laxmann, 1770). *Journal of Venomous Animal Toxins Including Tropical Diseases*, **15**, 146–156.

Yoshida, M. (1987). Predatory behavior of *Tetragnatha praedonia* (Araneae: Tetragnathidae). *Acta Arachnologica*, **35**, 57–75.

Zax, D. B., Armanios, D. E., Horak, S., Malowniak, C. and Yang, Z. T. (2004). Variation of mechanical properties with amino acid content in the silk of *Nephila clavipes*. *Biomacromolecules*, **5**, 732–738.

Zschokke, S. (1996). Early stages of orb web construction in *Araneus diadematus* Clerck. *Revue Suisse de Zoologie*, **2**, 709–720.

2

Flexibility in the foraging strategies of spiders

XIMENA J. NELSON AND ROBERT R. JACKSON

Although many spiders build prey-capture webs, spider foraging strategies include species that, instead of building webs, deploy silk in other ways for prey capture. Additionally, there are species that capture prey, either by ambush or by active pursuit, without making notable use of silk in the process. There are striking examples of predatory specialisation from spiders, particularly among the Salticidae, suggesting that assumptions about adaptive trade-offs, in which the small nervous systems of spiders might constrain their cognitive or sensory abilities, need to be carefully evaluated. Predatory versatility, whereby an individual spider adopts a conditional strategy with which it classifies prey into diverse categories, illustrates that an individual spider may be a poly-specialist, because it is polyphagic and at the same time it is highly specialised on more than one prey type. More generally, individual flexibility in spider behaviour has important implications concerning the cognitive capacities of predators that orchestrate their strategies using small nervous systems.

2.1   Introduction

At first glance, characterising spider foraging might appear straightforward. All spiders are predators, and most frequently the spider's prey is an insect. All spiders produce silk, which is often put to use as part of their predatory arsenal. Yet a closer look reveals staggering diversity – and it is not just variation between species that contributes to this diversity, as we also need to address variation within single species and even within individual spiders. This is because spider foraging strategies provide us with some of the most

Spider Behaviour: Flexibility and Versatility, ed. Marie Elisabeth Herberstein. Published by Cambridge University Press. © Cambridge University Press 2011.

remarkable examples of behavioural flexibility known in the animal kingdom. A first step towards appreciating what this means is to move beyond some of the oversimplifications and misunderstandings that have bedevilled the literature on spider foraging.

One of the myths we need to dispel is the notion that spiders are automatons, rigid in their behaviour and devoid of cognitive attributes. Another is the prevalent characterisation of spiders as generalist predators, as there are numerous examples of spiders making distinctive prey-choice decisions and deploying prey-capture tactics that are exquisitely effective at capturing particular types of prey.

We need to be careful when using the words 'generalist' and 'generalised', and especially their seeming opposites, 'specialist' and 'specialised'. Here we use the word specialised to mean something well designed for a specified task. This definition does not consider whether design is a product of natural selection or of learning, as this is a separate question. Sometimes it is convenient simply to call a spider a specialist instead of always, more correctly, specifying a trait of the spider and the task in the context of which the trait might be specialised.

To illustrate this, we will consider spiders that not only prey frequently on other spiders but also target spiders with distinctive prey-choice behaviour. Additionally, these spiders deploy prey-capture behaviour that is highly effective and specific at capturing spiders. Using these traits as our criteria, we will call these species 'specialised araneophagic spiders' or just 'araneophagic spiders', with 'specialised' being implicit. We will avoid applying the term araneophagy to instances of spiders occasionally eating other spiders.

Problems arise because there is an unfortunate and misleading habit in the literature of using specialised and generalised to describe a predator's natural diet (Berenbaum, 1996). Other terms are more appropriate for natural diet, including 'monophagic' for predators that feed mostly on one type of prey and 'polyphagic' for predators that feed often on a variety of prey types, but 'stenophagy' (narrow range of prey types in a natural diet) and 'euryphagy' (wide range of prey types) are better terms, as they encourage a more realistic expectation of finding that variation in diet breadth is on a continuum.

We also need to guard against uncritical, and often unacknowledged, application of trade-off ideas that are deeply engrained in the literature, often seeming to be used like axioms, or foregone conclusions. When applied to predators, trade-off hypotheses are sometimes called 'jack-of-all-trades' hypotheses, the core idea being that, for a predator, there is a cost associated with acquiring the specialised traits that make it especially effective at capturing one type of prey. This cost is usually envisaged as a loss in capacity to acquire the specialised

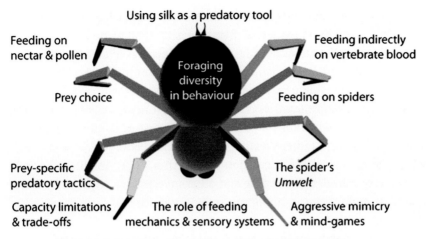

Using silk as a predatory tool

Feeding on
nectar & pollen

Feeding indirectly
on vertebrate blood

Foraging
diversity
in behaviour

Prey choice

Feeding on spiders

Prey-specific
predatory tactics

The spider's
Umwelt

Capacity limitations
& trade-offs

The role of feeding
mechanics & sensory systems

Aggressive mimicry
& mind-games

Figure 2.1 Overview of flexibility in spider foraging strategies.

tactics that will make it especially effective at capturing other types of prey: the jack of all trades is the master of none.

At some level, trade-offs during the evolution of predatory adaptation may be an unavoidable corollary of natural selection, with trade-offs due to learning specialised predatory behaviour being a consequence of a nervous system's limited computational capacity. Acknowledging this should not blind us to how there are important questions concerning the level at which trade-offs actually become particularly significant (Eberhard, 2007). These are questions to be answered by research considered on a case-by-case basis (Fry, 1996, Futuyma and Moreno, 1988, Wilson and Yoshimura, 1994), but too often intuition that trade-offs are of paramount importance (Whitlock, 1996) may encourage thinking that specialised predatory tactics go hand in hand with stenophagy or monophagy. In this chapter, we will try to encourage a different way of thinking about specialisation.

We will not attempt anything like encyclopaedic completeness in our review of foraging behaviour in spiders and instead rely on particular examples as case studies for focusing on specific issues related to flexibility (Figure 2.1). For example, sexual cannibalism, social foraging and kleptoparasitism are topics we will largely ignore, as these will be discussed in other chapters (Chapters 7, 8 and 10).

2.2   Investments required by extra-oral digestion

Spiders do not ingest solid food and, instead, by extra-oral digestion, convert solid prey tissue to liquid (Cohen, 1995). This means that distinctions between ingestion and digestion are blurred, with the prey's body becoming something like a temporary extension of the spider's stomach (Pollard, 1990). A distinctive consequence of extra-oral digestion is that, being unable to gulp its food down, a spider invests substantial time in the process of ingesting the prey it captures. Additional investments include the venom and silk used by the predator for immobilising prey (Malli *et al.*, 1999, Wigger *et al.*, 2002). For the spider, there may be substantial risks that these investments will be lost because of encounters with competitors or predators, or because of numerous potential interferences that are not intentionally directed at the feeding spider (e.g. a large animal brushing against the vegetation on which a spider might be sitting). Although rarely considered, the time and other investments required by extra-oral digestion might have an important influence on the foraging decisions of the spider.

If you turn a spider upside down and examine it carefully, you will readily see the coxae of the second pair of appendages (the pedipalps, or simply 'palps'). Known as the maxillae, palp coxae are large and have become morphologically specialised as tools for crushing prey when feeding. What is not very conspicuous is the spider's mouth. Situated between the maxillae, it is no more than a tiny pore. The spider's anteriormost appendages, known as the chelicerae, are the most conspicuous of the spider's mouthparts. Cheliceral shape and size varies tremendously among spiders and, in some instances, we have an understanding of how cheliceral structure is specialised for predation on specific types of prey. One of the most elegant examples comes from recent research on the ground-dwelling hunting spider genus *Dysdera* (Dysderidae). Several species in this genus appear to prey on woodlice (oniscophagy). Attacking prey defended by an armoured dorsal surface and their ability either to cling to the substrate or roll up to protect the soft ventral side can be problematic, but *Dysdera* have morphological adaptations correlated with their predatory behaviour. In *Dysdera*, it appears that the extent of elongation and curvature of the chelicerae is positively correlated with their choice of woodlice as prey: species with unmodified chelicerae are generalist predators that do not capture woodlice, species with partially modified chelicerae appear to be facultatively oniscophagous, while those *Dysdera* with extreme modifications appear to be almost obligately oniscophagous (Řezáč *et al.*, 2008).

Spider chelicerae always consist of two segments, a robust basal segment and a slender fang. Most spiders have venom glands in the basal segments, with these glands extending back into the body of some species (Figure 2.2), and venom ducts in their fangs that open at a hole on the tip of the fang (Foelix, 1996). Exceptions include *Myrmarachne*, a genus of ant-mimicking spiders. *Myrmarachne* males have particularly long chelicerae that have no venom ducts in their long, slender fangs (Pollard, 1994). The family Uloboridae is the

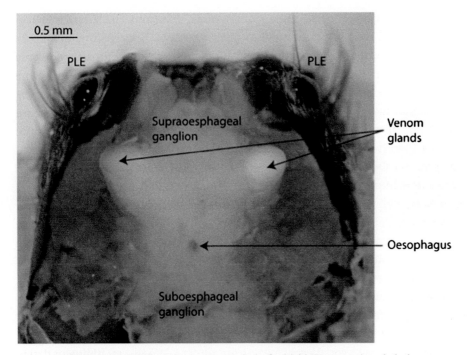

Figure 2.2 'Half frontal' view (posterior) of salticid (*Servaea* sp.) cephalothorax showing central nervous system (supraoesophageal and suboesophageal ganglia) and large venom glands. Supraoesophageal neuropil (fluffy white material) dominated by neurons used for processing input from eyes. Only PLE: (posterior lateral eyes) visible in this section through carapace. See also colour plate.

major exception to the rule of spiders being venomous predators, as both sexes of all species in this family are venomless. The uloborid's substitute for immobilising prey with venom is to wrap prey in silk, and to keep on wrapping until the prey disappears inside a silken cocoon (Weng *et al.*, 2006).

2.3   Silk use, behavioural categories and predatory versatility

The silk for which spiders are best known comes from a variety of glands in the posterior abdomen. The ducts from these glands open on spigots on special appendages (spinnerets) and, for some spiders, also on a spinning plate (the cribellum). The tasks for which spinneret and cribellum silk is deployed include, among other things, foraging. The best-known example of silk being put to use in foraging is, of course, in the building of prey-capture webs (see Chapter 3).

Web-building spiders normally rely heavily on interpreting movement and tension patterns (web signals) conveyed through the silk lines of their self-made webs (Krafft and Leborgne, 1979, Masters et al., 1986) and this specialised sensory system is also important for many spiders that make predatory forays into the webs of other spiders (Jackson, 1986). Spiders that do not use webs are generally called cursorial spiders or hunting spiders, yet many of these spiders build silk structures of one kind or another, even though their silk constructions are not normally called webs. For example, hunting spiders may spin cocoon-like (tubular) and tent-like nests. Often given the quaint name 'retreat' in the spider literature, nests typically function as resting, moulting, mating and oviposition sites (Foelix, 1996, Jackson, 1979), and they may also have a role in predation, blurring the distinction between a nest and a web. For example, prey inadvertently moving across nest silk may convey vibratory stimuli to the resident spider and trigger a predatory attack (e.g. Jackson and Macnab, 1989), with nest silk sometimes being sticky and comparable to the silk in prey-capture webs in its ability to detain prey (Hallas and Jackson, 1986).

It may often be convenient to envisage web-building spider and hunting spider as distinct categories, with every spider belonging to one or the other, but closer examination reveals a common, elementary type of predatory versatility. An individual hunting spider may shift between nest-based predation and predation initiated completely away from nests. Likewise, an individual web-building spider may shift between capturing prey in its web and initiating predation completely away from its web. Moreover, an individual spider may build its own prey-capture web, invade other spiders' webs and also capture prey completely away from webs (Jackson, 1986).

2.4   Flexibility based on chemoreception

Spider's sensory systems, what Barth (2002) called 'masterpieces of engineering', sit at the interface between environment and behaviour. Although the sensory systems of spiders vary considerably, we might say chemoreception is foremost for spiders, and for animals in general, as this is the most ancient sensory modality (Wyatt, 2003). In the spider literature, it is customary to distinguish between olfaction and contact chemoreception (Foelix, 1996). For both, the stimulus comes from specific compounds or blends of compounds, the distinction being that compounds targeted by olfaction are volatile. The spider's olfactory and contact-chemoreception systems are roughly analogous to what we call a sense of smell and a sense of taste, respectively, but with the spider using its legs and palps for smelling and tasting, as this is where its chemoreceptors tend to be concentrated (Foelix, 1970).

Often silk has an important role in conveying chemosensory information to conspecific individuals, including information about species, sex, maturity, virgin-mated status, and fighting ability (Clark and Jackson, 1994, 1995, Clark et al., 1999, Pollard et al., 1987, Roberts and Uetz, 2005; see Chapter 5). Besides web and nest silk, the silk that is relevant includes draglines, these being strands of silk trailed behind by a spider as it moves through the environment. However, it is particularly when we consider spiders that prey on other spiders that we see how silk-mediated chemosensory information can have an important role in foraging strategies.

For an example, we can look at *Portia fimbriata*, an araneophagic salticid spider (Salticidae) from the Australian and Asian tropics. When discussing *P. fimbriata*'s predatory behaviour, distinctive ecotypic variation makes it important to specify how in this single species populations from different areas are locally adapted to local prey. In the Queensland habitat of *P. fimbriata*, another salticid species, *Jacksonoides queenslandicus*, is especially abundant (Jackson, 1988) and it is one of the spiders for which this population of *P. fimbriata* has a prey-specific predatory strategy. How *P. fimbriata* responds to the odour and to the draglines of *J. queenslandicus* is an important part of this strategy (Jackson et al., 2002a).

One of *P. fimbriata*'s responses is to adopt a special posture, this posture being a component of a special style of stalking, called cryptic stalking. This stalking posture is an innate tactic specific to the Queensland *P. fimbriata* and specific to instances where the prey is *J. queenslandicus* (Jackson and Wilcox, 1998). Although all species in the genus *Portia* are unusual in appearance, in the field being easily mistaken by people, and apparently by other salticids, for a piece of detritus, *P. fimbriata*'s special posture when adopting cryptic stalking masks the outlines of its legs and palps, making *P. fimbriata*'s already un-spider-like appearance even more obscure. Chemical cues from *J. queenslandicus* also call up an innate search image for this particular prey species: these cues trigger selective visual attention by *P. fimbriata*, specifically to the appearance of *J. queenslandicus* (not prey in general, not spiders in general and not even salticids in general), with no prior experience of encountering *J. queenslandicus* being necessary (Jackson et al., 2002a).

Another effect of chemical cues from *J. queenslandicus* is to elicit what has been called speculative hunting by the Queensland *P. fimbriata* (Curio, 1976). This predatory tactic, which is performed without any prior exposure to *J. queenslandicus* (Clark et al., 2000), exploits how *J. queenslandicus*, like other salticids, tends to orient towards sudden movement in its vicinity. After contacting specifically the draglines of *J. queenslandicus*, and in the absence of any visual cue from the prey, *P. fimbriata* repeatedly leaps almost straight upward and then, when *J. queenslandicus* makes orientation movements, *P. fimbriata* locates its prey by sight.

2.5   Flexibility based on vision

Although the number is reduced in a minority of species, spiders generally have four pairs of eyes: the anterior median (AM), anterior lateral (AL), posterior median (PM), and posterior lateral (PL). The AM eyes are also called the principal eyes, with the remaining three pairs being collectively known as the secondary eyes. However, what spiders do with their eyes varies considerably and, in some instances, foraging strategies and specialised eye design are clearly interrelated. For example, *Deinopis* (Deinopidae) builds a highly specialised, expandable orb web (Coddington, 1986). Unlike other orb-web spiders that reside in their webs, *Deinopis* holds its web with its first two pairs of legs. When an insect comes close, *Deinopis* spreads its legs apart, expanding the web into a net that is then slung accurately over the prey (Austin and Blest, 1979, Getty and Coyle, 1996, Robinson and Robinson, 1971). *Deinopis* is nocturnal and yet net casting is a vision-based predatory strategy made possible by *Deinopis* having eyes of extreme sensitivity, or light-capturing ability. Sometimes called 'ogre-face spider', *Deinopis* has posterior median eyes that are significantly larger than those of other spiders. Shifted forward so that they face straight ahead, these eyes have fish-eye lenses (i.e. they have a field of view of about 180°) and large photoreceptors that enhance their ability to capture light, giving the eyes of *Deinopis* the distinction of being among the most efficient known nocturnal movement detectors (Blest and Land, 1977, Laughlin *et al.*, 1980).

However, vision based on good spatial acuity that allows an animal to resolve fine detail of shape and form is what we most often emphasise when we, as humans, think about vision. On the whole, spider eyes are not especially well designed for this type of vision (Land and Nilsson, 2002), but the spider family to which *P. fimbriata* and *J. queenslandicus* belong, the Salticidae, is distinctively different from the rest. With their unique, complex principal eyes (Blest *et al.*, 1990, Land, 1969a, 1969b, Williams and McIntyre, 1980), salticids see with spatial acuity exceeding, by a wide margin, that known for any other animals of similar size (Harland and Jackson, in press).

Defined as the minimum separation required before objects in a scene are seen as separate (McIlwain, 1996), spatial acuity – an eye's visual angle – is usually expressed in units of arc (degrees, radians or minutes), with smaller visual angles corresponding to better spatial acuity. The critical determinants of small visual angles are the quality of the image provided by the lens system and a receptor mosaic in the retina that can sample this image optimally (Land and Nilsson, 2002). The best visual angles known for salticid eyes (0.04°; Blest *et al.*, 1988, Williams and McIntyre, 1980) are an order of magnitude better than the best visual angle known for insects (0.4°; Labhart and Nilsson, 1995) and are, in fact, more similar to that of human eyes (0.007°; Kirschfeld, 1976), which alone are bigger than an entire jumping spider. Achieving this level of spatial acuity is based on the salticid's unique, specialised eye characteristics (Harland and Jackson, 2000a), including a fovea in the retina where the receptor mosaic is optimally structured for sampling a high-quality image projected by telephoto optics. Telephoto optics in the principal eyes is achieved by the eye tubes being long and slender, with a corneal lens at the front and a second lens at the rear, just in front of the retina (Williams and McIntyre, 1980). The fovea has a minute field of view (Blest *et al.*, 1990), but there is complex musculature on the eye tubes that orchestrates intricate patterns of side-to-side and rotary movement by which the retinas sample the large images rendered by the lens system (Land, 1969b).

The salticid's specialised eyes are critical for understanding much of what is particularly intriguing about salticid foraging strategies, including ability to plan ahead, solve problems flexibly, make decisions, and deploy prey-specific predatory tactics (Jackson and Pollard, 1996). The salticid's exceptional eyesight is also important for the researcher because realistic responses can be elicited by testing salticids with lures (dead prey mounted in a life-like posture) and animated virtual prey rendered from computer-generated three-dimensional drawings and then projected on spider-size monitors (Harland and Jackson, 2000b, 2002, Nelson and Jackson, 2006a). In this way, confounding variables that arise from prey behaviour and especially from prey response to the predator can be controlled for in experiments.

Recent research on *Evarcha culicivora* is an example. This East African salticid feeds indirectly on vertebrate blood by choosing blood-carrying female mosquitoes as preferred prey (Jackson *et al.*, 2005). From using lures and virtual mosquitoes in experiments, we know that *E. culicivora* can make these choices when restricted to using visual cues alone (Jackson *et al.*, 2005, Nelson and Jackson 2006a). Furthermore, *E. culicivora* chooses mosquitoes from the genus *Anopheles* in preference to other mosquitoes (Nelson and Jackson, 2006a). *Anopheles* is the mosquito genus to which all human malaria vectors belong (White, 1974) and *E. culicivora* is the only predator known to have an active preference for a human disease vector. Indeed, *E. culicivora* is the only predator known to choose mosquitoes of any genus as preferred prey and also the only predator known to choose prey on the basis of what the prey has been eating.

The characteristic resting posture (abdomen tilted upward) of *Anopheles* (Clements, 1999) is a principal feature by which *E. culicivora* identifies its preferred prey (Nelson and Jackson, 2006a) and the smaller juveniles (1–2 mm in body length) of *E. culicivora* also adopt a specialised *Anopheles*-specific predatory routine by which they exploit *Anopheles*' resting posture. These small juveniles are less likely to be dislodged when they attack a mosquito from underneath and, when they detect this posture by sight, they approach the mosquito from behind, move under the mosquito, and attack from underneath (Nelson *et al.*, 2005).

It is important to appreciate the experimental basis for these various conclusions. Although we know from field data that *E. culicivora* feeds especially often on blood-carrying mosquitoes (Wesolowska and Jackson, 2003), field data on diet do not suffice as evidence of the predator's decisions. Outcomes from encounters staged in the laboratory between this predator and living prey also encourage hypotheses about *E. culicivora*'s decisions, but we have to acknowledge that the living prey's behaviour is a potential confounding variable. The strong evidence for conclusions about this predator's decisions comes from the outcome of experiments in which, instead of living prey, lures or virtual prey were used. It is the exceptional eyesight of salticids that makes these experiments possible.

2.6   Searching for sensory–modality trade-offs

It is commonplace to think that the brains of very small animals, such as spiders, must be limited to functioning at a level that is vastly inferior to what any bird's or any mammal's much bigger brain can do. After all, the numbers of neurons that can be housed in a small body seem to be inevitably fewer than the number that can be housed in a larger body. This is a physical consequence of how neurons appear to be constrained to be at least 2 μm in diameter (Beutel *et al.*, 2005). Common sense may tell us that the computational power of a brain with fewer neurons will be less than that of a brain with more neurons, and yet many spiders have surprisingly, perhaps disturbingly, complex, flexible and cognitive behaviour (see Chapter 9).

With sensory systems, as with behaviour and cognition, it is tempting to think a spider will be subject to severe trade-offs. Compared with the sheer numbers of neurons available for processing sensory input in mammals, for example, it may seem to be a foregone conclusion that the spider's small nervous system will impose severe capacity limitations. Due to their extraordinary eyesight, the way salticids in particular have often been portrayed (Jackson, 1982) suggests that there is an unacknowledged assumption about sensory capacity limitations, which seems to encourage an expectation that salticids will rely almost exclusively on vision as the sensory input that guides their behaviour. Yet there have been numerous published studies demonstrating important roles of other sensory modalities. Research on salticid courtship, for example, suggests that multimodal and conditional signalling involving mechanoreception and chemoreception, in addition to vision, are common-place (e.g. Cross and Jackson, 2009a, Elias *et al.*, 2003, Jackson, 1977, Pollard *et al.*, 1987).

Of course, it can be argued that trade-offs must become important at some level with sensory systems, as with behaviour, but conclusions about the severity of trade-off effects need to be evidence based, not simply assumed. For an example related to foraging, we can return to *E. culicivora*, the salticid that chooses blood-carrying mosquitoes as preferred prey. Besides the innate ability to identify its preferred prey by sight alone, *E. culicivora* also has an olfactory system with which it can identify this same prey by smell, also without prior experience with this prey being required (Jackson *et al.*, 2005). Vision and olfaction also work together, with the scent of blood-carrying mosquitoes triggering selective visual attention to the appearance of this prey. Conversely, seeing blood-carrying mosquitoes triggers selective olfactory attention to the smell of blood-carrying mosquitoes (Cross and Jackson, 2009b). Here we have, in single individual spiders, specialised use of vision coexisting with specialised use of olfaction, with no obvious trade-off. Acknowledging that no compelling experimental evidence has shown trade-offs is not the same as concluding that there never are trade-offs, but it should at least make us wary of applying trade-off assumptions simplistically.

2.7   From aggressive mimicry to mind games

Prey often defend themselves by resembling something else – by mimicry (Edmunds, 1974). However, predators can also use mimicry as a predatory ploy and examples of this are referred to as aggressive mimicry (Edmunds, 1974). One of the interesting things about aggressive mimicry is how it makes sense only when we consider the sensory systems of both prey and predator.

Sensory traps, sensory exploitation, sensory drive, and receiver psychology (Christy, 1995, Endler and Basolo, 1998), along with aggressive mimicry, belong to the terminological menagerie that has accumulated in the literature. All of these terms can be applied to situations in which a predator interfaces with its prey's sensory biology, and the distinctions being made with these different terms are often rather subtle. In this chapter we will side-step these terminological issues and focus instead on how a predator's strategy can sometimes be likened to playing mind games with its prey (Jackson and Pollard, 1996, 1997).

Just over a century ago, von Uexküll (1909, 1957) considered how sensory systems, styles of behaviour and cognitive profiles are interrelated. No animals, including humans, have simple, direct access to an independent physical world, and instead they operate on the basis of a model of the world (Dawkins, 1996), or what von Uexküll called the animal's *Umwelt*. The animal's *Umwelt*, or 'self-world' (Schiller, 1957), can be envisaged as a product of sensory input, internal state and central processing, but it is not arbitrary. Natural selection ensures that the model is adaptive (Dennett, 1996, 2005, Harland and Jackson, 2004). In the context of communication, what Guilford and Dawkins (1991) called 'receiver psychology' comes close to what von Uexküll (1909) was hinting at when discussing an animal's *Umwelt*. It may also come close to what Minsky (1986) was suggesting with his famous expression 'minds are what brains do'.

Examples of aggressive mimicry taken from spider–ant interactions are particularly relevant in this respect. There are many spiders that, to people, resemble ants and are called ant mimics. We also have experimental evidence that predators that naturally avoid ants also avoid ant mimics, although they would normally prey on spiders (Nelson and Jackson, 2006b). This implies that ant mimics are convincing look-alikes of ants, even for non-human animals. On this basis, ant-like spiders are considered to be Batesian mimics, in which resemblance to well-defended animals enables harmless potential prey escape the dedicated attention of predators (Chapter 4).

As there has been a longstanding question of whether some spiders that look like ants are aggressive mimics of ants (Cushing, 1997), any instance of an ant-mimicking spider eating ants is interesting, but simply determining that an ant-mimicking spider eats ants is not evidence that the spider is an aggressive mimic of ants. In fact, ant-like appearance is unlikely to be salient to most ants, as ants rely much more strongly on chemoreception than on acute vision. In particular, ants often acquire a colony-specific chemical signature, based on hydrocarbons integrated into their cuticle, and rely on chemoreception of this signature for discriminating nestmates from alien intruders (Hölldobler and Wilson, 1990).

There is, however, a compelling example of a spider using, as a predatory ploy, resemblance to ants in the sensory modality that is especially salient to ants. *Cosmophasis bitaeniata* is an Australian salticid that preys on the eggs, larvae and pupae of *Oecophylla smaragdina* (Allan and Elgar, 2001). Called weaver ants because their nests are made from leaves folded together with silk, *O. smaragdina* is an especially formidable predator in its own right (Hölldobler, 1983), but *C. bitaeniata* enters the nest of these ants without being molested, protected by having acquired the colony-specific chemical signature of the ants (Elgar and Allan, 2004). *Cosmophasis bitaeniata* can be thought of as smelling like a 'wolf in sheep's clothing'. With the spider being detected and then misidentified by the ants, this is an example of a predator – the spider – adopting aggressive mimicry as a predatory ploy. However, this example differs from another example of aggressive mimicry where ant-like spiders provoke overt responses from their prey.

Myrmarachne melanotarsa is an ant-mimicking salticid that deploys its resemblance to ants not only as defence against ant-averse predators (Batesian mimicry), but also as a critical component of a predatory strategy with which it preys on the eggs and juveniles of other salticid species (Nelson and Jackson, 2009a). Besides being well defended against most salticids that might target them as potential prey, ants are also, for many spiders, especially dangerous predators (Nelson *et al.*, 2004) and salticids are known to identify and then avoid ants by their distinctive appearance (Nelson and Jackson, 2006b). For a salticid, a group of ants might be especially threatening and, as ants are social insects, salticids are likely to encounter a group of ants instead of a solitary ant.

Crematogaster is the particular ant that serves as *M. melanotarsa*'s model (Jackson *et al.*, 2008). Ant-averse salticid females often abandon their nests when there is an encounter with a group of *Crematogaster* or a group of *M. melanotarsa* (Nelson and Jackson, 2009a, 2009b), but the silk covering the eggs or juveniles left behind usually provides the progeny protection against being eaten by the ants. However, *M. melanotarsa*, being a spider, has little difficulty negotiating the silk and readily preys on the abandoned progeny. We can say that *M. melanotarsa*, like *C. bitaeniata*, is an aggressive mimic of ants, albeit in a different sensory modality. However, *C. bitaeniata*'s prey is the progeny of the ant, whereas *M. melanotarsa*'s prey is the progeny of an ant-averse salticid. Another key difference between these two examples of aggressive mimicry is that *C. bitaeniata* uses resemblance to ants as a method of *avoiding* an overt response, whereas *M. melanotarsa*'s strategy is based on *eliciting* a particular overt response – fleeing.

Using aggressive mimicry for eliciting overt responses is unique neither to the Salticidae nor to visual signals. For example, most species in the family Araneidae build orb webs, but there are some remarkable exceptions, including species that capture their prey using a single silk line (Yeargan, 1994). With one of its legs, the so-called bolas spider holds one end of the silk line that terminates in a sticky ball (the bolas). Bolas spiders sit in the vegetation and at night capture prey by whirling the silk line around, intersecting their prey, male moths, with the sticky ball, then reeling the moth in and eating it. The key to this tactic's success is that the spider emits chemicals that mimic those of female moths belonging to the same species as the male moths that are captured (Eberhard, 1977 Haynes *et al.*, 1996, Gemeno *et al.*, 2000, Stowe *et al.*, 1987). The male, normally being attracted to the odour (pheromones) of female moths, is lured to within striking distance of the bolas by the spider's simulation (an allomone) of this same odour. Bolas spiders also give us an example of predatory versatility (Curio, 1976), as the same individual bolas spider may, at different times, mimic pheromones of different moth species (Haynes *et al.*, 2002; see also Chapter 6).

There are also aggressive mimics that invade the webs of other spiders and, by producing web signals, solicit overt responses from the resident spider. At least six spider families give us examples of this (Jackson, 1992), but it is research on araneophagic salticids that most clearly demonstrates aggressive mimicry based on pronounced behavioural flexibility.

2.8   Araneophagic salticids

With more than 5200 described species and almost 570 genera (Platnick, 2010), the family Salticidae provides many predatory strategies to explore. Three primary taxa are currently recognised within this family (Lyssomaninae, Spartaeinae and Salticoida), with the salticoids accounting for the majority of species and with the lyssomanines and spartaeines being smaller groups that appear to have branched off early (Maddison and Hedin, 2003, Su *et al.*, 2007). It is especially the spartaeines that seem intent on surprising us with unusual predatory strategies. All of the examples of salticids using web signals as part of an aggressive-mimicry strategy come from five spartaeine genera (Su *et al.*, 2007). However, in the Spartaeinae, we also find other styles of araneo-phagy (Chapter 4), often with the same individual spider switching repeatedly between different araneophagic tactics.

Species from the genus *Portia* are the most thoroughly studied araneophagic spartaeines. Salticids in general are characterised as hunting spiders that, with-out using webs, detect their prey (primarily insects) by sight, stalk until close and then attack by leaping (Forster, 1982, Richman and Jackson, 1992). *Portia* also readily captures prey, including insects, away from webs, but the same individual of *Portia* will also build a large, three-dimensional prey-capture web (Jackson and Wilcox, 1998) and also prey on other spiders by invading their webs, where it adopts a highly flexible strategy based on an almost unlimited capacity to match aggressive-mimicry signalling to different prey species (Jackson and Hallas, 1986, Jackson and Wilcox, 1998, Tarsitano *et al.*, 2000).

The most straightforward examples of aggressive mimicry by *Portia* are instances in which the resident spider is not especially dangerous. In these instances, *Portia* uses leg and palp movements to simulate the struggles of a small insect entangled in the web and, in this way, lures the resident spider in, capturing it when close (Jackson and Blest, 1982). However, explaining what is actually happening quickly becomes more complicated when we consider pred-atory sequences in more detail and when we consider the large variety of spiders on which *Portia* preys.

The particular signals that are most effective vary between webs and also from spider to spider. As examples of adaptation to local prey, *Portia* sometimes initiates a predatory sequence with innate prey-specific signalling routines that appear to be especially effective against particular types of prey spider. *Portia* also derives signals by trial and error (Jackson and Wilcox, 1994). For example, *Portia* may, after entering the web of a spider species for which it does not have an innate signalling tactic, first present the resident spider with a kaleidoscope of different vibratory signals. When one of these signals eventually elicits an appropriate response from the resident spider, *Portia* stops varying its signals and concentrates on making the signal that elicits the appropriate response. The appropriate response might be, for example, the resident spider approaching *Portia* as though *Portia* were a small insect ensnared in the web, but communication between predator and prey is often more subtle than this.

For example, simply simulating the signals of the resident spider's prey can be problematic when the resident spider is fully capable of turning *Portia* into its next meal. In these cases, *Portia* may stalk slowly across the web, all the while making signals that keep the resident spider out in the open and avoiding signals that would provoke full-scale predatory attacks by the resident spider (Tarsitano *et al.*, 2000). However, *Portia* sometimes adopts more intricate strategies. For example, one of the dominant prey species of *Portia labiata* from Los Baños, in the Philippines, is *Scytodes pallida*, a spider that builds webs on the tops of leaves and preys especially on salticids (Li *et al.*, 1999). All species in the genus *Scytodes* spit a sticky gum on prey and on potential predators (Suter and Stratton, 2005). *Scytodes*' spit is a formidable weapon against *Portia*, as a spat-upon *Portia* is gummed down long enough for *Scytodes* to finish the job by wrapping *Portia* in silk and injecting venom. However, the Los Baños *P. labiata* has an innate strategy, absent from the repertoire of *P. labiata* that come from habitats in the Philippines where *S. pallida* is not found. This strategy includes taking detours to approach the spitting spider from behind and using its palps to make vibratory signals that keep *Scytodes* facing away (Jackson *et al.*, 1998), thereby minimising the likelihood of *P. labiata* becoming a target of a spitting attack.

All individuals of *S. pallida* are not the same and the predatory strategy of *P. labiata* is adjusted to account for some of this variation. For example, as *S. pallida* females carry their eggs in their mouths, they have to release their eggs to spit. Being reluctant to release their eggs, egg-carrying *S. pallida* females are less dangerous to *P. labiata* and, consistent with this, *P. labiata* prefers to prey on egg-carrying instead of eggless *S. pallida* (Li and Jackson, 2003). Furthermore, when the *S. pallida* female is carrying eggs, *P. labiata* is more willing to adopt the shorter head-on approach it avoids when *S. pallida* is eggless (Jackson *et al.*, 2002b).

It is important to appreciate that trial and error derivation of signals may almost always have a role when *Portia* encounters spiders in webs, regardless of whether *Portia* also has an innate routine for the particular spider it has encountered. When present, the role of innate routines seems to be something like getting a predatory sequence off to a good start, after which the sequence is completed by trial and error derivation of signals. Trial and error derivation of signals may also be critical for fine-tuning the sequence to the prey's response. For example, an eggless spitting spider approached from behind may suddenly turn and face *P. labiata* head on. When this happens, *P. labiata* usually stops making the signals that preceded this response and instead uses trial and error to derive other signals that subdue the spitting spider so that eventually it turns away (Jackson *et al.*, 2002b).

The word mimicry conjures up expectations of an easily identifiable model, but it is not always that simple. For example, when *Portia* produces signals that keep the resident spider out in the web, or eliciting escape behaviour (e.g. dropping out of the web) and rather than provoking a predatory attack, we might say the model being simulated is something in the web that is, to the resident spider, potentially salient but for now of uncertain identity. However, when specifying the model requires these sorts of subtleties and lengthy expressions, it may be more useful to forego specifying a model at all and instead to use the metaphor of 'mind games' as a way to emphasise how *Portia* uses signals to gain dynamic fine control over the resident spider's behaviour (Harland and Jackson, 2004, Jackson and Wilcox, 1998).

2.9   Ambushing spiders on tree trunks

Phaeacius, another spartaeine genus, illustrates an alternative way to be araneophagic. Instead of invading webs, *Phaeacius* is an ambush predator that lives on tree trunks (Jackson, 1990). Owing to markings, flattened body shape and specialised posture, *Phaeacius* blends in with its bark background. Other bark-dwelling salticid species are *Phaeacius*' preferred prey and, because these are prey with excellent eyesight, being highly camouflaged appears to be an especially important aspect of *Phaeacius*' predatory strategy (Li, 2000).

It might be tempting to envisage ambushing as a rather simple prey-capture routine, but *Phaeacius* disabuses us of that preconception. Each individual of *Phaeacius* has two basic predatory tactics in its repertoire. When prey is active and close by, *Phaeacius* remains quiescent until its prey comes to within striking distance and then attacks the prey with a sudden lunge. *Phaeacius*' other tactic, called insinuation, is adopted when prey is detected from a distance. Keeping its body close to the substrate, *Phaeacius* slowly moves in closer to the prey and, arriving near the prey, becomes quiescent again, ready for an ambush attack (Jackson, 1990). Besides salticids, *Phaeacius* ambushes other spiders and also insects, but insinuation is a salticid-specific tactic (Li *et al.*, 2003). The special posture and slow gait *Phaeacius* adopts apparently functions to compensate for the salticid's exceptional eyesight. *Phaeacius* also makes decisions based on information about the background and the prey's orientation, but only when the prey is a salticid. *Phaeacius* chooses to adopt insinuation specifically when the salticid is facing away and the background *Phaeacius* is on matches *Phaeacius'* markings (Li *et al.*, 2003).

2.10   Plants as spider food

Besides capturing living prey, some spiders also scavenge on already dead arthropods (Cramer, 2008, Sandidge, 2003). However, the most striking examples of non-predatory foraging versatility come from spiders that feed on plant material, particularly honeydew, nectar and pollen. Honeydew might be thought of as a mixed product, being of plant origin but passing through an insect before being ingested by the spider (Jackson *et al.*, 2008). For a web-building spider, pollen seems to reach the spider indirectly, as it collects in the web and is digested along with old web silk (Smith and Mommsen, 1984), but there are other spiders that feed on pollen directly when they visit flowers (Figure 2.3). Perhaps feeding on honeydew or pollen is uncommon, but there

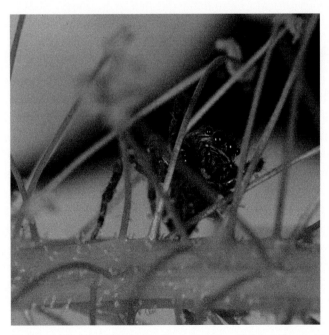

Figure 2.3 *Evarcha culicivora* feeding on pollen of *Hibiscus* flower. Note large anterior median eyes (characteristic of salticids). See also colour plate.

are now numerous records of spiders from many families feeding on nectar that they acquire by visiting flowers or extrafloral nectaries (Jackson *et al.*, 2001, Morse, 2006, Pollard *et al.*, 1995, Ruhren and Handel, 1999, Taylor and Bradley, 2009, Taylor and Foster, 1996, Taylor and Pfannenstiel, 2008, Vogelei and Greissl, 1989). *Evarcha culicivora* illustrates how a spider that has specialised prey-choice behaviour as a predator can also have specialised plant-choice behaviour as a nectivore. Besides feeding indirectly on vertebrate blood by choosing blood-carrying mosquitoes as preferred prey (Jackson *et al.*, 2005), this species also has an innate affinity for particular plants (Cross and Jackson, 2009b).

The most remarkable example of herbivory by a spider may come from *Bagheera kiplingi*, a Central American salticid that lives on acacia trees and exploits the well-known mutualistic relationship these plants have with ants (Hölldobler and Wilson, 1990). The acacia feeds the ants by growing specialised leaf tips, known as Beltian bodies that are loaded with protein and sugar. Ants feed on these trophic structures and the plant benefits because the ants drive away herbivores, the plant's enemies. *Bagheera kiplingi* has apparently become a specialised forager on Beltian bodies. Skilfully moving within the plant's foliage, it dodges the dangerous ants and snatches unguarded Beltian bodies. Radioisotope data imply that nutrition from Beltian bodies is the dominant component of this salticid's natural diet (Meehan *et al.*, 2009).

2.11   Conclusions and outlook

With the examples we present here, perhaps the single most striking impression is that there is a need for a better understanding of the level at which trade-offs and capacity limitations become important. Intuition about trade-offs and capacity limitations needs to be turned into explicit hypotheses that can be examined critically. As an important step towards this goal, we should be more careful about how we use terms like specialist and generalist. When considering natural diet, a predator can be positioned somewhere on a stenophagy–euryphagy continuum, with the continuum being defined by categories that are relevant to the researcher. Most often these are formal taxonomic categories (species, genus, family and so forth). However, concluding that a predator is stenophagic or monophagic is very different from concluding that a predator's prey-capture behaviour is especially adapted for the capture of the limited prey types in its diet. That particular conclusion requires research on the predator's actual behaviour.

It is conditional predatory strategies (predatory versatility) that forcefully remind us that the concepts of specialised and generalised behaviour are distinct from stenophagic or euryphagic natural diet. West-Eberhard (2003) voiced a similar warning after reviewing a much wider range of organisms and considering more than just predatory strategies. *Portia* is a striking example. Having a repertoire of prey-specific tactics, each tactic being specialised in a different way, each individual of *Portia* is euryphagic and at the same time specialised. Using West-Eberhard's term, spiders that use conditional predatory strategies are 'poly-specialists' a term that acknowledges that sometimes it is appropriate to say an individual predator is a specialist on one prey type and at the same time be a specialist on other prey types. As illustrated by *Portia*, the predator can be highly effective at using predatory behaviour that targets one type of prey and also be highly effective at using other predatory behaviour that targets other prey types. The jack-of-all-trades hypothesis appears to have minimal relevance for what is being considered. We seem to have an example that shows compellingly that being euryphagic in diet need not go hand in hand with generalised behaviour.

Acknowledgements

We gratefully acknowledge Marie Herberstein, John Prenter, Daniel Zurek, Sara Kross, Jutta Schneider, and Paul McDonald for commenting on the manuscript and, for financial support for much of the research reviewed in this manuscript, the Royal Society of New Zealand (Marsden Fund and James Cook Fellowship), the National Geographic Society and the Australian Research Council.

References

Allan, R. A. and Elgar, M. A. (2001). Exploitation of the green tree ant, *Oecophylla smaragdina*, by the salticid spider *Cosmophasis bitaeniata*. *Australian Journal of Zoology*, **49**, 129–137.

Austin, A. D. and Blest, A. D. (1979). The biology of two Australian species of dinopid spider. *Journal of Zoology, London*, **189**, 145–156.

Barth, F. G. (2002). Spider senses: technical perfection and biology. *Zoology*, **105**, 271–285.

Berenbaum, M. R. (1996). Introduction to the symposium: on the evolution of specialization. *American Naturalist*, **148** (Suppl.), S78–S83.

Beutel, R. G., Pohl, H. and Hunefeld, F. (2005). Strepsipteran brains and effects of miniaturization (Insecta). *Arthropod Structure and Development*, **34**, 301–313.

Blest, A. D. and Land, M. F. (1977). The physiological optics of *Dinopis subrufus* L. Koch: a fish-lens in a spider. *Proceedings of the Royal Society of London, B*, **196**, 197–222.

Blest, A. D., McIntyre, P. and Carter, M. (1988). A re-examination of the principal retinae of *Phidippus johnsoni* and *Plexippus validus* (Araneae: Salticidae): implications for optical modelling. *Journal of Comparative Physiology, A*, **162**, 47–56.

Blest, A. D., O'Carroll, D. C. and Carter, M. (1990). Comparative ultrastructure of Layer I receptor mosaics in principal eyes of jumping spiders: the evolution of regular arrays of light guides. *Cell and Tissue Research*, **262**, 445–460.

Christy, J. H. (1995). Mimicry, mate choice, and the sensory trap hypothesis. *American Naturalist*, **146**, 171–181.

Clark, R. J. and Jackson, R. R. (1994). Self recognition in a jumping spider: *Portia labiata* females discriminate between their own draglines and those of conspecifics. *Ethology, Ecology & Evolution*, **6**, 371–375.

Clark, R. J. and Jackson, R. R. (1995). Araneophagic jumping spiders discriminate between the draglines of familiar and unfamiliar conspecifics. *Ethology, Ecology & Evolution*, **7**, 185–190.

Clark, R. J., Harland, D. P. and Jackson, R. R. (2000). Speculative hunting by an araneophagic salticid spider. *Behaviour*, **137**, 1601–1612.

Clark, R. J., Jackson, R. R. and Waas, J. R. (1999). Draglines and assessment of fighting ability in cannibalistic jumping spiders. *Journal of Insect Behavior*, **12**, 753–766.

Clements, A. N. (1999). *The Biology of Mosquitoes*. Wallingford, UK: CABI Publishing.

Coddington, J. A. (1986). Orb webs in 'non-orb weaving' ogre-faced spiders (Araneae: Dinopidae): a question of genealogy. *Journal of Cladistics*, **2**, 53–67.

Cohen, A. C. (1995). Extra-oral digestion in predaceous terrestrial Arthropoda. *Annual Review of Entomology*, **40**, 85–103.

Cramer, K. L. (2008). Are brown recluse spiders *Loxosceles reclusa* (Araneae, Sicariidae) scavengers? The influence of predator satiation, prey size, and prey quality. *Journal of Arachnology*, **36**, 140–144.

Cross, F. R. and Jackson, R. R. (2009a). How cross-modality effects during intraspecific interactions of jumping spiders differ depending on whether a female-choice or mutual-choice mating system is adopted. *Behavioral Processes*, **80**, 162–168.

Cross, F. R. and Jackson, R. R. (2009b). A blood-feeding jumping spider's affinity for particular plants, *Lantana camara* and *Ricinus communis*. *New Zealand Journal of Zoology*, **36**, 75–80.

Curio, E. (1976). *The Ethology of Predation*. Berlin: Springer Verlag.

Cushing, P. E. (1997). Myrmecomorphy and myrmecophily in spiders: a review. *Florida Entomologist*, **80**, 165–193.

Dawkins, R. (1996). *Climbing Mount Improbable*. New York: W.W. Norton.

Dennett, D. C. (1996). *Kinds of Minds: Towards an Understanding of Consciousness*. New York: Simon and Schuster.

Dennett, D. C. (2005). *Sweet Dreams: Philosophical Obstacles to a Science of Consciousness*. Cambridge, MA: MIT Press.

Eberhard, W. G. (1977). Aggressive chemical mimicry by a bolas spider. *Science*, **198**, 1173–1175.

Flexibility in the foraging strategies of spiders 51

Eberhard, W. G. (2007). Miniaturized orb-weaving spiders: behavioural precision is not limited by small size. *Proceedings of the Royal Society of London, B*, **274**, 2203–2209.

Edmunds, M. (1974). *Defence in Animals: A Survey of Anti-Predator Defences*. London: Longman.

Elgar, M. A. and Allan, R. A. (2004). Predatory spider mimics acquire colony-specific cuticular hydrocarbons from their ant model prey. *Naturwissenschaften*, **91**, 143–147.

Elias, D. O., Mason, A. C., Maddison, W. P. and Hoy, R. R. (2003). Seismic signals in a courting male jumping spider (Araneae: Salticidae). *Journal of Experimental Biology*, **206**, 4029–4039.

Endler, J. A. and Basolo, A. L. (1998). Sensory ecology, receiver biases and sexual selection. *Trends in Ecology and Evolution*, **13**, 415–420.

Foelix, R. F. (1970). Chemosensitive hairs in spiders. *Journal of Morphology*, **132**, 313–334.

Foelix, R. F. (1996). *Biology of Spiders*, 2nd edn. Oxford, UK: Oxford University Press and New York: Georg Thieme Verlag.

Forster, L. M. (1982). Vision and prey-catching strategies in jumping spiders. *American Scientist*, **70**, 165–175.

Fry, J. D. (1996). The evolution of host specialization: are trade-offs overrated? *American Naturalist*, **148** (Suppl.), S84–S107.

Futuyma, D. J. and Moreno, G. (1988). The evolution of ecological specialization. *Annual Reviews of Ecology and Systematics*, **19**, 207–233.

Gemeno, C., Yeargan, K. V. and Haynes K. F. (2000). Aggressive chemical mimicry by the bolas spider *Mastophora hutchinsoni*: identification and quantification of a major prey's sex pheromone components in the spider's volatile emissions. *Journal of Chemical Ecology*, **26**, 1235–1243.

Getty, R. M. and Coyle, F. A. (1996). Observations on prey capture and anti-predator behaviors of ogre-faced spiders (*Deinopis*) in southern Costa Rica (Araneae, Deinopidae). *Journal of Arachnology*, **24**, 93–100.

Guilford, T. and Dawkins, M. S. (1991). Receiver psychology and the evolution of animal signals. *Animal Behaviour*, **42**, 1–14.

Hallas, S. E. A. and Jackson, R. R. (1986). Prey-holding abilities of the nests and webs of jumping spiders (Araneae, Salticidae). *Journal of Natural History*, **20**, 881–894.

Harland, D. P. and Jackson, R. R. (2000a). 'Eight-legged cats' and how they see: a review of recent work on jumping spiders (Araneae: Salticidae). *Cimbebasia*, **16**, 231–240.

Harland, D. P. and Jackson, R. R. (2000b). Cues by which *Portia fimbriata*, an araneophagic jumping spider, distinguishes jumping-spider prey from other prey. *Journal of Experimental Biology*, **203**, 3485–3494.

Harland, D. P. and Jackson, R. R. (2002). Influence of cues from the anterior medial eyes of virtual prey on *Portia fimbriata*, an araneophagic jumping spider. *Journal of Experimental Biology*, **205**, 1861–1868.

Harland, D. P. and Jackson, R. R. (2004). *Portia* perceptions: the *Umwelt* of an araneophagic jumping spider. In *Complex Worlds from Simpler Nervous Systems* (ed. F. R. Prete). Cambridge, MA: MIT Press, pp. 5–40.

Harland, D. P. and Jackson, R. R. (in press). How jumping spiders see the world. In *How Animals See the World: Behavior, Biology, and Evolution of Vision* (ed. O. Lazareva, T. Shimizu and E. Wasserman). Oxford, UK: Oxford University Press.

Haynes, K. F., Gemeno, C., Yeargan, K. V., Millar, J. G. and Johnson, K. M. (2002). Aggressive chemical mimicry of moth pheromones by a bolas spider: how does this specialist predator attract more than one species of prey? *Chemoecology*, **12**, 99–105.

Haynes, K. F., Yeargan, K. V., Millar, J. G. and Chastain, B. B. (1996). Identification of sex pheromone of *Tetanolita mynesalis* (Lepidoptera: Noctuidae), a prey species of bolas spider, *Mastophora hutchinsoni*. *Journal of Chemical Ecology*, **22**, 75–89.

Hölldobler, B. (1983). Territorial behavior in the green tree ant (*Oecophylla smaragdina*). *Biotropica*, **15**, 241–250.

Hölldobler, B. and Wilson, E. O. (1990). *The Ants*. Heidelberg, Germany: Springer Verlag.

Jackson, R. R. (1977). Courtship versatility in the jumping spider *Phidippus johnsoni* (Araneae: Salticidae). *Animal Behaviour*, **25**, 953–957.

Jackson, R. R. (1979). Nests of *Phidippus johnsoni* (Araneae, Salticidae): characteristics, pattern of occupation, and function. *Journal of Arachnology*, **7**, 47–58.

Jackson, R. R. (1982). The behavior of communicating in jumping spiders (Salticidae). In *Spider Communication: Mechanisms and Ecological Significance* (ed. P. N. Witt and J. S. Rovner). Princeton, NJ: Princeton University Press, pp. 213–247.

Jackson, R. R. (1986). Web building, predatory versatility, and the evolution of the Salticidae. In *Spiders: Webs, Behavior, and Evolution* (ed. W. A. Shear). Stanford, CA: Stanford University Press, pp. 232–268.

Jackson, R. R. (1988). The biology of *Jacksonoides queenlandicus*, a jumping spider (Araneae: Salticidae) from Queensland: intraspecific interactions, web-invasion, predators, and prey. *New Zealand Journal of Zoology*, **15**, 1–37.

Jackson, R. R. (1990). Ambush predatory behaviour of *Phaeacius malayensis* and *Phaeacius* sp. indet., spartaeine jumping spiders (Araneae: Salticidae) from tropical Asia. *New Zealand Journal of Zoology*, **17**, 491–498.

Jackson, R. R. (1992). Eight-legged tricksters: spiders that specialize at catching other spiders. *BioScience*, **42**, 590–598.

Jackson, R. R. and Blest, A. D. (1982). The biology of *Portia fimbriata*, a web-building jumping spider (Araneae, Salticidae) from Queensland: utilization of webs and predatory versatility. *Journal of Zoology, London*, **196**, 255–293.

Jackson, R. R. and Hallas, S. E. A. (1986). Capture efficiencies of web-building jumping spiders (Araneae, Salticidae): is the jack-of-all-trades the master of none? *Journal of Zoology, London*, **209**, 1–7.

Jackson, R. R. and Macnab, A. M. (1989). Display, mating and predatory behaviour of the jumping spider *Plexippus paykulli* (Araneae, Salticidae). *New Zealand Journal of Zoology*, **16**, 151–168.

Jackson, R. R. and Pollard, S. D. (1996). Predatory behavior of jumping spiders. *Annual Review of Entomology*, **41**, 287–308.

Jackson, R. R. and Pollard, S. D. (1997). Jumping spider mating strategies: sex among cannibals in and out of webs. In *The Evolution of Mating Systems in Insects and Arachnids* (ed. J. C. Choe and B. J. Crespi). Cambridge, UK: Cambridge University Press, pp. 340–351.

Jackson, R. R. and Wilcox, R. S. (1994). Spider flexibly chooses aggressive mimicry signals for different prey by trial and error. *Behaviour*, **127**, 21–36.

Jackson, R. R. and Wilcox, R. S. (1998). Spider-eating spiders. *American Scientist*, **86**, 350–357.

Jackson, R. R., Clark, R. J. and Harland, D. P. (2002a). Behavioural and cognitive influences of kairomones on an araneophagic spider. *Behaviour*, **139**, 749–775.

Jackson, R. R., Li, D., Fijn, N. and Barrion, A. T. (1998). Predator-prey interactions between aggressive-mimic jumping spiders (Salticidae) and araeneophagic spitting spiders (Scytodidae) from the Philippines. *Journal of Insect Behavior*, **11**, 319–342.

Jackson, R. R., Nelson, X. J. and Salm, K. (2008). The natural history of *Myrmarachne melanotarsa*, a social ant-mimicking jumping spider. *New Zealand Journal of Zoology*, **35**, 225–235.

Jackson, R. R., Nelson, X. J. and Sune, G. O. (2005). A spider that feeds indirectly on vertebrate blood by choosing female mosquitoes as prey. *Proceedings of the National Academy of Sciences of the USA*, **102**, 15 155–15 160.

Jackson, R. R., Pollard, S. D., Li, D. and Fijn, N. (2002b). Interpopulation variation in the risk-related decisions of *Portia labiata*, an araneophagic jumping spider (Araneae, Salticidae), during predatory sequences with spitting spiders. *Animal Cognition*, **5**, 215–223.

Jackson, R. R., Pollard, S. D., Nelson, X. J., Edwards, G. B. and Barrion, A. T. (2001). Jumping spiders (Araneae: Salticidae) that feed on nectar. *Journal of Zoology*, **255**, 25–29.

Kirschfeld, K. (1976). The resolution of lens and compound eyes. In *Neural Principles in Vision* (ed. F. Zettler and R. Weiler). Berlin: Springer Verlag, pp. 354–370.

Krafft, B. and Leborgne, R. (1979). Perception sensorielle et importance des phé nomènes vibratoires chez les araignées. *Journal de Psychologie*, **3**, 299–334.

Labhart, T. and Nilsson, D. E. (1995). The dorsal eye of the dragonfly *Sympetrum*: specializations for prey detection against the blue sky. *Journal of Comparative Physiology, A*, **176**(4), 437–453.

Land, M. F. (1969a). Structure of the retinae of the principal eyes of jumping spiders (Salticidae: Dendryphantinae) in relation to visual optics. *Journal of Experimental Biology*, **51**, 443–470.

Land, M. F. (1969b). Movements of the retinae of jumping spiders (Salticidae: Dendryphantinae) in response to visual stimuli. *Journal of Experimental Biology*, **51**, 471–493.

Land, M. F. and Nilsson, D. E. (2002). *Animal Eyes*. Oxford, UK: Oxford University Press.

Laughlin, S., Blest, A. D. and Stowe, S. (1980). The sensitivity of receptors in the posterior median eye of the nocturnal spider, *Dinopis*. *Journal of Comparative Physiology*, **141**, 53–65.

Li, D. (2000). Prey preferences of *Phaeacius malayensis*, a spartaeine jumping spider (Araneae: Salticidae) from Singapore. *Canadian Journal of Zoology – Revue Canadienne de Zoologie*, **78**, 2218–2226.

Li, D. and Jackson, R. R. (2003). A predator's preference for egg-carrying prey: a novel cost of parental care. *Behavioral Ecology and Sociobiology*, **55**, 129–136.

Li, D., Jackson, R. R. and Barrion, A. T. (1999). Parental and predatory behaviour of *Scytodes* sp., an araneophagic spitting spider (Araneae: Scytodidae) from the Philippines. *Journal of Zoology*, **247**, 293–310.

Li, D., Jackson, R. R. and Lim, L. M. M. (2003). Influence of background and prey orientation on an ambushing predator's decisions. *Behaviour*, **140**, 739–764.

Maddison, W. P. and Hedin, M. C. (2003). Jumping spider phylogeny (Araneae: Salticidae). *Invertebrate Systematics*, **17**, 529–549.

Malli, H., Kuhn-Nentwig, L., Imboden, H. and Nentwig, W. (1999). Effects of size, motility and paralysation time of prey on the quantity of venom injected by the hunting spider *Cupiennius salei*. *Journal of Experimental Biology*, **202**, 2083–2089.

Masters, W. M., Markl, H. S. and Moffat, A. M. (1986). Transmission of vibrations in a spider's web. In *Spiders: Webs, Behavior, and Evolution* (ed. W. A. Shear). Stanford, CA: Stanford University Press, pp. 47–69.

McIlwain, J. T. (1996). *An Introduction to the Biology of Vision*. Cambridge, UK: Cambridge University Press.

Meehan, C. J., Olson, E. J., Reudink, M. W., Kyser, K. T. and Curry, R. L. (2009). Herbivory in a spider through exploitation of an ant–plant mutualism. *Current Biology*, **19**, R892–R893.

Minsky, M. (1986). *The Society of Mind*. New York: Simon and Schuster.

Morse, D. H. (2006). Fine-scale substrate use by a small sit-and-wait predator. *Behavioral Ecology*, **17**, 405–409.

Nelson, X. J. and Jackson, R. R. (2006a). A predator from East Africa that chooses malaria vectors as preferred prey. *PLoS ONE*, **1**, e132.

Nelson, X. J. and Jackson, R. R. (2006b). Vision-based innate aversion to ants and ant mimics. *Behavioral Ecology*, **17**, 676–681.

Nelson, X. J. and Jackson, R. R. (2009a). An ant-like jumping spider that practises aggressive mimicry by deploying Batesian mimicry against ant-averse prey. *Biology Letters*, **5**, 755–757.

Nelson, X. J. and Jackson, R. R. (2009b). Collective Batesian mimicry of ant groups by aggregating spiders. *Animal Behaviour*, **78**, 123–129.

Nelson, X. J., Jackson, R. R., Edwards, G. B. and Barrion, A. T. (2004). Predation by ants on jumping spiders (Araneae: Salticidae) in the Philippines. *New Zealand Journal of Zoology*, **31**, 45–56.

Nelson, X. J., Jackson, R. R. and Sune, G. O. (2005). Use of *Anopheles*-specific prey-capture behavior by the small juveniles of *Evarcha culicivora*, a mosquito-eating jumping spider. *Journal of Arachnology*, **33**, 541–548.

Platnick, N. I. (2010). *The World Spider Catalogue*, Version 10.0. American Museum of Natural History, online at http://research.amnh.org/iz/spiders/catalog. Accessed 1/9/10.

Pollard, S. D. (1990). The feeding strategy of a New Zealand crab spider *Diaea* sp. indet. (Araneae, Thomisidae): post-capture decision rules. *Journal of Zoology, London*, **222**, 601–615.

Pollard, S. D. (1994). Consequences of sexual selection on feeding in male jumping spiders (Araneae: Salticidae). *Journal of Zoology, London*, **243**, 203–208.

Pollard, S. D., Beck, M. W. and Dodson, G. N. (1995). Why do male crab spiders drink nectar? *Animal Behaviour*, **49**, 1443–1448.

Pollard, S. D., Macnab, A. M. and Jackson, R. R. (1987). Communication with chemicals: pheromones and spiders. In *Ecophysiology of Spiders* (ed. W. Nentwig). Heidelberg, Germany: Springer Verlag, pp. 133–141.

Řezáč, M., Pekár, S. and Lubin, Y. (2008). How oniscophagous spiders overcome woodlouse armour. *Journal of Zoology, London*, **275**, 64–71.

Richman, D. B. and Jackson, R. R. (1992). A review of the ethology of jumping spiders (Araneae, Salticidae). *Bulletin of the British Arachnological Society*, **9**, 33–37.

Roberts, J. A. and Uetz, G. W. (2005). Information content of female chemical signals in the wolf spider, *Schizocosa ocreata*: male discrimination of reproductive state and receptivity. *Animal Behaviour*, **70**, 271–223.

Robinson, M. H. and Robinson, B. (1971). Predatory behavior of ogre-faced spider *Dinopis longipes* F. Cambridge (Araneae, Dinopidae). *American Midland Naturalist*, **85**, 85–96.

Ruhren, S. and Handel, S. N. (1999). Jumping spiders (Salticidae) enhance the seed production of a plant with extrafloral nectaries. *Oecologia*, **119**, 227–230.

Sandidge, J. S. (2003). Scavenging by brown recluse spiders. *Nature*, **426**, 30.

Schiller, C. (1957). *Instinctive Behavior*. New York: Hallmark Press.

Smith, R. B. and Mommsen, T. P. (1984). Pollen feeding in an orb-weaving spider. *Science*, **226**, 1330–1333.

Stowe, M. K., Tumlinson, J. H. and Heath, R. R. (1987). Chemical mimicry: bolas spiders emit components of moth prey species sex-pheromones. *Science*, **236**, 964–967.

Su, K. F. Y., Meier, R., Jackson, R. R., Harland, D. P. and Li, D. (2007). Convergent evolution of eye ultrastructure and divergent evolution of vision-mediated predatory behaviour in jumping spiders. *Journal of Evolutionary Biology*, **20**, 1478–1489.

Suter, R. B. and Stratton, G. E. (2005). *Scytodes vs. Schizocosa*: predatory techniques and their morphological correlates. *Journal of Arachnology*, **33**, 7–15.

Tarsitano, M. S., Jackson, R. R. and Kirchner, W. (2000). Signals and signal choices made by araneophagic jumping spiders while hunting the orb-weaving spiders *Zygiella x-notata* and *Zosis genicularis*. *Ethology*, **106**, 595–615.

Taylor, R. M. and Bradley, R. A. (2009). Plant nectar increases survival, molting, and foraging in two foliage wandering spiders. *Journal of Arachnology*, **37**, 232–237.

Taylor, R. M. and Foster, W. A. (1996). Spider nectarivory. *American Entomologist*, **42**, 82–86.

Taylor, R. M. and Pfannenstiel, R. S. (2008). Nectar feeding by wandering spiders on cotton plants. *Environmental Entomology*, **37**, 996–1002.

Vogelei, A. and Greissl, R. (1989). Survival strategies of the crab spider *Thomisus onustus* Walckenaer 1806 (Chelicerata, Arachnida, Thomisidae). *Oecologia*, **80**, 513–515.

von Uexküll, J. (1909). *Umwelt und Innenwelt der Tiere*. Berlin: Springer Verlag.

von Uexküll, J. (1957). A stroll through the worlds of animals and men: a picture book of invisible worlds. Reprinted 1957 in *Instinctive Behavior: The Development of a Modern Concept* (ed. C. H. Schiller). New York: International Universities Press.

Weng, J. L., Barrantes, G. and Eberhard, W. G. (2006). Feeding by *Philoponella vicina* (Araneae, Uloboridae) and how uloborid spiders lost their venom glands. *Canadian Journal of Zoology*, **84**, 1752–1762.

Wesolowska, W. and Jackson, R. R. (2003). *Evarcha culicivora* sp. nov., a mosquito-eating jumping spider from East Africa (Araneae: Salticidae). *Annales Zoologici*, **53**, 335–338.

West-Eberhard, M. J. (2003). *Developmental Plasticity and Evolution*. New York: Oxford University Press.

White, G. B. (1974). *Anopheles gambiae* complex and disease transmission in Africa. *Transactions of the Royal Society of Tropical Medicine and Hygiene*, **68**, 278–301.

Whitlock, M. C. (1996). The red queen beats the jack-of-all-trades: the limitations on the evolution of phenotypic plasticity and niche breadth. *American Naturalist*, **148** (Suppl.), S65–S77.

Wigger, E., Kuhn-Nentwig, L. and Nentwig, W. (2002). The venom optimisation hypothesis: a spider injects large venom quantities only into difficult prey types. *Toxicon*, **40**, 749–752.

Williams, D. S. and McIntyre, P. (1980). The principal eyes of a jumping spider have a telephoto component. *Nature*, **228**, 578–580.

Wilson, D. S. and Yoshimura, J. (1994). On the coexistence of specialists and generalists. *American Naturalist*, **144**, 692–707.

Wyatt, T. D. (2003). *Pheromones and Animal Behaviour*. Cambridge, UK: Cambridge University Press.

Yeargan, K. V. (1994). Biology of bolas spiders. *Annual Review of Entomology*, **39**, 81–99.

3

Spider webs: evolution, diversity and plasticity

MARIE E. HERBERSTEIN AND I-MIN TSO

The webs of spiders are the first things we notice, long before we recognise the occupant. Silk production and web building is a defining feature of all spiders, and certainly the trait they are best known for. The obvious diversity in different web types and structures has always fascinated; even Aristotle made attempts to define different web types. But it has not been until the latter half of the twentieth century that we have started to appreciate the level of diversity and plasticity in web-building behaviour, between individuals of the same species, and even within an individual from one day to the next. The recent work on silk composition and mechanics is starting to document similar levels of plasticity in response to a variety of extrinsic and intrinsic factors. We argue that that this underappreciated aspect of spider biology renders them superior models for studies investigating behavioural plasticity at the individual level.

3.1 Webs, silks and decorations

3.1.1 *The evolution of spider webs*

Spider webs fulfil a number of functions of which prey capture is clearly the best recognised and studied. But webs also provide a moulting and mating platform, a retreat from predators, a place to secure egg sacs, and in some cases a diving bell (e.g. *Argyroneta aquatica*; Schütz *et al.*, 2007). The reasons silk and webs evolved in the first place are still unresolved (Vollrath and Selden, 2007). Two current hypotheses propose that silk and webs either evolved for reproductive purposes such as the protection of eggs and the spermatophore (Shultz, 1987) or to protect the gills of early terrestrial spiders (Damen *et al.*, 2002). Several lines of

Spider Behaviour: Flexibility and Versatility, ed. Marie Elisabeth Herberstein. Published by Cambridge University Press. © Cambridge University Press 2011.

evidence are used to reconstruct the evolution of spider webs: fossil spiders (especially the structure of their spinnerets and spigots), fossilised silk and comparisons to extant spiders (Coddington and Levi, 1991, Vollrath and Selden, 2007).

The extant Liphistiidae (Mesothelae) are the sister group to all other spiders (mygalomorphs and araneomorphs). Yet, the earliest spider fossil from the Middle Devonian (385–380 MYA) shows similarities with the mygalomorphs based on the complexity of spigots (Shear et al., 1989, Vollrath and Selden, 2007). Nevertheless, both liphistiids and mygalomorphs utilise similar web structures. Both dig burrows into the soil and use silk to line these burrows. They sit in these tubes, often covered by a trapdoor, and pounce on prey wandering past. In order to increase their foraging area, they often extend silk threads from the burrow in a radial pattern (Coddington and Levi, 1991). As the evolution of these early spiders predates the evolution of flight in insects (Grimaldi and Engel, 2005), it may be reasonable to assume that the earliest spiders also resided in tubes with trip lines, preying on ground-dwelling arthropods.

The evolution of insect flight in the Carboniferous (354–290 MYA) is thought to be closely related to the evolution of aerial webs. Regrettably, there is no fossil evidence from that crucial time documenting the type of webs spiders might have been building (Vollrath and Selden, 2007). The discovery of a Permian (290–248 MYA) arachnid with an elongate spinneret similar to modern Dipluridae (Mygalomorphae) and Agelenidae (Araneomorphae) suggests the presence of funnel webs, perhaps similar to those of modern funnel-web spiders (Eskov and Selden, 2005).

The Triassic period (248–206 MYA) is characterised by a period of arthropod radiation, with the first records of true mygalomorphs and araneomorphs. The morphology of early araneomorphs suggests that they might belong within the extant Araneoidea (Selden et al., 1999, Vollrath and Selden, 2007). This has significant implication for the timeline of web evolution because extant araneoids construct aerial orb webs, suggesting that the origin of the orb web might be as early as the Triassic (Vollrath and Selden, 2007). Even though orb webs are built by two different spider clades, the Deinopoidea and the Araneoidea, it is now accepted that the orb web is monophyletic (Garb et al., 2006, Griswold et al., 1998).

The ancestral orb-web type was probably similar to that of the extant Deinopoidea: a horizontal orb constructed from cribellar silk (Bond and Opell, 1998, Griswold et al., 1998). Cribellar silk is a dry silk that derives its stickiness through thousands of fine silk strands that are brushed around larger axial silk fibres (Craig, 2003). The evolution of flagelliform silk that forms a coat of viscid glue around dry silk, as well as a vertical orb orientation, are key innovations that have contributed to the considerable diversification of the Araneoidea compared with the Deinopoidea (Bond and Opell, 1998). The fossil record of viscid silk enclosed in amber goes back to the early Cretaceous, around 130–110 MYA (Penalver *et al.*, 2006, Zschokke, 2003).

The orb web has long been considered the pinnacle of web evolution; however, it seems that 'the orb web has been an evolutionary base camp rather than a summit' (Griswold *et al.*, 1998:24). While it seems counterintuitive, less-symmetrical three-dimensional webs, such as the sheet webs of the Linyphiidae and the cob webs of the Theridiidae, have derived independently from the orb web (Blackledge *et al.*, 2009). The reason for the transition from the two-dimensional orb to a three-dimensional sheet is unclear. Several ideas have been proposed for such a change in capture function, such as a shift from intercepting flying prey to targeting jumping prey or walking prey (Griswold *et al.*, 1998). A protection from wasp predators (Blackledge *et al.*, 2003) is likely for linyphiid sheet webs, but less likely for theridiid webs (Eberhard *et al.*, 2008).

Finally, web building itself has been lost a number of times in all groups of spiders (Blackledge *et al.*, 2009). The most diverse clades of spiders (the RTA clade and the Araneoidea) shows the greatest proportion of web loss, suggesting radiation after abandoning substrate-bound hunting via webs (Blackledge *et al.*, 2009). For example, most wolf spiders (Lycosidae) are cursorial hunters without webs, although web building is considered ancestral with some genera still constructing sheet webs (Yoo and Framenau, 2006). Similarly, the most diverse families of spiders within the RTA clade, the jumping spiders (Salticidae) and crab spiders (Thomisidae), no longer build capture webs, with a few exceptions. The reason why so many derived species in most families have abandoned web building for a hunting strategy is not entirely resolved, but could include the risk of predation by predators that target the stationary web (Dippenaar-Schoeman and Jocqué, 1997).

3.1.2   Web diversity

The description of different web types below focuses on the function and structure of the web, rather than the phylogenetic relationships between them. Thus, similar-looking webs may be built by relatively unrelated groups of spiders (Blackledge *et al.*, 2009). It is generally assumed that similar structures reflect similar prey-capture function, but for the majority of spider webs, very little description of prey capture exists to verify this assumption. Our classification of web types is loosely based on Jocqué and Dippenaar-Schoeman's (2007) excellent key to spider webs.

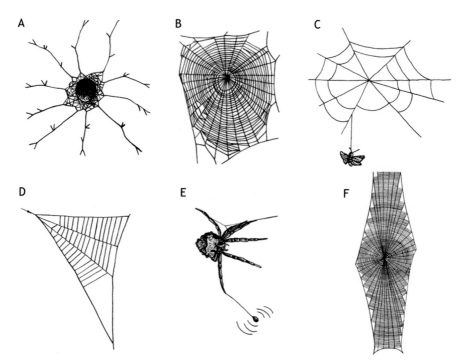

Figure 3.1 Examples of different web types found in the Araneae. (A) Tube web. (B) Orb web. (C) Reduced orb web built by *Cyrtarachne*. (D) Reduced orb web built by *Hyptiotes*. (E) Bolas spider with sticky bolas. (F) Ladder web by *Telaprocera*. (Redrawn from Jocqué and Dippenaar-Schoeman, 2007, by Monika Hänel with kind permission from Rudy Jocqué and Ansi Dippenaar-Schoeman.)

Substrate-defined webs

Tube webs and substrate-bound sheets

The main element of these types of web is a silk-lined retreat from which the spider forages by attacking passing prey (Figure 3.1A). Usually the spider does not venture far from this retreat. The silk retreat usually consists of a burrow dug into the soil or sometimes a tree hollow, as in the basal liphistiid or mygalomorph spiders, the haplogyne segestriid spiders (Segestriidae) or the araneomorph wolf spiders (Lycosidae). The entrance to this burrow may or may not be covered by a lid (Coddington and Levi, 1991, Murphy *et al.*, 2006, Shear, 1986). Structures such as trip lines, turrets, funnels or sheets that extend out from the burrow's entrance enhance the complexity of this type of web.

The vibrations created when prey trip over these structures alert the spider, thus extending the sensory radius of the animal (Coddington and Levi, 1991). The extensions from the retreat can be quite elaborate. The purse spider (*Atypus*, Mygalomorphae) extends the lip of the silk-lined retreat into a long sock-like tube that lies on the ground with the spider moving about within it. If an insect lands on top of this tube, the spider bites the prey through the tube (Coyle, 1986). The size of the substrate-bound sheets can also be substantial. For example, in the Dipluridae (Mygalomorphae), the sheet extending from the retreat funnel can cover an area up to 600 cm^2 (Coyle, 1986).

Orb webs

Undoubtedly, the best-known and most widely recognised web type is the orb web (Figure 3.1B). There are four main orb-web-building families in the Araneoidea and the Deinopoidea lineages: Uloboridae, Araneidae, Tetragnathidae and Nephilidae (Coddington and Levi, 1991, Garb *et al.*, 2006, Griswold *et al.*, 1998). The main elements of an orb web are the anchor threads, frame threads, radii and spirals. The anchor threads are attached to the substrate at anchor points. The frame threads, attached to the anchor threads, form the outline of the web. They act as a scaffold for the planar orb. The radial threads radiate out from a more or less central hub and the spiral threads are overlaid on top of the radials (Zschokke, 1999). While the radial and frame threads are always made from dry, non-viscid silk, the spirals may consist of dry cribellate silk (such as in the uloborids or deinopids) or viscid silk (such as in the araneids, tetragnathids and nephilids; Foelix, 1996). Typically the spider resides at the hub of the web, usually located in the centre of the web, from where it attacks entangled prey. There are some notable exceptions to this. For example, *Zygiella* sit in a retreat outside the orb, connected to the hub via a signal thread that allows the spider to detect vibrations in the web (Zschokke, 1999).

Orb-web derivatives

Among the orb-web-building families, many species no longer build the classical planar, two-dimensional orbs, but build derived webs, some of which bear no resemblance to the original orb. Orb webs are generally considered to be generalist traps, while their derived forms may represent prey specialisation (Griswold *et al.*, 1998) and/or increased access to food (Eberhard, 1990). These specialist derivatives are usually characterised by a reduction in the size and complexity of the original orb web. There are, however, some notable exceptions of additions and extensions to the classical orb design. We illustrate these trends using a few selected examples that are by no means intended to be exhaustive.

Reduced orb webs

An example of an obvious loss of complexity is the orb web constructed by *Cyrtarachne* (Araneidae). While the web is planar and circular containing radials and spirals, it contains far fewer radials and spirals (fewer than five spirals) compared with typical orb webs (Figure 3.1C). Instead, the stickiness and thickness of the spiral threads are substantially greater. These web and silk characteristics are thought to be an adaptation to capturing moth prey (Cartan and Miyashita, 2000). Ogre-faced spiders (Deinopidae) construct a miniature version of the web that vaguely resembles an orb, which they hold with their front legs and throw over passing prey (Robinson and Robinson, 1971).

In sector webs, the original circular orb web has simply been reduced to only a section of the web. In the case of *Nephilengys* (Nephilidae) the spider builds a 'semi orb web' without an upper web half. All radials and spirals vertically above the hub are absent and the hub of the web or sometimes a silk retreat is right at the upper frame threads (Japyassu and Ades, 1998, Kuntner, 2007). The web reduction follows an ontogenetic pattern as juvenile *Nephilengys* build classic complete circular orb webs and only adults lose the upper web half (Japyassu and Ades, 1998).

A more extreme loss of orb-web sections occurs in *Hyptiotes* (Uloboridae). Here the planar orb is reduced to a triangle with only three sectors consisting of four radials and the cribellate capture spiral (Opell, 1982). The spider positions itself at the attachment point of the web and assumes a monitoring position by pulling the web taut (Figure 3.1D). When the web intercepts an insect, the spider quickly lets go of the silk, jerking the web. The spider may repeatedly pull and let go of the web, entrapping the insect more thoroughly before subduing it (Opell, 1985, 1987). A similar triangular web is constructed by the Papua New Guinean genus *Pasilobus* (Araneidae; Robinson and Robinson, 1975 in Cartan and Miyashita, 2000). When an insect comes in contact with one of the very viscid spirals, the thread breaks off the radials at one end and the insect remains suspended by the spiral thread (Cartan and Miyashita, 2000).

Bolas spiders (e.g. the genus *Mastophora*, Araneidae) have reduced the orb web to just a horizontal line of silk from which the female hangs, swinging a viscid ball of silk suspended from a silk thread – the bolas (Figure 3.1E; Yeargan, 1994). Chapter 6 describes this form of prey capture in greater detail.

Extended orb webs

Even when the basic configuration of the orb web remains unchanged, some species extend the web above the horizontal orb (e.g. *Cyrtophora*, Araneidae) or in front and behind the vertical orb (e.g. *Nephila*, Nephilidae; *Argiope*, Araneidae; Baba and Miyashita, 2006, Higgins, 1992, Lubin, 1973, Uhl, 2008, I. M. Tso, C. Hou and L.-F. Chen, unpublished data). These barrier webs consist mostly of a three-dimensional tangle of non-viscid threads (Higgins, 1992, Lubin, 1975). Their function may include structural support for the actual orb web, especially when natural support structures (e.g. dense vegetation) are rare or in strong wind

(Lubin, 1975). Alternatively, the barrier web may function as an early detection system alerting the spider of an approaching predator (Higgins, 1992, Robinson and Robinson, 1973, Tso *et al.*, unpublished data) or knock down prey onto the horizontal orb of *Cyrtophora* (Tso *et al.*, unpublished data). Functionally, the horizontal orb of *Cyrtophora* is similar to aerial sheet webs (see below).

Several araneid (*Scoloderus*, *Cryptaranea* and *Telaprocera*) and nephilid genera (*Clitaetra*, *Herennia*) and a tetragnathid (*Tylorida* sp.) (Eberhard, 1975, Forster and Forster, 1985, Harmer and Framenau, 2009, Kuntner, 2005, Kuntner *et al.*, 2008b, Robinson and Robinson, 1972, Stowe, 1978) extend and elongate rather than reduce the typical circular orb web (Figure 3.1F). These 'ladder webs' are typified by a vertically elongated web-capture area often many times longer than wide. The result can be a web that spans more than a metre (Stowe, 1978). In *Scoloderus*, this web elongation may be an adaptation for prey specialisation on moths. As a moth is entangled in a viscid orb web, it may struggle free and tumble down off the web relatively easily as the scales on the wings detach. Whereas through vertical elongation, the web may eventually arrest the moth once all scales have been removed (Eberhard, 1975). Alternatively, extreme web elongation may be an adaptation to environments with limited horizontal space, such as when building the webs against tree trunks (Harmer, 2009, Harmer and Herberstein, 2009, Kuntner *et al.*, 2008b).

3-D aerial webs

Irregular 3-D webs

The webs of spiders in several unrelated araneomorph families (e.g. Theridiidae, Pholcidae, Desidae, Anapidae) have been described as irregular three-dimensional webs, but with the exception of the comb-footed spiders (Theridiidae; Agnarsson, 2004, Benjamin and Zschokke, 2002, Eberhard *et al.*, 2008) there have been few comparative studies of these irregular webs. Thus, more fine-scale definitions of these webs are likely to be proposed in the future. Moreover, while regular structures are not immediately obvious, several aspects of the web-building behaviour can follow very strict stereotyped patterns (Benjamin and Zschokke, 2003, 2004). For simplicity, we have categorised the irregular 3-D webs into three main types: webs with an obvious horizontal sheet (aerial sheet webs), webs lacking a pronounced sheet but with viscid trapping lines (gum-footed webs) and irregular webs lacking these viscid trapping lines (tangle webs).

Aerial sheet webs

A number of largely unrelated groups of araneomorph spiders construct horizontal aerial sheet webs (Figure 3.2A), including wolf spiders (Lycosidae),

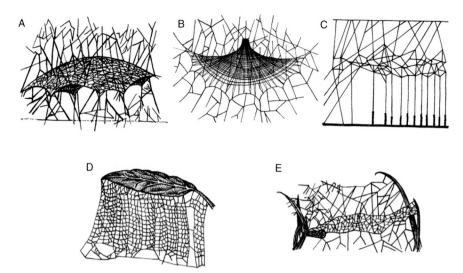

Figure 3.2 Examples of different web types found in the Araneae. (A) Sheet web. (B) Orb web build by *Cyrtophora*. (C) Gumfooted web. (D) Ladder-like tangle web build by Synotaxidae. (E) Irregular tangle web. (Redrawn from Jocqué and Dippenaar-Schoeman 2007, by Monika Hänel with kind permission from Rudy Jocqué and Ansi Dippenaar-Schoeman.)

sheet-web spiders (Linyphiidae), comb-footed spiders (Theridiidae), funnel-web spiders (Agelenidae) and hunting spiders (Pisauridae) (Arnedo *et al.*, 2009, Eberhard, 1990, Murphy *et al.*, 2006). In the Lycosidae and Pisauridae, however, web-building species are an exception in these largely cursorial families. Some daddy-longlegs spiders (Pholcidae) also build a delicate dome-shaped sheet (Japyassú and Macagnan, 2004). The general structure of this type of web consists of a primary horizontal sheet with the spiders either moving on top (e.g. Agelenidae, Lycosidae) or on the underside (e.g. Linyphiidae) of the sheet (Benjamin and Zschokke, 2004, Eberhard, 1990). There may be scaffolding silk threads above and/or below the primary sheet (Arnedo *et al.*, 2009, Benjamin and Zschokke, 2004). The function of these scaffolding threads is to support the sheet, and if located above the sheet they may also have a knock-down effect on flying insects (Benjamin and Zschokke, 2004, Benjamin *et al.*, 2002). Some linyphiid spiders build a second sheet below the primary sheet (Benjamin *et al.*, 2002). The funnel-web spiders (Agelenidae) incorporate a silk tube retreat into their sheet web (Eberhard, 1990) from which they attack prey captured on the sheet.

There is debate as to whether sheet webs, such as those built by linyphiid spiders, contain viscid silk similar to that found in some orb webs. The debate is based on the presence of globules in these sheet webs. However, it seems that while linyphiid spiders are able to produce viscid silk, this type of silk is used as a fast-drying cement (Benjamin *et al.*, 2002). The sheet webs built by Theridiidae and Pholcidae, however, may include viscid gumfoot lines that are used for prey capture (Eberhard *et al.*, 2008, Japyassú and Macagnan, 2004).

As already alluded to above, even though the araneid *Cyrtophora* builds an orb web, the horizontal arrangement of the orb along with the elaborate scaffolding threads above and below the orb suggest that it functions more like the aerial sheet webs (Figure 3.2B), knocking down prey onto the orb (Tso *et al.*, unpublished data).

Gumfooted webs

These types of webs are mostly found in the Theridiidae and the closely related Nesticidae. Their diversity is intriguing, with substantial inter- and intraspecific diversity and frequent convergences in web structure (Agnarsson and Coddington, 2006, Eberhard *et al.*, 2008). The basic elements of gumfooted webs are a supporting structure and several gumfoot lines that are under tension and viscid (Figure 3.2C). Often the web is built under some sort of cover such as a leaf or crevice and may contain a retreat (Benjamin and Zschokke, 2002, 2003, Griswold *et al.*, 1998). These webs typically target ambulatory prey that is lifted off the ground when it comes in contact and breaks the viscid and tensed gumfoot lines. Gumfooted webs range from several gumfoot lines suspended between two leaves to elaborate three-dimensional tangles with retreats (Eberhard *et al.*, 2008).

Tangle webs

This category, referring to a three-dimensional network of cribellate or ecribellate silk (Eberhard *et al.*, 2008) obviously welcomes many web types for which we lack a more refined definition for the moment. Some of these webs can be somewhat ladder-like such as in the Synotaxidae (Figure 3.2D). Others are quite irregular consisting of a maze of silk strands (Figure 3.2E), such as the daddy-longlegs spiders (Pholcidae; Benjamin and Zschokke, 2003, Eberhard *et al.*, 2008, Jocqué and Dippenaar-Schoeman, 2007).

3.1.3   Silk types

Spiders have a wide array of silk types used in various aspects of their biology. Other silk-producing animals, such as lepidopteran larvae, often use silk for very specific purposes (such as building cocoons) so their silk types are rather limited. By contrast spiders such as the Araneidae may have up to seven kinds of glands, which produce six types of silk and one type of glue.

The silks produced by the major ampullate glands are composed of proteins encoded by at least two genes (Hu *et al.*, 2006) and are used as a drag or safety line and for the construction of the web frame and the web radial (Foelix, 1996). The major ampullate silk has received most research attention. Consequently we have the most comprehensive information regarding the genetic basis (Hu *et al.*, 2006), physical properties (Vollrath, 2000), spinning processes (Chen *et al.*, 2006, Sponner, 2007, Vollrath and Knight, 2001), organisation (Sponner *et al.*, 2007) and even potential application (Sponner, 2007) for major ampullate silk.

Minor ampullate glands produce silk used for the temporary capture spiral (Vollrath, 2000) and this silk type is composed of products from at least two genes (Colgin and Lewis, 1998). Flagelliform glands produce the supporting core silk for the capture spiral of the araneid orb webs. This silk core is subsequently coated with sticky droplets produced by the aggregate glands (Higgins *et al.*, 2001). While major ampullate gland silks have high tensile strength and are thought to absorb the kinetic energy of insects impacting the web, the function of the spiral silks is to retain prey through their viscosity and elasticity (Vollrath, 2000). The physical properties of the flagelliform silks are thought to be generated by the underlying genes (Hayashi and Lewis, 1998) and the modulation by aggregate gland secretions (Hu *et al.*, 2006).

The major function of aciniform gland silk is for wrapping prey (Foelix, 1996). In certain spiders products of this gland are also used to construct web decorations (Peters, 1993). Hayashi *et al.* (2004) found that the major component of this silk, the aciniform spidroin 1 (AcSp1), was divergent from other silk proteins and was composed of highly similar repeat units. Although in aciniform silk the crystal-forming components seem to be relatively few, this silk's toughness was 50% greater than that of major ampullate silks (Hayashi *et al.*, 2004).

In female spiders, tubuliform glands produce silks that are used in constructing the egg sac (Vollrath, 2000). The major gene encoding tubuliform silk protein is *TuSp1* (Garb and Hayashi, 2005, Huang *et al.*, 2006). The phenomenon that the repeat units from 12 orbicularian species were highly similar (on both an intra-individual and interspecific basis) suggested a concerted evolution pattern in this silk protein (Garb and Hayashi, 2005). Finally, products of pyriform glands are a type of glue that attaches the dragline to the substrate while spiders are moving, or as a glue substance to unite silk strands together during web construction (Foelix, 1996).

3.1.4   *Decoration types*

Many diurnal orb-web spiders (at least 22 genera from five families; Herberstein *et al.*, 2000a) decorate their webs with various objects after completing the orb. Researchers have reported two major forms of web decorations: those composed entirely of silk and those incorporating non-silk materials. The shape and arrangement of these silk decorations vary between species

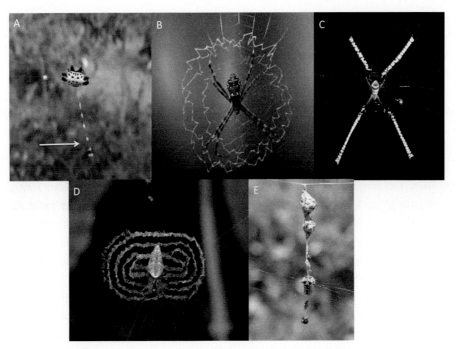

Figure 3.3 Examples of different decoration types found in orb-web spiders. (A) Silk tufts (white arrow) in *Gasteracantha* (photo credit: F. Gawryszewski). (B) Discoid decoration in *Argiope mascordi* (photo credit: G. Pappas). (C) Cruciate decorations in *Argiope keyserlingi* (photo credit: M. Herberstein). (D) Spiral decorations in *Cyclosa mulmeinensis* (photo credit: D. Li). (E) Egg-sac decoration in *Cyclosa* (photo credit: I. M. Tso). See also colour plate.

(Figure 3.3). For example, adult *Argiope savignyi* (Araneidae) sometimes cover the hub of the web with a silk disc (Levi, 1968). In other *Argiope* species, adult spiders spin zig-zag silk bands arranged either vertically (e.g. *Argiope aurantia*) or diagonally (e.g. *Argiope argentata*) (Levi, 1968). Some spiders, such as *Lubinella morobensis* (Lubin, 1986), *Octonoba varians* (Uloboridae) and *Cyclosa sedeculata* (Araneidae) (Yaginuma, 1986) spin concentric silk bands around the hub. Finally, *Gasteracantha cancriformis*, and *Micrathena sexspinosa* (Araneidae) spin silk tufts – or 'silken dots' – at various positions in the webs (Nentwig and Heimer, 1987). Non-silk decorations include prey remains, plant material and egg sacs that are incorporated into the web (Herberstein *et al.*, 2000a).

Over the past century, many studies have aimed to identify the functions for web decorations, especially for those made entirely out of silk. The functional hypotheses are almost as diverse as the form and composition of decorations (Bruce, 2006, Herberstein *et al.*, 2000a, Théry and Casas, 2009). These hypotheses can be divided into two major categories: non-visual and visual functions.

Probably the oldest non-visual idea is that web decorations are involved in web structural stability. By introducing the term *stabilimentum* in 1895, Simon first asserted a web-stabilising function for web decorations (Simon, 1895; see also Robinson and Robinson, 1970). By applying silk decorations after the web was completed, a spider might use them to adjust the tension of the web. However, the decoration silks are loosely placed on webs rather than tightly uniting two adjacent radial silks (Foelix, 1996), and therefore it is unlikely that decorations function to adjust web tension. Nevertheless, there is some experimental evidence that the spiral-shaped decorations of uloborids do change the tension in the radials, thus improving prey detection for the spider at the hub (Watanabe, 2000).

Humphreys (1992) showed that the dense, disc-shaped decorations can help regulate the body temperature of spiders by shading the spider from the sunlight (Humphreys, 1992). However, other types of decorations (crosses, lines or tufts) may not be very effective in shading the spider. Nentwig and Rogg (1988) compared *Argiope* webs with and without linear decorations and found no significant difference in spider body temperature (Nentwig and Rogg, 1988). A more recent non-visual hypothesis proposes that silk decorations might function to regulate aciniform silk gland activity (Tso, 2004, Walter *et al.*, 2008a). Since aciniform gland silk is used for prey wrapping as well as for decoration building, the silk reserve of this gland might be quite variable and consequently result in inconsistent building and shape polymorphism of silk decorations. In support of this hypothesis, researchers have shown that factors such as frequency of prey-wrapping events (Tso, 2004) or moulting (Walter *et al.*, 2008a) affected the spiders' silk gland physiological conditions and generate predictable decoration-building patterns.

Another group of studies consider spider web decorations as a visual signal that influences the interactions between spiders, prey and predators. Among the visual functions, attracting prey, protecting the spiders from predators and advertising the presence of webs are the three most popularly accepted ones (Bruce, 2006, Herberstein *et al.*, 2000a). The prey attraction function of silk decorations has been empirically demonstrated by field and laboratory experiments in several spider genera: *Cyclosa* (Tso, 1998b); *Octonoba* (Watanabe, 1999); *Araneus* (Bruce *et al.*, 2004); *Argiope* with discoid (Li, 2005, Li *et al.*, 2004); linear (Tso, 1996, 1998a); or cruciate form decorations (Blamires *et al.*, 2008, Bruce *et al.*, 2001, Cheng and Tso, 2007, Craig, 1991, Craig and Bernard, 1990). Despite the wealth of studies supporting a prey attraction function for many decorating orb-web spiders, there are also results and observations that are not consistent with such a function (Blackledge and Wenzel, 1999, Eberhard, 2007, 2008, Nakata, 2009).

As for the anti-predator hypothesis, the supporting evidence is mostly derived from correlation studies or enclosure experiments. Lubin (1975) reported that the frequencies of decorated webs built by *Argiope* spiders in Daphne and Santa Cruz islands in Galapagos were negatively correlated with the abundance of vertebrate predators (Lubin, 1975). Schoener and Spiller (1992) found that among various size classes of *A. argentata* in the Bahamas, medium-sized spiders decorated their webs most frequently. They thus suggested that the cruciate form decorations might render the medium-sized spiders looking larger, thereby deterring gape-limited lizards (Schoener and Spiller, 1992). In an enclosure experiment, Horton (1980) showed that blue jays (*Cyanocilla cristata*) attacked *Argiope* spiders less frequently when spiders were on decorated webs, suggesting that these birds might have learned to avoid sticky webs by associating them with decorations (Horton, 1980). Blackledge and Wenzel (2001) also showed that in enclosures, *A. trifasciata* on undecorated webs were more likely to be captured by predatory mud-dauber wasps.

In the case of the web advertisement hypothesis, there is relatively little supporting evidence. Eisner and Nowicki (1983) found that the damage rate of webs with attached dummy decorations were lower than those without. In a field experiment, Blackledge and Wenzel (1999) showed that webs built by *A. aurantia* with linear decorations were less likely to be damaged than undecorated webs.

One problem in assigning one or multiple functions for silk decorations is the phenomenon that in many species the frequency and shape of decorations are highly inconsistent and polymorphic (Starks, 2002). If silk decorations have a strong selective benefit (for example, by either attracting prey or deterring predators) why do not spiders build them consistently? Clearly, the discussion over the function of silk decorations is far from resolved, making this a very exciting area of research.

The function of non-silk decoration has received less attention, with some exceptions. For example, some species of *Nephila* (Nephilidae) store consumed prey on their barrier webs and use silk to assemble them into a conspicuous band (Griffiths *et al.*, 2003). Laboratory studies suggest that these bands of prey caracasses could serve as food caches (Champion de Crespigny *et al.*, 2001) and that the decaying prey carcasses were attractive to saprophagous insects (Bjorkman-Chiswell *et al.*, 2004). Nevertheless, field studies found that their presence had no significant effects on survival or growth of spiders (Griffiths *et al.*, 2003).

Different species of *Cyclosa* spiders (Uloboridae), conversely, incorporate a diverse array of objects such as prey remains, egg sacs and plant detritus into the webs (Marples, 1969, Yaginuma, 1986). The function of *Cyclosa* non-silk web decorations has traditionally been hypothesised as camouflaging the spiders (Eberhard, 1973, 2003). Recent studies demonstrated that these decorations might be conspicuous anti-predator devices, which function as decoys to distract predators. Webs with such devices actually attracted more wasps to approach the webs (Tan and Li, 2009) and received more wasp attacks (Chou *et al.*, 2005, Tseng and Tso, 2009). However, the chromatic (Chou *et al.*, 2005) and morphological resemblance (Tseng and Tso, 2009) of these decorations to spiders redirect the wasp attacks away from the spider.

3.2   Genetic basis for variation

3.2.1   *Genetically based variation in silk*

Despite the considerable diversity in silk types and silk glands, especially among the orb-web spiders, most genetic studies focus on one to two silk types produced by a limited number of species. Most of the studies focus on dragline silks produced by the major ampullate glands, perhaps because such silks and glands are relatively easily obtained from spiders and therefore ample material and physiological studies are available as background information for genetic studies. During the past two decades, several species of the large orb-web spider genus *Nephila* (Nephilidae) have been used in many silk genetic studies. Members of this genus are quite large and are rather abundant in tropical/subtropical regions of Asia, America and Africa (Harvey *et al.*, 2007). The handling ease and availability might explain why *Nephila* spiders are widely used in these studies. However, in certain temperate regions where *Nephila* spiders are not readily available researchers switch to locally abundant orb-web spiders such as *Araneus* and *Argiope* (Araneidae). Very recently, studies on gumfooted webs, such as those built by *Latrodectus* spiders (Theridiidae) generated some major breakthroughs such as the first report of full-length major ampullate gene sequence from a non-orb-web spider (Ayoub *et al.*, 2007).

So far, we can only address the genetic basis of silk variation based on major ampullate silks as other silk types have not been studied to the same extent. Major ampullate silks are composed of the products of at least two genes: major ampullate spidroin 1 (MaSp1) (Xu and Lewis, 1990) and major ampullate spidroin 2 (MaSp2) (Hinman and Lewis, 1992). The architectures of both gene products are characterised by an internal region containing highly repetitive peptide motifs flanked by relatively conserved and non-repetitive C and N termini (Winkler and Kaplan, 2000). The repetitive region of MaSp1 contains poly (GA), poly (A) and poly (GGX) motifs (G, glycine; A, alanine; X, any amino acids; Xu and Lewis, 1990). Among these motifs, poly (GA) and poly (A) are major components of the β-sheet crystal structure (Gosline *et al.*, 1999) and they are regarded as being responsible for the tensile strength of the silk (Winkler and Kaplan, 2000). The GGX repeat regions might form helix structures that function as linkages between crystalline and non-crystalline portions of the molecule or function to align protein molecules in the silk (Hayashi *et al.*, 1999). The repetitive region of MaSp2, by contrast, exhibits GPGXX and GPGQQ motifs (P, proline; Q, glutamine). These motifs form β-turn spirals of the dragline silk and thus are responsible for the extensibility of the silk (Hayashi *et al.*, 1999). The non-repetitive C-terminal of MaSp1 might be involved in the liquid/crystalline phase transition. It might function to maintain solubility of spidroin molecules, or to form disulfide bonds to stabilise the alignment of neighbouring peptides (Sponner *et al.*, 2005c). The function of the non-repetitive N-terminal of MaSp1 is still not clear, but it might be involved in molecular conformation, or serve as a signal during the secretion of spidroins into the lumen of the major ampullate gland (Rising *et al.*, 2006).

Many orb-web (Araneidae and Nephilidae) and non-orb-web spiders (Theridiidae) spiders were shown to alter silk amino acid composition and/or material properties under various environmental conditions (see Section 3.3.1). Given the known molecular construct of major ampullate silks, what might be the genetic mechanisms generating such variations? Empirical evidence from a very limited array of spider species suggests that mechanisms generating variation in major ampullate silk could occur at two stages of the silk production pathway: during gene expression/post-transcriptional editing or at the silk protein assembly stage. There are three major hypothesised mechanisms responsible for silk variation, described below.

Post-transcriptional editing hypothesis

Craig *et al.* (2000) found that the amino acid composition of dragline silk differed when *Argiope argentata* fed on different types of prey. They were the first to propose that either a different way of post-transcriptional editing or differential expression of multiple gene systems might be the underlying genetic mechanisms (Craig *et al.*, 2000). The post-transcriptional editing hypothesis initially seemed plausible, because Hayashi and Lewis (2000) reported that the flagelliform silk of araneid orb-web spiders is expressed by a single locus (the *Flag* gene) with multiple exons and introns. Beckwitt *et al.* (1998) found that different forms of partial MaSp1 sequences could be amplified from cDNA and genomic DNA of *Nephila clavipes*. They suggested that different sequences obtained from different individual spiders represented allelic variants of MaSp1, rather than different members of a gene family. Tai *et al.* (2004) found inter- and intra-individual variations in MaSp1 sequences in *Nephila pilipes*. The variations existed in both non-repetitive C-terminal and repetitive regions, and therefore were unlikely to be allelic variants. All these results suggested that in araneid orb-web spiders MaSp1 exhibits several forms in one individual, a phenomenon that is congruent with the post-transcription editing hypotheses proposed by Craig *et al.* (2000).

Silk gene differential expression hypothesis

Another hypothesis proposed by Craig *et al.* (2000) is that silk variation is mediated through differential expression of a multiple gene system. This idea is supported by the realisation of the major ampullate silk gene molecular constructs. Recently, the full-length major ampullate gland silk genes were reported for the first time from a non-araneid spider. Ayoub *et al.* (2007) obtained the full length MaSp1 and MaSp2 genes from a widow spider, *Latrodectus hesperus* (Theridiidae). Both genes are unusually large (>10 kb) and are composed of a single exon. The study by Ayoub and Hayashi (2008) on widow spiders further confirmed that MaSp1 was encoded by multiple loci. Although a multilocus encoding system of major ampullate silk genes was proposed to function primarily to increase spidroin production (Ayoub and Hayashi, 2008), such a system also can potentially generate variation in silk protein compositions through differential expression of different loci. Guehrs *et al.* (2008) subjected *N. clavipes* to starvation and found that the dragline silk became stiffer, less elastic and contained less MaSp2 protein. Such a result indicates that orb-web spiders may adjust the relative expression of MaSp1 and MaSp2 genes according to their nutritional condition. Since MaSp2 protein is energetically more costly to produce (Craig, 2003), under starvation the depletion of certain essential chemicals may lead to a reduction of MaSp2 production (Guehrs *et al.*, 2008), and consequently generate changes in dragline silk mechanical properties. Some researchers further suggested that during silk production the quantity of MaSp2 is fine-tuned to modulate the rigidity and elasticity of dragline silks (Guehrs *et al.*, 2008, Liu *et al.*, 2008, Porter *et al.*, 2005). On the molecular level, how spiders regulate synthesis of MaSp2 (or MaSp1) proteins is currently not clear. One possibility is by modulating certain gene-specific transcription factors (Ayoub *et al.*, 2007). Alternatively, a reduction in MaSp2 protein synthesis could be achieved by controlling the synthesis pathway of key amino acids (such as proline) of MaSp2 (Guehrs *et al.*, 2008). Further studies are needed to see whether changes in foraging conditions could lead to concentration changes in certain transcription factors, or composition variations in key amino acids in silk-producing epithelial cells.

Silk protein assembly hypothesis

Silk chemical composition does not seem to be the sole determinant of its mechanical properties. Recent empirical evidence indicates that how different silk proteins are assembled may also greatly affect the material properties of major ampullate silks. Liao *et al.* (2009) subjected *Cyclosa mulmeinensis* to different wind intensities but the same foraging condition. Major ampullate silks produced by spiders receiving different wind treatments did not differ in diameter or amino acid composition, but those receiving strong wind produced much stronger silks. Such results indicated that at least in certain orb-web spiders variation in the silk mechanical properties does not have to involve differential expression of different silk genes. Liao *et al.* (2009) suggested that wind disturbance might have affected silk properties at the protein assembling rather than the gene expression stage. The mechanical properties of major ampullate silk are not only determined by relative amounts of MaSp1 and MaSp2 proteins, but also by how they are assembled (Sponner *et al.*, 2005b). During the spinning process, orb-web spiders seem to be able to adjust the relative amount of MaSp1 and MaSp2 gene products and their arrangement pattern in the silk (Sponner *et al.*, 2005a). MaSp1 molecules that were arranged more homogeneously seemed to facilitate the formation of crystalline areas in major ampullate silk and thus enhance the silk mechanical property (Sponner *et al.*, 2005b). Conversely, owing to the biochemical nature of the MaSp2 molecule this protein is proposed to interfere with MaSp1 molecule alignment and thus may affect crystalline formation (Sponner *et al.*, 2005b). Theoretically, it is much faster to adjust major ampullate silk mechanical properties by physiologically rearranging MaSp1 and MaSp2 molecules than by genetically altering the expression patterns of these two genes.

Other influences on silk assembly include the nature of the spinning process itself and the pH within the silk duct. The spinning process (such as reeling speed) of major ampullate silk has a profound influence on the arrangement of molecular chains and consequently affects the mechanical properties of the silk (Liu *et al.*, 2008). In addition, some researchers hypothesised that spiders may be able to physiologically manipulate the pH within the silk gland duct to determine where in the duct the liquid/solid phase transformation occurs. Such pH modulation can potentially influence the conformation of MaSp2 molecules, which in turn affects their interactions with MaSp1 molecules and consequently influences crystalline structure formation (Sponner, 2007).

3.2.2   *Genetically based variation in web-building behaviour*

Variation in web-building behaviour and consequently web structure between species has long been recognised (Wiehle, 1928) and has stimulated a prolific and dynamic field of research. However, interpreting the source of this variation has been difficult. What aspect of web-building behaviour is genetically determined and how much of variation in webs can be attributed to non-genetic influences such as experience, environmental conditions or other aspects of behavioural flexibility?

The literature on this topic is clearly biased towards orb webs (see also Eberhard, 1990), probably because the relatively simple two-dimensional web with its regular and geometric elements (radials and spiral) is easily quantified and compared. Nevertheless, recent work on non-orb webs is starting to address this bias (Benjamin and Zschokke, 2002, 2003, 2004, Eberhard *et al.*, 2008).

Web-building behaviour and the resulting web structure clearly has a significant genetic component: freshly hatched spiders do not require any prior experience to construct their species-specific webs. Even when these spiderlings are deprived of any web-building experience by confining them to a small glass tube until they are adult, they build appropriate webs (Heiling and Herberstein, 1999, Reed *et al.*, 1970). Early interpretations of web-building behaviour suggested that species-specific design patterns were almost exclusively limited to genetic control (Savory, 1952, Witt and Baum, 1960). However, this view was soon challenged by observations of substantial variation within species that obscured any species-specific web patterns (Eberhard, 1988, 1990, Heiling and Herberstein, 2000, Sherman, 1994).

Due to this substantial flexibility, web-building behaviour and the resulting web structure is unlikely to be a reliable taxonomic tool to distinguish between closely related species but it has been used for higher taxonomic identification and for phylogenetic analyses (Blackledge *et al.*, 2009, Eberhard, 1990, Kuntner *et al.*, 2008a). Implicit in this is that gross differences in webs, say between different families of web-building spiders, are innate and stereotyped based on a genetic component. However, while the research into behavioural flexibility has been prolific (see below), we lack detailed understanding of the genetic influences on web-building behaviour. Witt *et al.* (1972), referring to an unpublished study, argue that individuals show high repeatability in web architecture between consecutive webs and that this repeatability extends to full sibs, but clearly we need more studies of this kind to understand how much genes contribute to web building.

Extreme web forms can be useful in untangling how much genetic control, as opposed to behavioural flexibility, contributes to species-specific webs. Large-scale orb-web extensions or reductions are often a result of prey or habitat specialisations (Eberhard, 1990, Harmer and Herberstein, 2009, Stowe, 1978, Stowe *et al.*, 1987) and thus assumed to be largely under genetic control. However, a recent study on vertically elongated ladder webs revealed that by changing ecological conditions (in this case the available horizontal space) even extreme web forms revert to more typical orb-web structures (Harmer, 2009, Harmer and Herberstein, 2009). It is therefore not clear at what level genetic-based differences between species are responsible for specific web designs.

3.2.3   Genetically based variation in silk decorations

Several observations suggest that there is a genetic basis for the type of silk decoration and an individual's propensity to build them. There are some clear species-specific patterns in the shape of silk decorations. Tuft decorations only seem to be constructed by *Gasteracantha* (Araneidae), spiral-shaped decorations are mostly found in uloborid spiders, while the best studied genus *Argiope* (Araneidae) constructs discoid, linear and cruciate decorations (Bruce, 2006, Herberstein *et al.*, 2000a). The conspicuous ontogenetic shift in decorating behaviour between juvenile and adult spiders as well as reported differences in the rate of decorating behaviour between conspecific populations also suggests a genetic basis for this behaviour (Herberstein *et al.*, 2000a). However, only one study to date has investigated whether the propensity to decorate is inherited. Craig and colleagues (2001) set up pedigrees of *Argiope argentata*, a species with great variability among adults in whether or not to decorate the web. They found that an individual's decorating behaviour is influenced by the behaviour of its parents. The high mortality costs as opposed to the substantial foraging benefits of web decorations in *A. argentata* seem to maintain the polymorphic expression of this behaviour (Craig *et al.*, 2001).

3.3   Plasticity in web building

3.3.1   Plasticity in silk

Intraspecific variation in silk properties

Studies on interpopulation variation in silk properties are quite limited, and exclusively focus on major ampullate silks and to a lesser extent the glue substances of sticky spirals (the product of the aggregate gland). Consequently, in the sections below, we use the general term 'silk' to describe major ampullate silk, unless we specify a different silk type.

The first report of interpopulation silk property variation comes from Craig *et al.* (2000). They found that dragline silks obtained from *Argiope argentata* (Araneidae) of 13 Caribbean islands exhibited variation in the percentage of glycine and serine. Tso *et al.* (2005) surveyed the dragline silk amino acid compositions of nine *Nephila pilipes* (Nephilidae) populations in Taiwan and found significant spatial variation. Among various populations, the percentage of amino acids in silk could differ as much as 37% in glutamine, 25% in proline and 17% in alanine. Tso *et al.* (2005) also surveyed the prey composition of four of the nine populations and found a significant difference in relative abundance of insect orders. They suggested that the spatial heterogeneity of different prey types might be responsible for the observed interpopulation variation in silk protein of *N. pilipes*. Subsequent manipulative studies conducted (discussed in next section) confirmed that spiders adjust silk amino acid and even its physical properties when encountering different prey types.

Intra-individual plasticity in silk properties

The structural and material properties of the silk incorporated into webs largely determine how effectively prey are stopped and retained by webs (Craig, 1987, Denny, 1976, Gosline *et al.*, 1986). There is growing evidence that spiders can adjust the performance of webs by actively controlling many aspects of silk performance (Guinea *et al.*, 2005, Pan *et al.*, 2004). Empirical evidence accumulated so far shows that orb-web spiders under certain abiotic and biotic conditions exhibit plasticity in various properties of major ampullate silk and aggregate gland products.

Major ampullate silk plasticity induced by abiotic factors

Araneid and nephilid orb-web spiders have long been known to be able to adjust silk mechanical properties in response to various abiotic environmental factors. Garrido *et al.* (2002) found that *Argiope trifasciata* (Araneidae) produced dragline silk that resisted larger loads while climbing vertically, compared with climbing horizontally. Similarly, Pan *et al.* (2004) found that *Araneus ventricosus* (Araneidae) produced dragline silk with higher ultimate strength when the distance between the web and ground was greater. Furthermore, when spiders descended from a height, the physical properties of the draglines produced at the start differed from those produced at the latter stage of the descent (Ortlepp and Gosline, 2004). Currently it is not clear how such mechanical property changes are generated. However, an increase in silk diameter might be an efficient and prompt way of enhancing silk mechanical property. Vollrath and Köhler (1996) reported that when the body weight of a web-building *Araneus diadematus* (Araneidae) was artificially increased, the spiders initially increased the diameter of the radial threads and subsequently doubled or tripled the number of radial threads in the orb web. The diameter of silk is controlled by valves in the gland (Ortlepp and Gosline, 2004). These valves are under neural control, allowing spiders to actively manipulate the diameters of fibres spun under different conditions (Garrido *et al.*, 2002). Because the breaking force of a fibre is directly proportional to its cross-sectional area, even small changes in fibre diameter would greatly alter the physical performance of webs.

Reeling speed and strong wind have been shown to significantly influence the physical properties of silk. As the reeling speed increased so did the strength of the silk (Ortlepp and Gosline, 2004, Pérez-Rigueiro *et al.*, 2005). Such strength enhancement might result from a more orientated arrangement of spidroin molecules when the silk threads are pulled out at a greater speed (Knight *et al.*, 2000, Madsen *et al.*, 1999, Riekel *et al.*, 1999). Liao *et al.* (2009) found that persistent wind induced the small orb-web spider *Cyclosa mulmeinensis* (Araneidae) to produce silk of higher strength, extensibility, toughness, ultimate tension and breaking energy. Since this species inhabits seashore areas, such plasticity can potentially reduce web damage caused by winds. Liao *et al.* (2009) suggest that perhaps *C. mulmeinensis* changes silk mechanical property by physiologically altering the arrangement pattern of MaSp1 and MaSp2 proteins. Future experiments using spidroin-specific antibodies might be able to reveal whether such a mechanism really exists.

Major ampullate silk property affected by biotic factors

Madsen *et al.* (1999) were the first to report that food quantity could significantly affect the mechanical property of silk. When the nephilid orb-web spider *Nephila edulis* was starved for about a month the breaking elongation of the silk significantly decreased. In addition to hunger level, prey type is another biotic factor known to effectively induce plasticity in various physical properties of silks. When the diet of *Argiope keyserlingi* (Araneidae) was changed from bees to crickets the proportion of serine in silk changed significantly (Craig *et al.*, 2000). However, since serine is not the major property-determining amino acid in silk, the ecological significance of such a change is not clear. Tso *et al.* (2005) conducted a similar manipulative study by feeding nephilid orb-web spiders (*N. pilipes*) with either high kinetic energy prey (crickets) or low kinetic energy prey (flies). The silk of the cricket-fed spiders contained significantly higher percentages of proline but lower alanine. These changes were predicted to have a strong effect on the physical performance of silk because they were major components of secondary structures determining mechanical properties in silk (Hayashi *et al.*, 1999, Winkler and Kaplan, 2000). To test this hypothesis, Tso *et al.* (2005) used FTIR spectroscopy to examine the percentage of secondary structures in the silk protein. The different amino acid composition induced by a diet of crickets did indeed result in significantly higher percentages of proline- and glutamine-rich β-turns and lower alanine-rich β-sheet structures of silk.

Recent studies further demonstrate that orb-web and non-orb-web spiders are able to adjust silk mechanical properties when they encounter different prey types. *Nephila pilipes* fed crickets produced webs with greater structural stiffness than did spiders fed flies (Tso *et al.*, 2007). This was achieved primarily by altering the diameter of the silk threads, for cricket-fed spiders spun threads with 30% greater cross-sectional area than those spun by fly-fed spiders. Silk plasticity is also seen in spiders building 3-D prey-capture devices such as cob webs. Boutry and Blackledge (2008) fed common house spider *Parasteatoda tepidariorum* (Theridiidae) either high or low kinetic energy prey (cricket versus pillbug). The supporting threads of webs constructed by cricket-fed spiders were thicker, stiffer, tougher and broke at higher loads.

However, in other studies, prey type had a significant effect on mechanical properties but little effect on the amino acid composition of silk. Tso *et al.* (2007) found that silk produced by *N. pilipes* fed with crickets or flies did not differ in amino acid composition, even though the mechanical properties differed significantly. Zax *et al.* (2004) deprived alanine and glycine from diets of *N. clavipes* and found a significant decrease in silk stress and strain. However, the treatment had little effect on the amino acid composition of the silk. These results suggest that orb-web spiders seem to be flexible in how they adjust silk proteins in response to the prey environment, sometimes exhibiting a strong response and at other times producing silk that is remarkably similar in amino acid composition even in different prey environments. This may occur in part because spiders have alternative mechanisms by which they can influence the mechanical performance of their silks, such as the structural changes in the diameters of threads, or translational changes in silk protein composition.

Plasticity in aggregate gland products

Araneid and nephilid orb-web spiders also exhibit plasticity in substances produced by aggregate glands. This gland produces glue, pigments or low molecular weight organic compounds that modulate physical properties of flagelliform silks and maintain stickiness of glue. Craig *et al.* (1996) subjected *N. clavipes* to different light conditions and found that viscid silks produced by individuals kept in bright light contained more yellow pigments than those kept in a dim light environment. Many herbivore and pollinator insects have innate preferences for yellow colours (Heuschen *et al.*, 2005) and not surprisingly, yellow pigments are quite common in flowers and pollen of angiosperms that exploit this colour preference (Lunau, 1995). Thus, under bright light conditions with good visibility, spiders actively incorporated yellow pigments on viscid silks that attracted insect prey. In dim light conditions with low visibility, spiders reduced pigment production, which is likely to reduce the metabolic and material costs (Craig *et al.*, 1996).

Higgins *et al.* (2001) reported that low molecular weight (LMW) organic compounds of viscid spirals in *N. clavipes* changed significantly when spiders were moved from field to laboratory. They suggested that diet variation might have induced the production of different LMW organic compounds by the aggregate glands. Similarly, starvation in *Argiope trifasciata* caused significant changes in LMW composition in viscid droplets. The quantity of substances that were less readily synthesised (such as choline, isethionate and N-acetyltaurine) were more likely to be affected by starvation and replaced by readily synthesised ones (such as GABamide and glycine) (Townley *et al.*, 2006). Indirect evidence for plasticity in aggregate gland products comes from seasonal variation in the stickiness of the viscid spirals in the araneid orb-web spiders *Argiope* (Opell *et al.*, 2009). Seasonal changes in quantity of silk reserves, or low availability of resources due to reproductive needs, might be the reasons for the observed temporal variation.

Currently, it is not clear whether spiders will fine-tune the composition of LMW organic compounds in viscid spirals when encountering different prey types. However, the study by Opell *et al.* (2009) showed that in *Argiope trifasciata* and *A. aurantia* the capture spirals in the outer parts of the orb had a greater stickiness per viscous droplet volume than those in the inner parts. Such non-random distribution of orb stickiness might endow the spider with more time to reach prey retained further away from the hub. Opell *et al.* (2009) also suggested that the variation in sticky substance composition might be caused by depletion of the available substance during web construction (orb-web spiders usually begin sticky spiral laying from the outer web part then proceed inward). Further research could examine whether individual spiders can adjust the stickiness of sticky spirals when encountering different prey and the consequences (such as catching efficiency) of this plasticity.

3.3.2   *Plasticity in web-building behaviour and web structure*

'Web-building behaviour does not seem a fruitful ground for investigating plasticity in the spider nervous system' (Reed *et al.*, 1970). Reed's conclusion reflected the prevailing sentiments about the cognitive abilities and behavioural flexibilities of invertebrates such as spiders. However, early work by Witt (1963), challenged these preconceptions and stimulated a dynamic field of research into behavioural flexibility in web building and the resulting web structure that continues to elicit exciting discourse today.

Over the years, the interpretations of web-building plasticity have undergone several paradigm shifts (Heiling and Herberstein, 2000). An early fruitful approach was to place web-building behaviour within a mechanistic context where spiders feed environmental information (e.g. gravity) as well as kinaesthetic information (e.g. leg length) into a web-building algorithm (Krink and Vollrath, 1997, 1998, Vollrath, 1992). Variation in the input generates variation in the output, the web. The landmark study by Peter Sherman (1994) stimulated considerable research activity in interpreting webs within an optimal foraging framework that interprets flexibility as a trade-off between costs and benefits of foraging and trade-offs with other activities, such as reproduction (Blackledge, 1998, Blackledge and Zevenbergen, 2007, Blamires *et al.*, 2007, Herberstein *et al.*, 2000b, Higgins, 1995, Pasquet *et al.*, 1999, Venner *et al.*, 2000). Finally, the influence of spider experience and learning has recently contributed to interpretations of web-building flexibility (Chmiel *et al.*, 2000, Heiling and Herberstein, 1999, Venner *et al.*, 2000).

Extent of intraspecific and intra-individual flexibility

Several web characteristics can vary either between individuals of the same species and population or within an individual over time. These include where to construct the web in the first place, the amount of silk incorporated in the web, the arrangement of silk within the web and the rate of web relocation. Variation in the arrangement of silk is best quantified in orb webs due to the regular and symmetric nature of the web and may include the number and spacing of radials and spirals (Zschokke, 1999).

Variation in the above listed web variables may be substantial. For example, some individual spiders may relocate their webs every day while others remain at a given web site for up to three weeks (Gillespie and Caraco, 1987, Nakata and Ushimaru, 1999). Within an individual spider, the size of the web and the number of spirals and radials incorporated into the web can vary by more than 150% over just three consecutive webs (Eberhard, 1988). Moreover the individual behaviour of sheet-web spiders (Linyphiidae) revealed a complete absence of any stereotypic behaviour during web construction, which is contrary to orb-web spiders (Araneoidea) and, in part, cob-web spiders (Benjamin and Zschokke, 2004, Zschokke, 1996a). Considering these non-trivial differences within and between individuals, significant research effort has gone into identifying factors that might be responsible for causing them.

Ontogenetic factors

Changes in web size and web structure during an individual's development can include gradual modifications or quite abrupt steps that lack intermediate forms (Japyassu and Ades, 1998). As spiders increase in size and weight, the web and the amount of silk generally also increases (Heiling and Herberstein, 1998, Ward and Lubin, 1993, Witt *et al.*, 1972). In some species this overall web increase is not allometric but may be associated with structural changes, such as greater web asymmetry in orb webs (Eberhard, 1990, Herberstein and Heiling, 1999). More dramatic ontogenetic changes include the loss of entire web sections, such as the upper orb-web half in *Nephilengys* (Japyassu and Ades, 1998) or the cessation of web building altogether in mature spiders (Kaston, 1972).

As spiders mature, they also gain experience in web building and prey capture. Thus, they may enlarge those web sections that are particularly successful in prey capture, such as the lower web half of orb webs (Heiling and Herberstein, 1999). Similarly, they may respond to frequent web damage to only one side of the web by shifting the web away from the source of damage (Chmiel *et al.*, 2000). Both these examples suggest that web-building spiders have a spatial memory of their webs and events that occur within the web (prey capture, damage) and adjust their web-building behaviour accordingly.

Abiotic factors

Environmental conditions such as temperature, light levels, humidity and available space can all influence web size and structure. Vollrath and colleagues (1997) comprehensibly examined the effects of available space, humidity, wind and temperature on web size and architecture of the orb-web spider *Araneus diadematus* (Araneidae). Some of the behavioural responses of the spiders were quite predictable. For example, the spiders adjusted web size and web symmetry (vertical top-to-bottom symmetry) to the available space. Interestingly, when space was limited, the spiders built smaller webs but with more spiral turns (Vollrath *et al.*, 1997). Web size and mesh size are likely to influence prey capture success, and may therefore reflect a foraging strategy to maximise prey capture under spatial constraints. Alternatively, the observed response may reflect the available silk in the silk glands (Vollrath *et al.*, 1997). The response to wind was slightly different: webs were also smaller but with fewer spiral turns, resulting in a wider mesh, presumably to reduce the surface area of the web and hence stress and breakage (Vollrath *et al.*, 1997). A recent study has confirmed this response in *Cyclosa* (Araneidae) showing that the modified web structure actually reduces wind drag (Liao *et al.*, 2009).

Other web-building responses by the spiders were not entirely intuitive. For example, under lower temperatures, *A. diadematus* did not adjust web size, but decreased the number of spiral turns, resulting in a wider mesh (Vollrath *et al.*, 1997). It has been suggested that under lower temperatures larger insect prey are more likely to be active and a large mesh is more suitable for such prey. Alternatively, the wider mesh may be the result of spiders moving more slowly during web construction at lower temperatures (Vollrath *et al.*, 1997). However, it is not likely that the response to temperature is linear, but rather reflects an optimum and preferred temperature range (Barghusen *et al.*, 1997). Under lower humidity, *A. diadematus* built smaller webs with fewer spiral turns. The lack of humidity may have limited the production of the aqueous coat of the viscid spiral or the spiders tailored their webs to specific prey under these environmental conditions (Vollrath *et al.*, 1997). A different study found that orb-web spiders (*Argiope*, Araneidae) decrease web size under bright light conditions, presumably to reduce exposure to visually hunting predators during web construction (Herberstein and Fleisch, 2003).

These examples of abiotic influences on web-building behaviour are far from exhaustive, but they do highlight how sensitive and responsive web-building spiders can be to even slight environmental changes. What is still lacking is a more holistic method that manipulates multiple environmental variables simultaneously to reflect a more natural situation. Such an approach may also reveal how spiders prioritise the potential constraints and costs of each abiotic variable.

Biotic factors

Spiders may dynamically adjust their webs according to the type of prey active in the environment, the spider's nutritional and reproductive state, the presence of predators or the presence of conspecifics. While we cannot provide an exhaustive review here, our aim is to highlight some studies that exemplify the influence of biotic factors on web-building behaviour.

The ability to predict and respond to prevailing prey conditions without having to sample them first may entail a selective advantage. The construction and material costs of a web are significant and a web with an ill-suited architecture (e.g. arrangement of the capture spiral) may miss out on important prey-capture opportunities. The South American orb-web spider *Parawixia bistriata* (Araneidae) usually builds small webs with a fine capture mesh at night, capturing small flies. The web-building behaviour changes dramatically during the onset of the wet season, resulting in additional diurnal webs that are larger with a wider mesh. These webs are better suited at capturing swarming termites during the wet season. Impressively, the spider changes its behaviour *before* having captured its first termite, presumably responding to environmental cues that predict the swarming event (Sandoval, 1994).

The response of spiders to their own nutritional state is expected to follow a bell curve: when individuals are highly food deprived, they lack the necessary energy to produce silk and construct the web and hence the web is expected to be small. Similarly, when individuals are highly satiated, webs are expected to be also small as spiders divert time and energy to reproduction and predator avoidance. At intermediate nutritional levels web-building behaviour and hence the web is increased to maximise prey-capture opportunities (Higgins, 1995). These predictions are supported by empirical data in a variety of different spiders (Herberstein *et al.*, 2000b, Higgins, 1995, Pasquet *et al.*, 1999, Sherman, 1994). In addition to changes in overall web size, spiders also vary specific web elements. For example, in the western black widow (*Latrodectus hesperus*), deprived spiders built more gumfoot lines that are likely to increase prey capture while satiated spiders built more support lines that may provide protection against predation (Blackledge and Zevenbergen, 2007, Zevenbergen *et al.*, 2008).

The influence of predators on web-building behaviour has not yet been examined extensively. In the orb-web spider *Argiope versicolor* (Araneidae), individuals exposed to the predator cues of the araneophagic jumping spider *Portia* (see also

Chapter 4) reduced web size and silk incorporated into the web (Li and Lee, 2004). Presumably, a reduction in web-building activity reduces the exposure to this predator. The predator cue in this case was olfactory and the test spiders did not have to experience a predatory attack to respond (Li and Lee, 2004).

The presence of conspecifics may have variable effects on web-building behaviour. Western black widow spiders (*Latrodectus hesperus*) initiated web building earlier and built larger webs that incorporate more silk in the presence of a conspecific individual. The presence of a conspecific may indicate a high quality foraging site, or the potential for competition. In either case, increasing web-building behaviour is likely to be advantageous in this situation (Salomon, 2007). In the orb-web spider *Zygiella x-notata*, however, conspecifics seem to limit the space available for web construction. When the competitor is removed, individuals with small webs increase their webs in response to the newly available space (Leborgne and Pasquet, 1987).

3.3.3   Plasticity in web decorations

For most taxa of decorating spiders the occurrence and form of decorations are relatively consistent and predictable. However, in the best-studied araneid genus *Argiope*, the decoration-building behaviour is quite unpredictable and inconsistent. While in most *Argiope* species juveniles build discoid decorations, individual adults tend to decorate webs inconsistently on a daily basis. To appropriately address the functions of silk decorations built by *Argiope* spiders, we must first understand how such inconsistency is involved in the functioning of decorations. If decorating webs has selective advantages for *Argiope* spiders, why do they perform this behaviour in such an unpredictable way? Therefore, understanding the mechanisms that generate this plasticity is essential and empirical studies conducted so far have identified several proximate and ultimate mechanisms.

Argiope *decoration plasticity: proximate mechanisms*

Earlier efforts attempting to identify the non-genetic proximate factors generating predictable *Argiope* decoration plasticity were not successful. Nentwig and Rogg (1988) performed laboratory manipulations and field observations to evaluate the effects of numerous abiotic and biotic factors on decoration building of *A. argentata*. They found only factors such as extreme temperatures, moulting and age to be influential and concluded that decoration building in *Argiope* spiders might reflect a response to stress (Nentwig and Rogg, 1988). However, several studies conducted after the 1990s showed that certain abiotic and biotic factors were able to generate predictable effects on *Argiope* spiders' decoration building. Elgar *et al.* (1996) found that the intensity of ambient light has a negative effect on the size of decorations built by *Argiope aetherea*, although both field surveys and laboratory experiments conducted by (Nentwig and Rogg, 1988) found this factor to be unimportant. Since decorations may attract insects to webs and thus can be considered as part of the foraging effort, several studies predicted that the size of decorations and past foraging success was negatively related (Blackledge, 1998, Herberstein *et al.*, 2000b, Tso, 1999). The food treatments used in these studies did generate significant effects, but the results were inconsistent with the predictions. Food deprivation had either no (Tso, 1999) or a negative effect (Blackledge, 1998, Herberstein *et al.*, 2000b), while food satiation enhanced decoration building. These results suggest that decoration building in *Argiope* spiders cannot simply be regarded as a form of foraging response and other factors must also be involved in the proximate control of this behavioural trait.

Peters (1993) suggested that the content of the decoration silk-producing gland (aciniform gland) may be one of the key factors influencing the tendency to build decorations. The silk produced in the aciniform gland is also used to wrap prey (Foelix, 1996). Since the amount of silk reserve in other silk glands greatly affects the size of orb webs (Eberhard, 1988, Zschokke, 1996b), perhaps the size of decorations is determined by the amount of silk reserve in the aciniform gland, which in turn is affected by the intensity of prey wrapping. Tso (2004) tested this hypothesis by manipulating the aciniform gland reserve of *A. aetheroides* and showed that a depletion of silk reserve significantly decreases the size of decorations. Tso (2004) proposed that stochastic prey abundance and capture success might influence the amount of silk reserve in the aciniform silk glands and thus affect the size of decorations in subsequent webs. Walter *et al.* (2008b) also demonstrated that various *Argiope* species responded to artificially induced web changes by increasing web decoration size. They suggested that web decorations might physiologically serve to regulate aciniform gland activity; that is, building larger decorations may elevate gland activity and vice versa. In addition, moulting activities might also affect decoration building in *Argiope* spiders as subadult *A. keyserlingi* greatly increase decoration size when they are about to undergo their final moult. The large-sized decorations might serve as storage of aciniform silk protein and spiders that ingest and recycle these silk proteins after moulting have a readily available silk reserve to wrap prey (Walter *et al.*, 2008a).

Argiope decoration plasticity: ultimate mechanisms

Studies conducted during the past few decades successfully identified the benefit and cost of web-decorating behaviour, and from this empirical evidence we can now attempt to address decoration plasticity from an ultimate perspective. Interpreting *Argiope* web decorations as visual signals that lure prey has received much support, and has been demonstrated in species such as *A. argentata* (Craig,

1991, Craig and Bernard, 1990), *A. trifasciata* (Tso, 1996) *A. keyserlingi* (Bruce *et al.*, 2001, Herberstein, 2000), *A. versicolor* (Li *et al.*, 2004), *A. aurantia* (Tso, 1998a) and *A. aemula* (Cheng and Tso, 2007). Results of several recent studies, however, demonstrated that decorating webs imposes the cost of increased predation risk, at least during certain developmental stages. Bruce *et al.* (2001) found that praying mantids were more likely to approach decorated webs than undecorated ones irrespective of whether there were spiders on the webs or not. Similarly, jumping spider predators also use silk decorations to locate the position of *Argiope* prey (Seah and Li, 2001). In a laboratory experiment, Li and Lee (2004) showed that in the presence of jumping spider predators, *Argiope* spiders decreased not only the building frequency but also the size of decorations. In a field experiment, Cheng and Tso (2007) found that medium-sized *A. aemula* on decorated webs received far more wasp attacks than those on undecorated webs. Therefore, the risk of exposure to predators may prevent spiders from consistently decorating their webs. Moreover, the cost of learning by prey may also select against consistent building of decorations. Since decorations are visible to insects (Blamires *et al.*, 2008, Bruce *et al.*, 2005) and since some hymenopteran predators use them to locate the spiders, it is possible that prey of spiders also learn to associate decorations with danger. Although the colour signals and shape of decorations might be similar to the general pattern of pollinator food resources (Biesmeijer *et al.*, 2005, Prokopy and Owens, 1983), insects that were attracted and trapped by decorated webs learned to avoid them after escaping the web once (Craig, 1994). Therefore, from an ultimate perspective the inconsistent building and shape polymorphism of decorations can be regarded as trade-offs between opposing selection pressures.

In conclusion, we suggest that both ultimate and proximate factors are involved in *Argiope* silk decoration-building plasticity. Co-occurrence of opposing selective pressures mediated by the cognitive behaviour of prey and predators, and the complicated interactions between genetic make-up, stochastic prey abundance, hunger level and aciniform gland regulatory activities result in the observed inconsistent occurrence and form polymorphism. Future studies should examine whether the relative strengths of these selection pressures and proximate factors might be responsible for the observed variation in different *Argiope* populations and species.

3.4   Conclusions and outlook

The intense work on web-building behaviour and silk production over the last few decades has uncovered an unexpected level of variability and flexibility in spiders. We have a reasonable handle on identifying proximate and ultimate mechanisms to explain variation in web size and structure, but are limited by a taxonomic bias on orb-web spiders, although this is slowly being addressed. Understanding variation in web-decorating behaviour is proving to be more difficult with many opposing results and unexplained variation. While opposing selection pressure on this behaviour can partly help resolve these controversies, systematic tests of multiple functional hypotheses will ultimately provide the most unambiguous answers. Research on the plasticity in silk composition and mechanics is currently only scratching the surface of the underlying potential. The lack of comparative data, both in terms of different species as well as silk types is likely to be addressed in the next few years, as more sequencing information is becoming available. This rapidly expanding area of research will be of particular interest to the material sciences and efforts to synthesise the superior mechanical properties of spider silk. Silks, spider webs and web-building behaviour continue to fascinate and inspire researchers. Their extraordinary variability and plasticity only amplifies the appeal of spiders as research models.

Acknowledgements

We thank Paul Selden, Samuel Zschokke, Aaron Harmer, Rudy Jocqué, Jutta Schneider and Suresh Benjamin for helpful feedback on earlier drafts of this chapter, and Rudy Jocqué and Ainsi Dippenaar-Schoeman for permission to utilise their web illustrations.

References

Agnarsson, I. (2004). Morphological phylogeny of cobweb spiders and their relatives (Araneae, Araneoidea, Theridiidae). *Zoological Journal of the Linnean Society*, **141**, 447–626.

Agnarsson, I. and Coddington, J. (2006). Notes on web and web plasticity and description of the male of *Achaearanea hieroglyphica* (Mello-Leitao) (Araneae, Theridiidae). *Journal of Arachnology*, **34**, 638–641.

Arnedo, M., Hormiga, G. and Scharff, N. (2009). Higher-level phylogenetics of linyphiid spiders (Araneae, Linyphiidae) based on morphological and molecular evidence. *Cladistics*, **25**, 231–262.

Ayoub, N. A. and Hayashi, C. Y. (2008). Multiple recombining loci encoding MaSp1, the primary constituent of dragline silk, in widow spiders (*Latrodectus*: Theridiidae). *Molecular Biology and Evolution*, **25**, 277–286.

Ayoub, N. A., Garb, J. E., Tinghitella, R. M., Collin, M. A. and Hayashi, C. Y. (2007). Blueprint for a high-performance biomaterial: full-length spider dragline silk genes. *PLoS ONE*, **2**, e514.

Baba, Y. and Miyashita, T. (2006). Does individual internal state affect the presence of a barrier web in *Argiope bruennichii* (Araneae: Araneidae)? *Journal of Ethology*, **24**, 75–78.

Barghusen, L. E., Claussen, D. L., Anderson, M. S. and Bailer, A. J. (1997). The effects of temperature on the web-building behaviour of the common house spider, *Achaearanea tepidariorum*. *Functional Ecology*, **11**, 4–10.

Beckwitt, R., Arcidiancono, S. and Stote, R. (1998). Evolution of repetitive proteins: spider silks from *Nephila clavipes* (Tetragnathidae) and *Araneus bicentenarius* (Araneidae). *Insect Biochemistry and Molecular Biology*, **28**, 121–130.

Benjamin, S. P. and Zschokke, S. (2002). Untangling the tangle-web: web construction behavior of the comb-footed spider *Steatoda triangulosa* and comments on phylogenetic implications (Araneae: Theridiidae). *Journal of Insect Behavior*, **15**, 791–809.

Benjamin, S. P. and Zschokke, S. (2003). Webs of theridiid spiders: construction, structure and evolution. *Biological Journal of the Linnean Society*, **78**, 293–305.

Benjamin, S. and Zschokke, S. (2004). Homology, behaviour and spider webs: web construction behaviour of *Linyphia hortensis* and *L. triangularis* (Araneae: Linyphiidae) and its evolutionary significance. *Journal of Evolutionary Biology*, **17**, 120–130.

Benjamin, S. P., Düggelin, M. and Zschokke, S. (2002). Fine structure of sheet-webs of *Linyphia triangularis* (Clerck) and *Microlinyphia pusilla* (Sundevall), with remarks on the presence of viscid silk. *Acta Zoologica – Stockholm*, **83**, 49–59.

Biesmeijer, J. C., Giurfa, M., Koedam, D., *et al.* (2005). Convergent evolution: floral guides, stingless bee nest entrances, and insectivorous pitchers. *Naturwissenschaften*, **92**, 444–450.

Bjorkman-Chiswell, B. T., Kulinski, M. M., Muscat, R. L., *et al.* (2004). Web-building spiders attract prey by storing decaying matter. *Naturwissenschaften*, **91**, 245–248.

Blackledge, T. A. (1998). Stabilimentum variation and foraging success in *Argiope aurantia* and *Argiope trifasciata* (Araneae, Araneidae). *Journal of Zoology*, **246**, 21–27.

Blackledge, T. A. and Wenzel, J. W. (1999). Do stabilimenta in orb webs attract prey or defend spiders? *Behavioral Ecology*, **10**, 372–376.

Blackledge, T. A. and Wenzel, J. W. (2001). Silk mediated defense by an orb web spider against predatory mud-dauber wasps. *Behaviour*, **138**, 155–171.

Blackledge, T. A. and Zevenbergen, J. M. (2007). Condition-dependent spider web architecture in the western black widow, *Latrodectus hesperus*. *Animal Behaviour*, **73**, 855–864.

Blackledge, T. A., Coddington, J. and Gillespie, R. G. (2003). Are three-dimensional spider webs defensive adaptations? *Ecology Letters*, **6**, 13–18.

Blackledge, T. A., Scharff, N., Coddington, J. A., *et al.* (2009). Reconstructing web evolution and spider diversification in the molecular era. *Proceedings of the National Academy of Sciences of the USA*, **106**, 5229–5234.

Blamires, S. J., Hochuli, D. F. and Thompson, M. B. (2008). Why cross the web: decoration spectral properties and prey capture in an orb spider (*Argiope keyserlingi*) web. *Biological Journal of the Linnean Society*, **94**, 221–229.

Blamires, S. J., Thompson, M. B. and Hochuli, D. F. (2007). Habitat selection and web plasticity by the orb spider *Argiope keyserlingi* (Argiopidae): do they compromise foraging success for predator avoidance? *Austral Ecology*, **32**, 551–563.

Bond, J. E. and Opell, B. D. (1998). Testing adaptive radiation and key innovation hypotheses in spiders. *Evolution*, **52**, 403–414.

Boutry, C. and Blackledge, T. A. (2008). The common house spider alters the material and mechanical properties of cobweb silk in response to different prey. *Journal of Experimental Zoology*, **309**A, 542–552.

Bruce, M. (2006). Silk decorations: controversy and consensus. *Journal of Zoology*, **269**, 89–97.

Bruce, M. J., Heiling, A. M. and Herberstein, M. E. (2004). Alternative foraging strategies in the orb-web spider '*Araneus*' *eburnus* (Araneidae, Araneae). *Annales Zoologici Fennici*, **41**, 563–575.

Bruce, M. J., Heiling, A. M. and Herberstein, M. E. (2005). Spider signals: are web decorations visible to birds and bees? *Biology Letters*, **1**, 299–302.

Bruce, M. J., Herberstein, M. E. and Elgar, M. A. (2001). Signalling conflict between prey and predator attraction. *Journal of Evolutionary Biology*, **14**, 786–794.

Cartan, C. and Miyashita, T. (2000). Extraordinary web and silk properties of *Cyrtarachne* (Araneae, Araneidae): a possible link between orb-webs and bolas. *Biological Journal of the Linnean Society*, **71**, 219–235.

Champion de Crespigny, F. E., Herberstein, M. E. and Elgar, M. A. (2001). Food caching in orb-web spiders (Araneae: Araneoidea). *Naturwissenschaften*, **88**, 42–45.

Chen, X., Shao, Z. Z. and Vollrath, F. (2006). The spinning processes for spider silk. *Soft Matter*, **2**, 448–451.

Cheng, R. C. and Tso, I. M. (2007). Signaling by decorating webs: luring prey or deterring predators? *Behavioral Ecology*, **18**, 1085–1091.

Chmiel, K., Herberstein, M. E. and Elgar, M. A. (2000). Web damage and feeding experience influence web site tenacity in the orb-web spider *Argiope keyserlingi* Karsch. *Animal Behaviour*, **60**, 821–826.

Chou, I. C., Wang, P. H., Shen, P. S. and Tso, I. M. (2005). A test of prey-attracting and predator defence functions of prey carcass decorations built by *Cyclosa* spiders. *Animal Behaviour*, **69**, 1055–1061.

Coddington, J. A. and Levi, H. W. (1991). Systematics and evolution of spiders (Araneae). *Annual Review of Ecology and Systematics*, **22**, 565–592.

Colgin, M. A. and Lewis, R. V. (1998). Spider minor ampullate silk proteins contain new repetitive sequences and highly conserved non-silk-like 'spacer regions'. *Protein Science*, **7**, 667–672.

Coyle, F. A. (1986). The role of silk in prey capture by nonaraneomorph spiders. In *Spiders: Webs, Behavior, and Evolution* (ed. W. A. Shear). Stanford, CA: Stanford University Press.

Craig, C. L. (1987). The ecological and evolutionary interdependence between web architecture and web silk spun by orb web weaving spiders. *Biological Journal of the Linnean Society*, **30**, 135–162.

Craig, C. L. (1991). Physical constraints on group foraging and social evolution: observations on web-spinning spiders. *Functional Ecology*, **5**, 649–654.

Craig, C. L. (1994). Limits to learning: effects of predator pattern and colour on perception and avoidance-learning by prey. *Animal Behaviour*, **47**, 1087–1099.

Craig, C. L. (2003). *Spiderwebs and Silk*. Oxford, UK: Oxford University Press.

Craig, C. L. and Bernard, G. D. (1990). Insect attraction to ultraviolet-reflecting spider webs and web decorations. *Ecology*, **71**, 616–623.

Craig, C. L., Reikel, C., Herberstein, M. E., *et al.* (2000). Evidence for diet effects on the composition of silk proteins produced by spiders. *Molecular Biology and Evolution*, **17**, 1904–1913.

Craig, C. L., Weber, R. S. and Bernard, G. D. (1996). Evolution of predator-prey systems: spider foraging plasticity in response to the visual ecology of prey. *American Naturalist*, **147**, 205–229.

Craig, C. L., Wolf, S. G., Davis, J. L. D., Hauber, M. E. and Maas, J. L. (2001). Signal polymorphism in the web-decorating spider *Argiope argentata* is correlated with reduced survivorship and the presence of stingless bees, its primary prey. *Evolution*, **55**, 986–993.

Damen, W. G. M., Saridaki, T. and Averof, M. (2002). Diverse adaptations of an ancestral gill: a common evolutionary origin for wings, breathing organs, and spinnerets. *Current Biology*, **12**, 1711–1716.

Denny, M. (1976). The physical properties of spider's silk and their role in the design of orb-webs. *Journal of Experimental Biology*, **65**, 483–506.

Dippenaar-Schoeman, A. S., and Jocqué, R. (1997). *African Spiders: An Identification Manual*. Handbook 9. Pretoria: Agricultural Research Council Plant Protection Research Institute.

Eberhard, W. G. (1973). Stabilimenta on the webs of *Uloborus diversus* (Araneae: Uloboridae) and other spiders. *Journal of Zoology*, **171**, 367–384.

Eberhard, W. G. (1975). The 'inverted ladder' orb web of *Scoloderus* sp. and the intermediate orb of *Eustala* (?) sp. Araneae: Araneidae. *Journal of Natural History*, **9**, 93–106.

Eberhard, W. G. (1988). Behavioral flexibility in orb web construction: effects of supplies in different silk glands and spider size and weight. *Journal of Arachnology*, **16**, 295–302.

Eberhard, W. G. (1990). Function and phylogeny of spider webs. *Annual Review of Ecology and Systematics*, **21**, 341–372.

Eberhard, W. G. (2003). Substitution of silk stabilimenta for egg sacs by *Allocyclosa bifurca* (Araneae: Araneidae) suggests that silk stabilimenta function as camouflage devices. *Behaviour*, **140**, 847–868.

Eberhard, W. G. (2007). Stabilimenta of *Philoponella vicina* (Araneae: Uloboridae) and *Gasteracantha cancriformis* (Araneae: Araneidae): evidence against a prey attractant function. *Biotropica*, **39**, 216–220.

Eberhard, W. G. (2008). *Araneus expletus* (Araneae, Araneidae): another stabilimentum that does not function to attract prey. *Journal of Arachnology*, **36**, 191–194.

Eberhard, W. G., Agnarsson, I. and Levi, H. W. (2008). Web forms and the phylogeny and theridiid spiders (Araneae: Theridiidae): chaos from order. *Systematics and Biodiversity*, **6**, 415–475.

Eisner, T. and Nowicki, S. (1983). Spider web protection through visual advertisment: role of the stabilimentum. *Science*, **219**, 185–187.

Elgar, M. A., Allan, R. A. and Evans, T. A. (1996). Foraging strategies in orb-spinning spiders: ambient light and silk decorations in *Argiope aetherea* Walckenaer (Araneae: Araneoidea). *Australian Journal of Ecology*, **21**, 464–467.

Eskov, K. Y. and Selden, P. (2005). First record of spiders from the Permian period (Araneae: Mesothelae). *Bulletin of the British Arachnological Society*, **13**, 111–116.

Foelix, R. F. (1996). *Biology of Spiders*, 2nd edn. Oxford, UK: Oxford University Press.

Forster, C. M. and Forster, R. R. (1985). A derivative of the orb web and its evolutionary significance. *New Zealand Journal of Zoology*, **12**, 455–465.

Garb, J. E. Dimauro, T., Vo, V. and Hayashi, C. Y. (2006). Silk genes support the single origin of orb webs. *Science*, **312**, 1762.

Garb, J. E. and Hayashi, C. Y. (2005). Modular evolution of egg case silk genes across orb-weaving spider superfamilies. *Proceedings of the National Academy of Sciences of the USA*, **102**, 11 379–11 384.

Garrido, M. A., Viney, C. and Pérez-Rigueiro, J. (2002). Active control of spider silk strength: comparison of drag line spun on vertical and horizontal surfaces. *Polymer*, **43**, 1537–1540.

Gillespie, R. G. and Caraco, T. (1987). Risk-sensitive foraging strategies of two spider populations. *Ecology*, **68**, 887–899.

Gosline, J. M., Demont, M. E. and Denny, M. W. (1986). The structure and properties of spider silk. *Endeavour*, **10**, 37–43.

Gosline, J. M., Guerette, P. A., Ortlepp, C. S. and Savage, K. N. (1999). The mechanical design of spider silks: from fibroin sequence to mechanical function. *Journal of Experimental Biology*, **202**, 3295–3303.

Griffiths, B. V., Holwell, G. I., Herberstein, M. E. and Elgar, M. A. (2003). Frequency, composition and variation in external food stores constructed by orb-web spiders: *Nephila edulis* and *Nephila plumipes* (Araneae: Araneoidea). *Australian Journal of Zoology*, **51**, 119–128.

Grimaldi, D. A. and Engel, M. S. (2005). *Evolution of Insects*. Cambridge, UK: Cambridge University Press.

Griswold, C. E., Coddington, J. A., Hormiga, G. and Scharff, N. (1998). Phylogeny of the orb-web building spiders (Araneae, Orbiculariae: Deinopoidea, Araneoidea). *Zoological Journal of the Linnean Society*, **123**, 1–99.

Guehrs, K. H., Schlott, B., Grosse, F. and Weisshart, K. (2008). Environmental conditions impinge on dragline silk protein composition. *Insect Molecular Biology*, **17**, 553–564.

Guinea, G. V., Elices, M., Pérez-Rigueiro, J. and Plaza, G. R. (2005). Stretching of supercontracted fibers: a link between spinning and the variability of spider silk. *Journal of Experimental Biology*, **208**, 25–30.

Harmer, A. (2009). Elongated orb-webs of Australian ladder-web spiders (Araneidae: *Telaprocera*) and the significance of orb-web elongation. *Journal of Ethology*, **27**, 453–460.

Harmer, A. M. and Herberstein, M. E. (2009). Taking it to extremes: what drives extreme web elongation in Australian ladder web spiders (Araneidae: *Telaprocera maudae*)? *Animal Behaviour*, **78**, 499–504.

Harmer, A. M. T. and Framenau, V. W. (2009). *Telaprocera* (Araneae: Araneidae), a new genus of Australian orb-web spiders with highly elongated webs. *Zootaxa*, **1956**, 59–80.

Harvey, M. S., Austin, A. D. and Adams, M. (2007). The systematics and biology of the spider genus *Nephila* (Araneae: Nephilidae) in the Australasian region. *Invertebrate Systematics*, **21**, 407–451.

Hayashi, C. Y. and Lewis, R. V. (1998). Evidence from flagelliform silk cDNA for the structural basis of elasticity and modular nature of spider silk. *Journal of Molecular Biology*, **275**, 773–784.

Hayashi, C. Y. and Lewis, R. V. (2000). Molecular architecture and evolution of a modular spider silk protein gene. *Science*, **287**, 1477–1479.

Hayashi, C. Y., Blackledge, T. A. and Lewis, R. V. (2004). Molecular and mechanical characterization of aciniform silk: uniformity of iterated sequence modules in a novel member of the spider silk fibroin gene family. *Molecular Biology and Evolution*, **21**, 1950–1959.

Hayashi, C. Y., Shipley, N. H. and Lewis, R. V. (1999). Hypotheses that correlate the sequence, structure, and mechanical properties of spider silk proteins. *International Journal of Biological Macromolecules*, **24**, 271–275.

Heiling, A. M. and Herberstein, M. E. (1998). The web of *Nuctenea sclopetaria* (Araneae, Araneidae): relationship between body size and web design. *Journal of Arachnology*, **26**, 91–96.

Heiling, A. M. and Herberstein, M. E. (1999). The role of experience in web-building spiders (Araneidae). *Animal Cognition*, **2**, 171–177.

Heiling, A. M. and Herberstein, M. E. (2000). Interpretations of orb-web variability: a review of past and current ideas. *Ekologia – Bratislava*, **19**, 97–106.

Herberstein, M. E. (2000). Foraging behaviour in orb-web spiders (Araneidae): do web decorations increase prey capture success in *Argiope keyserlingi* Karsch, 1878? *Australian Journal of Zoology*, **48**, 217–223.

Herberstein, M. E. and Fleisch, A. F. (2003). Effect of abiotic factors on the foraging strategy of the orb-web spider *Argiope keyserlingi* (Araneae: Araneidae). *Austral Ecology*, **28**, 622–628.

Herberstein, M. E., and Heiling, A. M. (1999). Asymmetry in spider orb webs: a result of physical constraints? *Animal Behaviour*, **58**, 1241–1246.

Herberstein, M. E., Craig, C. L., Coddington, J. A. and Elgar, M. A. (2000a). The functional significance of silk decorations of orb-web spiders: a critical review of the empirical evidence. *Biological Reviews*, **75**, 649–669.

Herberstein, M. E., Craig, C. L. and Elgar, M. A. (2000b). Foraging strategies and feeding regimes: web and decoration investment in *Argiope keyserlingi* Karsch (Araneae: Araneidae). *Evolutionary Ecology Research*, **2**, 69–80.

Heuschen, B., Gumbert, A. and Lunau, K. (2005). A generalized mimicry system involving angiosperm flower colour, pollen and bumblebees' innate colour preferences. *Plant Systematics and Evolution*, **252**, 121–137.

Higgins, L. (1992). Developmental changes in barrier web structure under different levels of predation risk in *Nephila clavipes* (Araneae, Tetragnathidae). *Journal of Insect Behavior*, **5**, 635–655.

Higgins, L. E. (1995). Direct evidence for trade-offs between foraging and growth in a juvenile spider. *Journal of Arachnology*, **23**, 37–43.

Higgins, L. E., Townley, M. A., Tillinghast, E. K. and Rankin, M. A. (2001). Variation in the chemical composition of orb webs built by the spider *Nephila clavipes* (Araneae, Tetragnathidae). *Journal of Arachnology*, **29**, 82–94.

Hinman, M. B. and Lewis, R. V. (1992). Isolation of a clone encoding a second dragline silk fibroin. *Nephila clavipes* dragline silk is a two-protein fiber. *Journal of Biological Chemistry*, **267**, 19 320–19 324.

Horton, C. C. (1980). A defensive function for the stabilimenta of two orb weaving spiders (Araneae: Araneidae). *Psyche*, **87**, 13–20.

Hu, X., Vasanthavada, K., Kohler, K., *et al.* (2006). Molecular mechanisms of spider silk. *Cellular and Molecular Life Sciences*, **63**, 1986–1999.

Huang, W., Lin, Z., Sin, Y. M., *et al.* (2006). Characterization and expression of a cDNA encoding a tubuliform silk protein of the golden web spider *Nephila antipodiana*. *Biochimie*, **88**, 849–858.

Humphreys, W. F. (1992). Stabilimenta as parasols: shade construction by *Neogea* sp. (Araneae: Araneidae, Argiopinae) and its thermal behaviour. *Bulletin of the British Arachnological Society*, **9**, 47–52.

Japyassú, H. and Macagnan, C. (2004). Fishing for prey: the evolution of a new predatory tactic among spiders (Araneae, Pholcidae). *Revista de Etologia*, **6**, 79–94.

Japyassu, H. F. and Ades, C. (1998). From complete orb to semi-orb webs: developmental transitions in the web of *Nephilengys cruentata* (Araneae: Tetragnathidae). *Behaviour*, **135**, 931–956.

Jocqué, R. and Dippenaar-Schoeman, A. S. (2007). *Spider Families of the World*. Tervuren, Belgium: Royal Museum for Central Africa.

Kaston, B. J. (1972). Web making by young *Peucetia viridans* (Hentz) (Araneae: Oxyopidae). *Notes of the Arachnologists of the Southwest*, **3**, 6–7.

Knight, D. P., Knight, M. M. and Vollrath, F. (2000). Beta transition and stress-induced phase separation in the spinning of spider dragline silk. *International Journal of Biological Macromolecules*, **27**, 205–210.

Krink, T. and Vollrath, F. (1997). Analysing spider web-building behaviour with rule-based simulations and genetic algorithms. *Journal of Theoretical Biology*, **185**, 321–331.

Krink, T. and Vollrath, F. (1998). Emergent properties in the behaviour of a virtual spider robot. *Proceedings of the Royal Society of London, B*, **265**, 2051–2055.

Kuntner, M. (2005). A revision of *Herennia* (Araneae: Nephilidae: Nephilinae), the Australasian 'coin spiders'. *Invertebrate Systematics*, **19**, 391–436.

Kuntner, M. (2007). A monograph of *Nephilengys*, the pantropical 'hermit spiders' (Araneae, Nephilidae, Nephilinae). *Systematic Entomology*, **32**, 95–135.

Kuntner, M., Coddington, J. A. and Hormiga, G. (2008a). Phylogeny of extant nephilid orb-weaving spiders (Araneae, Nephilidae): testing morphological and ethological homologies. *Cladistics*, **24**, 147–217.

Kuntner, M., Haddad, C. R., Aljancic, G. and Blejec, A. (2008b). Ecology and web allometry of *Clitaetra irenae*, an arboricolous African orb-weaving spider (Araneae, Araneoidea, Nephilidae). *Journal of Arachnology*, **36**, 583–594.

Leborgne, R. and Pasquet, A. (1987). Influences of aggregative behavior on space occupation in the spider *Zygiella x-notata* (Clerck). *Behavioral Ecology and Sociobiology*, **20**, 203–208.

Levi, H. W. (1968). The spider genera *Gea* and *Argiope* in America (Araneae: Araneidae). *Bulletin of the Museum of Comparative Zoology*, **136**, 319–352.

Li, D. (2005). Spiders that decorate their webs at higher frequency intercept more prey and grow faster. *Proceedings of the Royal Society of London, B*, **272**, 1753–1757.

Li, D. and Lee, W. S. (2004). Predator-induced plasticity in web-building behaviour. *Animal Behaviour*, **67**, 309–318.

Li, D., Lim, M. L. M., Seah, W. K. and Tay, S. L. (2004). Prey-attraction as a possible function of discoid stabilimenta of juvenile orb-spinning spiders. *Animal Behaviour*, **68**, 629–635.

Liao, C.-P., Chi, K.-J. and Tso, I. M. (2009). The effects of wind on trap structural and material properties of a sit-and-wait predator. *Behavioral Ecology*, **20**, 1194–1203.

Liu, Y., Sponner, A., Porter, D. and Vollrath, F. (2008). Proline and processing of spider silks. *Biomacromolecules*, **9**, 116–121.

Lubin, Y. D. (1973). Web structure and function: the non-adhesive orb-web of *Cyrtophora moluccensis* (Doleschall) (Araneae: Araneidae). *Forma et Functio*, **6**, 337–358.

Lubin, Y. D. (1975). Stabilimenta and barrier webs in the orb webs of *Argiope argentata* (Araneae, Araneidae) on Daphne and Santa Cruz Islands, Galapagos. *Journal of Arachnology*, **2**, 119–126.

Lubin, Y. D. (1986). Web building and prey capture in the Uloboridae. In *Spiders: Webs, Behavior, and Evolution* (ed. W. A. Shear). Stanford, CA: Stanford University Press.

Lunau, K. (1995). Notes on the colour of pollen. *Plant Systematics and Evolution*, **198**, 235–252.

Madsen, B., Shao, Z. Z. and Vollrath, F. (1999). Variability in the mechanical properties of spider silks on three levels: interspecific, intraspecific and intraindividual. *International Journal of Biological Macromolecules*, **24**, 301–306.

Marples, B. J. (1969). Observations on decorated webs. *Bulletin of the British Arachnological Society*, **1**, 13–18.

Murphy, N. P., Framenau, V., Donnellan, S. C., *et al.* (2006). Phylogenetic recronstruction of the wolf spiders (Araneae: Lycosidae) using sequences from the 12S rRNA, 28S rRNA, and NADH1 genes: implications for classification, biogeography, and the evolution of web building behavior. *Molecular Phylogenetics and Evolution*, **38**, 583–602.

Nakata, K. (2009). To be or not to be conspicuous: the effects of prey availability and predator risk on spider's web decoration building. *Animal Behaviour*, **78**, 1255–1260.

Nakata, K. and Ushimaru, A. (1999). Feeding experience affects web relocation and investment in web threads in an orb-web spider, *Cyclosa argenteoalba. Animal Behaviour*, **57**, 1251–1255.

Nentwig, W. and Heimer, S. (1987). Ecological aspects of spider webs. In *Ecophysiology of Spiders* (ed. W. Nentwig). Berlin: Springer Verlag.

Nentwig, W. and Rogg, H. (1988). The cross stabilimentum of *Argiope argentata* (Araneae: Araneidae): nonfunctional or a nonspecific stress reaction? *Zoologischer Anzeiger*, **221**, 246–266.

Opell, B. D. (1982). Post-hatching development and web production of *Hyptiotes cavatus* (Hentz) (Araneae, Uloboridae). *Journal of Arachnology*, **10**, 185–191.

Opell, B. D. (1985). Web-monitoring forces exerted by orb-web and triangle-web spiders of the family Uloboridae. *Canadian Journal of Zoology*, **63**, 580–583.

Opell, B. D. (1987). Changes in web-monitoring forces associated with web reduction in the spider family Uloboridae. *Canadian Journal of Zoology*, **65**, 1028–1034.

Opell, B. D., Lipkey, G. K., Hendricks, M. L. and Vito, S. T. (2009). Daily and seasonal changes in the stickiness of viscous capture threads in *Argiope aurantia* and *Argiope trifasciata* orb-webs. *Journal of Experimental Zoology*, **311**A, 217–225.

Ortlepp, C. S. and Gosline, J. M. (2004). Consequences of forced silking. *Biomacromolecules*, **5**, 727–731.

Pan, Z. J., Li, C. P. and Xu, Q. (2004). Active control on molecular conformations and tensile properties of spider silk. *Journal of Applied Polymer Science*, **92**, 901–905.

Pasquet, A., Leborgne, R. and Lubin, Y. (1999). Previous foraging success influences web building in the spider *Stegodyphus lineatus* (Eresidae). *Behavioral Ecology*, **10**, 115–121.

Penalver, E., Grimaldi, D. A. and Delclos, X. (2006). Early Cretaceous spider web with its prey. *Science*, **312**, 1761.

Pérez-Rigueiro, J., Elices, M., Plaza, G., Real, J. I. and Guinea, G. V. (2005). The effect of spinning forces on spider silk properties. *Journal of Experimental Biology*, **208**, 2633–2639.

Peters, H. M. (1993). Über das Problem der Stabilimente in Spinnennetzen. *Zoologische Jahrbücher, Abteilung Physiologie*, **97**, 245–264.

Porter, D., Vollrath, F. and Shao, Z. (2005). Predicting the mechanical properties of spider silk as a model nanostructured polymer. *The European Physical Journal, E*, **16**, 199–206.

Prokopy, R. J. and Owens, E. D. (1983). Visual detection of plants by herbivorous insects. *Annual Review of Entomology*, **28**, 337–364.

Reed, C. F., Witt, P. N., Scarboro, M. B. and Peakal, D. B. (1970). Experience and the orb web. *Developmental Psychobiology*, **3**, 251–265.

Riekel, C., Muller, M. and Vollrath, F. (1999). In situ X-ray diffraction during forced silking of spider silk. *Macromolecules*, **32**, 4464–4466.

Rising, A., Hjalm, G., Engstrom, W. and Johnson, J. (2006). N-terminal nonrepetitive domain common to dragline, flagelliform, and cylindriform spider silk proteins. *Biomacromolecules*, **7**, 3120–3124.

Robinson, M. H. and Robinson, B. (1970). The stabilimentum of the orb web spider, *Argiope argentata*: an improbable defence against predators. *Canadian Entomologist*, **102**, 641–655.

Robinson, M. H. and Robinson, B. (1971). The predatory behavior of the ogre-faced spider *Dinopis longipes* F. Cambridge (Araneae: Dinopidae). *American Midland Naturalist*, **85**, 85–96.

Robinson, M. H. and Robinson, B. (1972). The structure possible function and origin of the remarkable ladder web built by a New Guinea orb-web spider. *Journal of Natural History*, **6**, 687–694.

Robinson, M. H. and Robinson, B. (1973). Ecology and behavior of the giant wood spider *Nephila maculata* (Fabricius) in New Guinea. *Smithsonian Contributions to Zoology*, **149**, 1–76.

Salomon, M. (2007). Western black widow spiders express state-dependent web-building strategies tailored to the presence of neighbours. *Animal Behaviour*, **73**, 865–875.

Sandoval, C. P. (1994). Plasticity in web design in the spider *Parawixia bistriata*: a response to variable prey type. *Functional Ecology*, **8**, 701–707.

Savory, T. H. (1952). *The Spider's Web*. London: Warne.

Schoener, T. W. and Spiller, D. A. (1992). Stabilimenta characteristics of the spider *Argiope argentata* on small islands: support of the predator-defense hypothesis. *Behavioural Ecology and Sociobiology*, **31**, 309–318.

Schütz, D., Taborsky, M. and Drapela, T. (2007). Air bells of water spiders are an extended phenotype modified in response to gas composition. *Journal of Experimental Zoology*, **307**A, 549–555.

Seah, W. K. and Li, D. (2001). Stabilimenta attract unwelcome predators to orb-webs. *Proceedings of the Royal Society of London, B*, **268**, 1553–1558.

Selden, P. A., Anderson, J. M., Anderson, H. M. and Fraser, N. C. (1999). Fossil araneomorph spiders from the Triassic of South Africa and Virginia. *Journal of Arachnology*, **27**, 401–414.

Shear, W. A. (1986). The evolution of web-building behavior in spiders: a third generation of hypotheses. In *Spiders: Webs, Behavior, and Evolution* (ed. W. A. Shear). Stanford, CA: Stanford University Press.

Shear, W. A., Palmer, J. M., Coddington, J. A. and Bonamo, P. M. (1989). A Devonian spinneret: early evidence of spiders and silk use. *Science*, **246**, 479–481.

Sherman, P. M. (1994). The orb-web: an energetic and behavioural estimator of spiders' dynamic foraging and reproductive strategies. *Animal Behaviour*, **48**, 19–34.

Shultz, J. W. (1987). The origin of the spinning apparatus in spiders. *Biological Reviews*, **62**, 89–113.

Simon, E. (1895). *Historie Naturelle des Araignées*. Paris: Roset.

Sponner, A. (2007). Spider silk as a resource for future biotechnologies. *Entomological Research*, **37**, 238–250.

Sponner, A., Schlott, B., Vollrath, F., Unger, E., Grosse, F. and Weisshart, K. (2005a). Characterization of the protein components of *Nephila clavipes* dragline silk. *Biochemistry*, **44**, 4727–4736.

Sponner, A., Unger, E., Grosse, F. and Weisshart, K. (2005b). Differential polymerization of the two main protein components of dragline silk during fibre spinning. *Nature Materials*, **4**, 772–775.

Sponner, A., Vater, W., Monajembashi, S., *et al.* (2007). Composition and hierarchical organisation of a spider silk. *PLoS ONE*, **2**, e998.

Sponner, A., Vater, W., Rommerskirch, W., *et al.* (2005c). The conserved C termini contribute to the properties of spider silk fibroins. *Biochemical, Biophysical Research Communication*, **338**, 897–902.

Starks, P. T. (2002). The adaptive significance of stabilimenta in orb-web: a hierarchical approach. *Annales Zoologici Fennici*, **39**, 307–315.

Stowe, M. K. (1978). Observations of two nocturnal orb weavers that build specialised webs: *Scoloderus cordatus* and *Wixia ectypa* (Araneae, Araneidae). *Journal of Arachnology*, **6**, 141–146.

Stowe, M. K., Tumlinson, J. H. and Heath, R. R. (1987). Chemical mimicry: bolas spiders emit components of moth prey species sex pheromones. *Science*, **236**, 964–967.

Tai, P. L., Hwang, G. Y. and Tso, I. M. (2004). Interspecific sequence conservation and intra-individual sequence variation in a spider silk gene. *International Journal of Biological Macromolecules*, **34**, 295–301.

Tan, E. J. and Li, D. Q. (2009). Detritus decorations of an orb-weaving spider, *Cyclosa mulmeinensis* (Thorell): for food or camouflage? *Journal of Experimental Biology*, **212**, 1832–1839.

Théry, M. and Casas, J. (2009). The multiple disguises of spiders: web colour and decorations, body colour and movement. *Philosophical Transactions of the Royal Society, B*, **364**, 471–480.

Townley, M. A., Tillinghast, E. K. and Neefus, C. D. (2006). Changes in composition of spider orb web sticky droplets with starvation and web removal, and synthesis of sticky droplet compounds. *Journal of Experimental Biology*, **209**, 1463–1486.

Tseng, L. and Tso, I. M. (2009). A risky defence by a spider using conspicuous decoys resembling itself in appearance. *Animal Behaviour*, **78**, 425–431.

Tso, I. M. (1996). Stabilimentum of the garden spider *Argiope trifasciata*: a possible prey attractant. *Animal Behaviour*, **52**, 183–191.

Tso, I. M. (1998a). Isolated spider web stabilimentum attracts insects. *Behaviour*, **135**, 311–319.

Tso, I. M. (1998b). Stabilimentum-decorated webs spun by *Cyclosa conica* (Araneae, Araneidae) trapped more insects than undecorated webs. *Journal of Arachnology*, **26**, 101–105.

Tso, I. M. (1999). Behavioral response of *Argiope trifasciata* to recent foraging gain: a manipulative study. *American Midland Naturalist*, **141**, 238–246.

Tso, I. M. (2004). The effect of food and silk reserve manipulation on decoration-building of *Argiope aetheroides*. *Behaviour*, **141**, 603–616.

Tso, I. M., Chiang, S. Y. and Blackledge, T. A. (2007). Does the giant wood spider *Nephila pilipes* respond to prey variation by altering web or silk properties? *Ethology*, **113**, 324–333.

Tso, I. M., Wu, H. C. and Hwang, I. R. (2005). Giant wood spider *Nephila pilipes* alters silk protein in response to prey variation. *Journal of Experimental Biology*, **208**, 1053–1061.

Uhl, G. (2008). Size dependent occurrence of different types of web decorations and a barrier web in the tropical spider *Argiope argentata* (Fabricius 1775) (Araneae Araneidae). *Tropical Zoology*, **21**, 97–108.

Venner, S., Pasquet, A. and Leborgne, R. (2000). Web-building behaviour in the orb-weaving spider *Zygiella x-notata*: influence of experience. *Animal Behaviour*, **59**, 603–611.

Vollrath, F. (1992). Analysis and interpretation of orb spider exploration and web-building behavior. *Advances in the Study of Behavior*, **21**, 147–197.

Vollrath, F. (2000). Strength and structure of spiders' silks. *Reviews in Molecular Biotechnology*, **74**, 67–83.

Vollrath, F. and Knight, D. P. (2001). Liquid crystalline spinning of spider silk. *Nature*, **410**, 541–548.

Vollrath, F. and Köhler, T. (1996). Mechanics of silk produced by loaded spiders. *Proceedings of the Royal Society of London, B*, **263**, 387–391.

Vollrath, F. and Selden, P. (2007). The role of behavior in the evolution of spiders, silks, and webs. *Annual Review of Ecology, Evolution, and Systematics*, **38**, 819–846.

Vollrath, F., Downes, M. and Krackow, S. (1997). Design variability in web geometry of an orb-weaving spider. *Physiology and Behavior*, **62**, 735–743.

Walter, A., Elgar, M. A., Bliss, P. and Moritz, R. F. A. (2008a). Molting interferes with web decorating behavior in *Argiope keyserlingi* (Araneae, Araneidae). *Journal of Arachnology*, **36**, 538–544.

Walter, A., Elgar, M. A., Bliss, P. and Moritz, R. F. A. (2008b). Wrap attack activates web-decorating behavior in *Argiope* spiders. *Behavioral Ecology*, **19**, 799–804.

Ward, D. and Lubin, Y. (1993). Habitat selection and the life history of a desert spider, *Stegodyphus lineatus* (Eresidae). *Journal of Animal Ecology*, **62**, 353–363.

Watanabe, T. (1999). Prey attraction as a possible function of the silk decoration of the uloborid spider *Octonoba sybotides*. *Behavioral Ecology*, **10**, 607–611.

Watanabe, T. (2000). Web tuning of an orb-web spider, *Octonoba sybotides*, regulates prey-catching behaviour. *Proceedings of the Royal Society of London, B*, **267**, 565–569.

Wiehle, H. (1928). Beitrage zur Biologie der Araneen, insbesondere zur Kentnis des Radnetzbaues. *Zeitschrift fuer Morphologie und Oekologie der Tiere*, **11**, 115–151.

Winkler, S. and Kaplan, D. L. (2000). Molecular biology of spider silk. *Reviews in Molecular Biotechnology*, **74**, 85–93.

Witt, P. N. (1963). Environment in relation to the behaviour of spiders. *Archives of Environmental Health*, **7**, 4–12.

Witt, P. N. and Baum, R. (1960). Changes in orb webs of spiders during growth (*Araneus diadematus* Clerck and *Neoscona vertebrata* McCook). *Behaviour*, **16**, 309–318.

Witt, P. N., Rawlings, J. O. and Reed, C. F. (1972). Ontogeny of web-building behavior in two orb-weaving spiders. *American Zoologist*, **12**, 443–454.

Xu, M. and Lewis, R. V. (1990). Structure of a protein superfiber: spider dragline silk. *Proceedings of the National Academy of Sciences of the USA*, **87**, 7120–7124.

Yaginuma, T. (1986). *Spiders of Japan in Colour*. Osaka: Hoikusha Publishing Company.

Yeargan, K. V. (1994). Biology of bolas spiders. *Annual Review of Entomology*, **39**, 81–99.

Yoo, J.-S. and Framenau, V. W. (2006). Systematics and biogeography of the sheet-web building wolf spider genus *Venonia* (Araneae: Lycosidae). *Invertebrate Systematics*, **20**, 675–712.

Zax, D. B., Armanios, D. E., Horak, S., Malowniak, C. and Yang, Z. T. (2004). Variation of mechanical properties with amino acid content in the silk of *Nephila clavipes*. *Biomacromolecules*, **5**, 732–738.

Zevenbergen, J. M., Schneider, N. K. and Blackledge, T. A. (2008). Fine dining or fortress? Functional shifts in spider web architecture by the western black widow *Latrodectus hesperus*. *Animal Behaviour*, **76**, 823–829.

Zschokke, S. (1996a). Early stages of orb web construction in *Araneus diadematus* Clerck. *Revue Suisse de Zoologie*, **2**, 709–720.

Zschokke, S. (1996b). Factors influencing the size of orb web in *Araneus diadematus*. In *Sixteenth European Colloquium of Arachnology* (ed. M. Zabka). Siedlce, Poland: Wyzsa Szkola Rolniczo-Pedagogiczna.

Zschokke, S. (1999). Nomenclature of the orb-web. *Journal of Arachnology*, **27**, 542–546.

Zschokke, S. (2003). Palaeontology: spider-web silk from the Early Cretaceous. *Nature*, **424**, 636–637.

4

Flexible use of anti-predator defences

XIMENA J. NELSON AND ROBERT R. JACKSON

Belonging to a size category that makes them vulnerable to a wide variety of predators, spiders have evolved a bewildering array of anti-predator adaptations, which can be clustered under two broad categories, primary and secondary defence. Primary defences are ploys by which the spider avoids provoking pursuit by, and interaction with, the predator. Camouflage and masquerade are especially common examples. Secondary defences come into play once an interaction with a predator is under way, and these are the defences that have been most thoroughly studied. However, elements of anti-predator defence may often be integrated into other aspects of the spider's biology. Cues from predators may influence a spider's decision to move away from a habitat, and may also influence the decisions spiders make in the context of courtship, mating and oviposition. Anti-predator defences are sometimes subject to local adaptation by different populations within single species, and considerable flexibility in anti-predator ploys may be evident even at the level of the individual spider. Although vertebrates are often predators of spiders, anti-predator flexibility may have evolved primarily when the predator is another spider or an insect. Spider–spider encounters in particular have a way of blurring the distinction between anti-predator and predatory behaviour. Tremendous opportunity remains for research on the anti-predator defences of spiders, but perhaps the major challenge for future researchers will be to devise and carry out experiments that demonstrate the efficacy in the field of anti-predator defences that have thus far been studied primarily in the laboratory.

4.1 Introduction

When reviewing the anti-predator defences of spiders 15 years ago, Cloudsley-Thompson (1995) warned that 'Only a fool would attempt to review

Spider Behaviour: Flexibility and Versatility, ed. Marie Elisabeth Herberstein. Published by Cambridge University Press. © Cambridge University Press 2011.

a topic as wide as anti-predator defences in spiders, because, to provide a balanced account, it is necessary to discuss many important aspects of the subject in a rather superficial manner' (p. 92). A recent surge in publications on anti-predator defence gives this warning even more force today and, for this review, we will not attempt a comprehensive coverage of this literature. As a more modest goal, we use case studies to illustrate how in spiders flexibility is expressed in anti-predator defence.

Predatory sequences consist of five stages, beginning with predators detecting prey, followed by prey identification, attack (or approach and then attack), capture, and finally eating their prey (Lima and Dill, 1990). There are examples of prey having defences that interfere with the predator's routine at each stage, though we need not name these. It is, however, useful to distinguish between what Edmunds (1974) called primary and secondary defence. In casual terms, prey use primary defence for keeping out of trouble and secondary defence for getting out of trouble. Although secondary defence comes into play during interactions between predators and prey, the efficacy of primary defence relies on the prey not providing the predator with the cues that would normally initiate an interaction.

A basic type of individual flexibility is evident as soon as we define primary defence and secondary defence, as spiders generally depend on both. Another aspect of flexibility is that characteristics of spiders that function in anti-predator defence may often have other functions (e.g. predatory) at the same time. Definitions such as primary and secondary defence make it easier to make distinctions, discuss mechanisms by which defence is achieved, and understand how defences evolved. Nevertheless, real-life examples of anti-predator defence tend to be messy, often seeming to defy our efforts to categorise phenomena with terminology. In this chapter, with our emphasis on flexibility, the messy character of real-life examples is our primary interest.

4.2   The predators of spiders

Like insects, spiders sit in about the middle of the range of body size known for animals (Gullan and Cranston, 2000) and consequently are an appropriate prey size for a great range of predators. Determining exactly what potential predators have the greatest impact on spiders is no easy task. More than a half century ago, Bristowe (1941) made one of the first, and still one of the most exhaustive, attempts at such an overview. However, our interest is not simply in the predators that eat lots of spiders but instead in the predators to which spiders might be most likely to evolve flexible defence mechanisms. For example, many predatory vertebrates, especially insectivorous species, may prey heavily on spiders (Spiller and Schoener, 1998, 2001). Bristowe (1941) concluded that birds in particular impact strongly on spider populations and this conclusion is supported by modern ecological research (e.g. Gunnarsson, 2007, Oxford and Gillespie, 1998). However, birds or other vertebrates do not appear to be primary predators for which flexible defence behaviour has evolved.

Among spiders, flexible use of anti-predator defence may have evolved especially against predatory arthropods, including not only predatory insects but also other spiders. Here, the predator can be a species from the same spider family, or even individuals of the same species. Part of what makes these examples interesting is that they can be considered in the context of intraguild predation: the predatory spider can also become a meal for its own prey, and the predator and the prey may be potential competitors for yet other prey (Hurd and Eisenberg, 1990, Kindlmann and Houdková, 2006, Moya-Laraño and Wise, 2007, Polis and Strong, 1996). Our interest in these examples is in how the intertwined relationships between predator and prey in intraguild systems may be especially conducive to the evolution of anti-predator flexibility.

4.3   Camouflage

Sometimes primary defence is based on the ability to go unnoticed by the predator, but it can also be based on the predator detecting the prey and then misidentifying it as something else. Blending in with the background, often called camouflage, is usually considered in visual terms, but the possibility of camouflage in other sensory modalities (e.g. having odour that blends in with the ambient odour in the environment) should also be considered (Ruxton, 2009).

The basis for considering that a spider 'blends in' is most often the difficulty researchers have in seeing a spider against a background. While useful as steps towards formulating hypotheses, these impressions are no substitute for evidence that the apparent camouflage works against natural predators, as exemplified by camouflage based on coloration. For example, human colour vision is based on visual receptors maximally sensitive to wavelengths corresponding to three primary colours: red, green and blue (Gregory, 1998). However, the relevant perspective is that of the spider's natural predators. Many of these, such as wasps and birds, are sensitive to ultraviolet (UV) light, and some are insensitive to red light (Briscoe and Chittka, 2001, Cuthill et al., 2000, Kelber et al., 2003, Lim and Li, 2006, Osorio and Vorobyev, 2008). For a predator that uses colour vision based in part on UV or is insensitive to red, we cannot simply assume that a spider that appears camouflaged or conspicuous to us is comparably camouflaged or conspicuous to the predator (Heiling et al., 2003, Théry, 2007, Théry and Casas, 2009). This warning applies not just to colour vision, but to other aspects of vision (Land and Nilsson, 2002), such as motion detection and spatial resolution.

Being tightly linked to predator-specific sensory systems, the efficacy of camouflage may vary considerably depending on the predator (Ruxton *et al.*, 2004, Zylinski *et al.*, 2009), but an understanding of how camouflage use might be based on the interaction of different predators and habitats is lacking. Moreover, flexibility in camouflage may be expressed in non-obvious ways. For example, ambient lighting and the relative positions of both predator and prey probably influence the efficacy of vision-based camouflage (Cott, 1940, Kiltie, 1988, Speed *et al.*, 2005), suggesting that camouflage may be an especially inviting topic for research on predator–prey coevolution and anti-predator flexibility. Yet, at this stage, there is not a lot that can be said beyond acknowledging the potential of research aimed at testing hypotheses about flexible use of camouflage by spiders and indicating that there are some particularly enticing candidates for research on how spiders use camouflage. For example, species belonging to several families have independently evolved mechanisms for reversibly changing their body coloration in response to background colour and local lighting conditions (Gabritchvesky, 1927, Oxford and Gillespie, 1998, Théry and Casas, 2009), and these may be especially likely to make flexible use of camouflage (Hanlon *et al.*, 2009, Stuart-Fox and Moussali, 2009).

4.4   Masquerade

We can distinguish between camouflage, which functions by rendering the prey hard to detect, and masquerade (Cloudsley-Thompson, 1995, Stevens, 2007), also called 'special protective resemblance' (Poulton, 1890), which renders the prey hard to identify specifically as prey. The everyday word for resemblance is mimicry, although there are various special types of mimicry that have technical definitions in biology (Stevens, 2007, Vane-Wright, 1980, Wickler, 1968). However, leaving the simple term mimicry unencumbered by formal definition makes it easier to specify how the resemblance we call masquerade differs from other types of resemblance we will consider later (aggressive mimicry and Batesian mimicry).

Portia, an unusual genus in the spider family Salticidae, illustrates how anti-predator defences sometimes defy the somewhat simplistic categorisations encouraged by our well-defined terms. Salticids are often characterised as not using webs for prey capture, but *Portia* builds prey-capture webs and also invades the webs of other spiders (Harland and Jackson, 2004). In order to understand how *Portia* interacts with other spiders in webs we have to appreciate that what salticids see is extraordinarily rich in detail because, uniquely, these spiders have complex principal eyes that support spatial acuity exceeding that of other animals of comparable size (Harland and Jackson, in press). Web-building spiders,

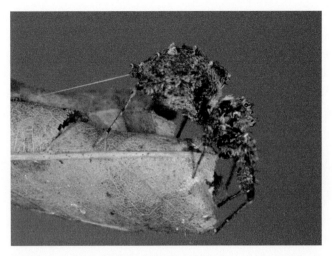

Figure 4.1 Detritus-like salticid *Portia fimbriata* standing at the door of the nest (rolled up dead leaf) of a female *Euryattus* sp. See also colour plate.

by contrast, excel at interpreting movement and tension patterns (web signals) conveyed through the silk lines of their self-made webs (Krafft and Leborgne, 1979) and often it is appropriate to consider the spider's web as an integral part of its sensory apparatus. This means that a spider invading another spider's web can be envisaged as not only entering the arena in which the resident spider normally captures prey, but also as walking directly into the resident spider's sensory system (Jackson and Pollard, 1997).

Although the distinctions made by the terms camouflage and masquerade are useful, deciding how much activity tips the balance away from camouflage and towards masquerade is difficult. *Portia*'s appearance may not be especially relevant to the resident spider in a web, but we can assume that *Portia*, whether in or out of webs, is potential prey for numerous predators that rely on vision. However, *Portia*'s appearance is unusual. Webs are often cluttered with detritus, such as mouldy, broken pieces of dead leaves. Having a body covered in a fine, low-contrast patchwork of browns, softened by fringes of hair (Figure 4.1), *Portia* is a convincing detritus mimic (Jackson and Blest, 1982, Wanless, 1978). A quiescent *Portia* tends to blend in (camouflage) when close to detritus in a web. When not close to detritus or when active, even near detritus, *Portia* is more likely to stand out as a distinct object, all the while being misidentified as only a piece of detritus rather than as potential prey (i.e. now it is more appropriate to say *Portia* is masquerading as a piece of detritus). In situations like this, a better perspective is to envisage a camouflage–masquerade continuum and accept that there will be many examples for which both terms are applicable.

How *Portia* walks is also interesting. Out of context, on a laboratory bench, *Portia*'s walking gait appears overacted, even comical. With its eight legs waving about in a slow, jerky manner, *Portia* is reminiscent of a robot in a 1950s' science fiction movie (Harland and Jackson, 2004). In nature, however, *Portia*'s stepping gait makes sense as an example of motion camouflage (Théry and Casas, 2009, Troscianko *et al.*, 2009) because exaggerated, hesitating motion creates an impression of no more than dapples of sunlight filtering through the canopy and flickering on a piece of detritus.

4.5   Limb loss as flexible secondary defence

Forfeiting an appendage (i.e. autotomy: an ability to lose one or more limbs with minimal trauma) can be an important mechanism by which a spider avoids being killed (Fleming *et al.*, 2007, Roth and Roth, 1984) and, as might be expected of a spider that forages in other spiders' webs, *Portia* is especially prone to autotomy of legs when attacked by its intended prey (Jackson and Blest, 1982). Especially distinctive ways in which leg loss functions in anti-predator defence can be found in pholcids (Pholcidae), spiders that are notable for their very long legs. The best way for a predator to secure a pholcid is to grab hold of the pholcid's body, but these spiders' long legs tend to get in the way. When a predator grabs a leg, the pholcid flees, losing a leg but saving its life. The lost leg may go on functioning for several seconds, making distinctive twitching movements that appear to distract the predator while the pholcid moves out of harm's way (Johnson and Jakob, 1999).

In most other examples, the lost leg probably becomes immediately inert and leg loss seems to provide protection primarily by giving the spider that loses the leg time to flee before the predator releases the leg and attacks the leg's owner (Formanowicz, 1990). However, concluding that the outcome for the predator is simply a failed foraging effort might sometimes be misleading. Although rarely considered, predator–prey sequences that end with prey losing a leg might sometimes be more accurately envisaged as instances in which predators acquire a non-trivial meal (the prey's leg) while the prey, although suffering injury, escapes with its life. How serious the injury is for the spider that loses the leg is not always clear. There is evidence in some instances of impaired running speed, diminished success in contests with same-sex conspecific individuals, and reduced attractiveness to the opposite sex during courtship (Amaya *et al.*, 2001, Taylor and Jackson, 2003, Uetz *et al.*, 1996). Juvenile spiders might regenerate lost legs, but several successive moults might be needed before regaining a full-size normal leg, and there may be costs related to the regeneration process (Wrinn and Uetz, 2007). Yet what is most striking is how often costs to the autotomised spider have been looked for but not found and, when found, are not especially pronounced (Amaya *et al.*, 2001, Apontes and Brown, 2005, Brautigam and Persons, 2003, Brueseke *et al.*, 2001, Johnson and Jakob, 1999, Riechert, 1988; but see Lutzy and Morse, 2008, Wrinn and Uetz, 2007). This research suggests that leg loss may reveal an elementary type of anti-predator flexibility based on morphology.

Like spiders, harvestmen (Opiliones) are arachnids with eight legs and readily lose legs to predators, with the cost of losing a leg for a harvestmen sometimes seeming to be minimal. This has been the rationale for what is called the spare-legs hypothesis (Guffey, 1998, 1999), a hypothesis that may sometimes be applicable to spiders as well as harvestmen (Johnson and Jakob, 1999). This hypothesis should not be interpreted as a proposal that an anti-predator advantage accounts for the origin of many legs, but having especially many legs might, nonetheless, provide an elementary kind of morphological flexibility that makes leg loss especially viable as a defence for these animals, at least against some predators.

Formanowicz (1990) examined the survival value of leg autotomy in *Kukulcania hibernalis* (Filistatidae) when confronted with two predators that use very different predatory tactics: scorpions and centipedes. Scorpions tend to grasp the spider's leg and are slower at injecting venom (stinging) than centipedes, which are apt to grasp the spider's body and quickly and repeatedly inject venom by biting. Spiders did not survive encounters with centipedes and did not autotomise legs during these encounters. However, several spiders survived encounters with scorpions, and of those that did survive, significantly more autotomised a leg than did not.

However, another more direct way in which autotomy and flexibility may be related has been only rarely considered. After a close encounter with a predator, a spider may use behaviour to compensate for the loss of a leg. For example, *Holocnemus pluchei*, a pholcid, normally uses its first pair of legs when probing at prey that land in the web but, after losing these legs, these spiders switch to probing with the second pair (Johnson and Jakob, 1999).

4.6   Aposematism and Batesian mimicry

Aposematism is a term for an anti-predator defence strategy that seems to be almost the antithesis of camouflage (Ruxton *et al.*, 2004). In the classic examples, aposematic prey make themselves conspicuous and identifiable to potential predators by deploying specialised warning signals (e.g. bright colours). These signals communicate to potential predators that the aposematic prey's defences are dangerous. For example, the aposematic prey may be able to defend itself by using venom.

That some spiders might be aposematic may appear likely, as most spiders have venom (Foelix, 1996) and the toxicity of some spider venoms to potential predators may be considerable (Vetter and Visscher, 1998). Some species in the theridiid genus *Latrodectus* (widow spiders) are especially noteworthy because their neurotoxic venom (Rash and Hodgson, 2002) has considerable potency to various vertebrates (Kaston, 1970) and they often have bright red markings contrasting sharply with their jet-black abdomens (Garb *et al.*, 2004), suggestive of a function as a warning signal (Vetter and Visscher, 1998). Nevertheless, the kind of evidence needed for concluding that these spiders use aposematism as an anti-predator defence is lacking. When we consider *Latrodectus*' venom in the context of aposematism, there is a striking absence of clear evidence of *Latrodectus* routinely making use of venom as secondary defence against predators. Bees and wasps are classic examples of venom-supported aposematism and, unlike *Latrodectus*, these insects aggressively inject venom that causes immediate and severe pain. We cannot rule out the possibility that *Latrodectus* uses its venom aggressively in defence against some of its natural predators, but the absence of evidence makes this mere speculation. As for why humans react adversely to *Latrodectus* venom, the explanation may lie in the vagaries of venom chemistry (Vetter and Isbister, 2008) rather than in how *Latrodectus* defends itself.

The secondary defence we know more about in *Latrodectus* is based on using silk instead of venom. When attacked, widow spiders sometimes defend themselves by applying silk onto the face of a vertebrate predator, causing the predator to stop and groom while the spider gains an opportunity to flee (Vetter, 1980). Perhaps red markings warn predators that, should they attack, they will get a face full of silk. Corroboration of this hypothesis would give evidence that *Latrodectus* is aposematic, but this would not be venom-based aposematism.

Batesian mimics are palatable prey species that deceive predators by advertising (signalling) like an aposematic prey species. We do have experimental evidence for Batesian mimicry in spiders, but only if we adopt a liberal attitude towards what qualifies as a model in a Batesian-mimicry system. In the classic examples of Batesian mimicry, the mimic's model is aposematic. Many spiders mimic ants (Cushing, 1997) and many potential predators of spiders seem to be averse to attacking ants, as ants are notorious for having formidable defences, including ability to harm potential predators by biting, stinging or spraying formic acid. Being social insects, ants are all the more dangerous because they can mount communal attacks on would-be predators (Hölldobler and Wilson, 1990). Ants also have a distinctive appearance, but calling an ant aposematic can be problematic because it seems unlikely that the origin of the ant's general appearance (e.g. a slender body, narrow waist, erratic style of locomotion and distinctive way of waving antennae) evolved as anti-predator defence. Yet, origin notwithstanding, predators often respond to ant-like appearance as a warning (i.e. a cue for avoidance; Nelson and Jackson, 2006) and to disqualify ant mimicry as examples of Batesian mimicry purely on the basis of hypotheses about the origin of the ant's general appearance seems to place unwarranted emphasis on a distinction that is irrelevant to the predator. However, in the context of this chapter, instead of these terminological issues, our interest is in how ant mimicry illustrates flexibility.

Animals that mimic ants in appearance are called myrmecomorphic and those that eat ants are myrmecophagic. Among spiders there are hundreds of myrmecomorphic species, including all species in the salticid genus *Myrmarachne*, these being spiders that resemble ants behaviourally as well as morphologically (Cushing, 1997). Most salticids appear to avoid attacking ants, and ant-averse salticids are deceived by the mimics' resemblance to ants (Nelson and Jackson, 2006). As ant-averse salticids often eat other salticids (Jackson and Pollard, 1996), confusing these predators works for *Myrmarachne* as an anti-predatory ploy (Batesian mimicry). However, it is not just ant-averse salticids that are fooled by *Myrmarachne*, but also myrmecophagic species. When myrmecophagic salticids respond to *Myrmarachne* as though they really were ants, the mimic may simply trade one predator for another (Nelson *et al.*, 2006a). However, some species of *Myrmarachne* have a way out of this predicament. Once the ant-like salticid detects the unwanted attentions of an ant-eating salticid, it stops acting like an ant by changing its usual ant-like posture and pattern of movement, thereby informing the ant-eating predator that it is not really an ant. The posture adopted by *Myrmarachne* is typical of displays towards conspecifics, and in fact is a posture commonly adopted by salticids during intraspecific interactions. It is tempting to conclude that these so-called erect leg postures communicate to the myrmecophagic salticid that it is in fact facing another salticid, but specific evidence for this is lacking (Nelson *et al.*, 2006b).

Ant-eating salticids are not the only special predation risk for *Myrmarachne* because, for ant resemblance to function effectively as Batesian mimicry, it may be important for ant-mimicking spiders to live in close proximity to the ants they resemble (myrmecophily). *Myrmarachne assimilis*, for example, faithfully resembles and lives in close association with *Oecophylla smaragdina*, dangerous ants that will not only kill unwary individuals of *M. assimilis* that come too close, but will also eat the eggs of *M. assimilis* females (Nelson and Jackson, 2008, Nelson *et al.*, 2004). Females of *M. assimilis*, like those of many salticid species, lay their eggs inside cocoon-like silk nests. Salticid nest silk may often function in part as a barrier that interferes with access to eggs by potential predators,

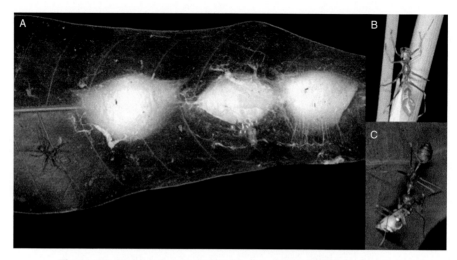

Figure 4.2 (A) Adult female ant-like *Myrmarachne assimilis* (body length, 7 mm) on mango leaf with crèche (three silk nests joined together) serving as defence against egg-eating ants. (B) Slim red body, modified to make the spider appear to have a head, thorax and abdomen, like an ant, instead of cephalothorax and abdomen, like a spider. Slender forelegs, held in characteristic posture, resemble ant's antennae. (C) *Oecophylla smaragdina*, ant model for *M. assimilis*, holding dead jumping spider in its jaws. See also colour plate.

including ants, but an isolated egg-holding nest of *M. assimilis* is not very effective at deterring *O. smaragdina*. *Myrmarachne assimilis* females solve this problem by coming together and clustering their egg-holding nests (Figure 4.2) so that the combined mass of silk makes an ant-proof crèche or 'childcare' (Nelson and Jackson, 2008).

Ants and spiders are both especially abundant in many habitats, and these are particularly interesting animals to consider in the context of intraguild predation (Moya-Laraño and Wise, 2007). Perhaps it is not surprising that some spiders have evolved ant-specific anti-predator defences and that some spiders have evolved ant-specific prey-capture behaviour. However, ant-specific coping mechanisms of spiders extend beyond straightforward predator–prey adaptation and include, for example, adjustments in spider mating behaviour.

4.7   Practising safe sex in the presence of predators

The courtship and mating behaviour of the salticid *Phintella piatensis* has characteristics that appear to function as defence against ants. Although this species does not resemble ants, it is myrmecophilic, and the ants with which it associates include *O. smaragdina*. Unwary individuals of *P. piatensis* fall victim to this particularly fearsome ant (Nelson *et al.*, 2004). However, the nests of *P. piatensis* are unusually dense, and inside its nest *P. piatensis* enjoys considerable protection from ants. Besides being oviposition sites and shelters when quiescent, the nests of *P. piatensis* (and other salticids) are sites for courtship and mating (Jackson and Pollard, 1997). Experiments have shown that *P. piatensis* pairs tend to mate inside nests when they can see ants in the vicinity, and that this behaviour reduces their otherwise considerable risk of being killed by ants. If ants are not seen in the vicinity of the nest, spiders are more inclined to mate outside. This is an unusually pronounced example of a prey species' mating decisions being influenced by perceived risk of predation (Nelson and Jackson, 2009).

For animals in general, the trend is for males to be more active than females in courtship. Courtship signals often make the male conspicuous to the female (Andersson, 1994; Chapter 7), but may also make males more conspicuous to predators (Jennions *et al.*, 2001, Kotiaho, 2001, Zuk and Kolluru, 1998). Among spiders, the clearest examples of this come from wolf spiders (Lycosidae), which, like salticids, often adopt conspicuous courtship displays. There is considerable evidence that courtship signals make lycosid males vulnerable to predators (Kotiaho *et al.*, 1998, Lindström *et al.*, 2006, Roberts and Uetz, 2008, Roberts *et al.*, 2006, Scheffer *et al.*, 1996) and there is also evidence that lycosid males, upon detecting cues from potential predators, assess risk and, based on this, make adjustments to their courtship behaviour (Pruden and Uetz, 2004, Taylor *et al.*, 2005).

Perhaps the clearest illustration of the level of detail concerned in risk assessment during courtship comes from a recent study on the lycosid *Schizocosa ocreata* with a simulated bird predator (Lohrey *et al.*, 2009). Males of *S. ocreata* have conspicuous hair tufts on their forelegs and during courtship they vigorously wave these legs. In laboratory experiments, males adjusted their courtship behaviour in response to bird calls, to playback of the seismic (substrate vibration) signals that imitated birds pecking at the ground, and to a shadow from a cardboard cut-out shaped like a bird and moved overhead as a simulation of a flying bird. Moreover, the courting male's specific response to these different cue types seemed to be fine-tuned to the nature of the threat. Courting males fled when the stimulus was the shadow of a bird flying overhead, and they froze (i.e. stopped courting and remained quiescent) when the stimuli were vocalisations or seismic cues. A bird pecking at the ground or making calls might be close by and this is a situation in which freezing may be the optimal response. However, a bird passing overhead will tend to be more distant, leaving time for the lycosid to flee and seek shelter (Lohrey *et al.*, 2009).

4.8   Flexible defence in webs

Although spiders are better known for being solitary predators, there is a sizable minority of species that naturally aggregate. In addition to functions related to foraging and reproduction, anti-predator defence has been proposed as an explanation for group living in spiders (Whitehouse and Lubin, 2005; Chapter 8), with the mechanisms proposed often being related to safety in numbers. For example, an individual spider's chances of survival may be higher when in a group than when solitary because predators have difficulty singling out and attacking any one prey individual in a crowd, or because the predator ignores an individual in a crowd after having reached satiation eating its neighbours. For an individual spider in a group, another advantage, known as the early-warning effect, depends on sharing information either actively or passively, with web silk making this defence mechanism especially efficient. There are also instances where individual spiders in groups join forces and, as a group, deploy defences that are beyond the capability of an individual acting alone. For illustrating each of these defence strategies, we will rely on some particularly well-researched case studies.

Uetz and co-workers have extensively investigated the social defences of *Metepeira incrassata* (Araneidae), a Mexican orb-web spider species. Individuals of this species live in web complexes that can be populated by tens to thousands of individual spiders within their individual, but interconnected, orb webs (Rayor and Uetz, 1990). Findings from early studies of how these spiders respond during wasp attacks suggest a selfish-herd effect (Hamilton, 1971), with individual spiders seeking safety from predators by moving as close as possible to the centre of the group (Rayor and Uetz, 1990, 1993). However, the signature of a selfish-herd mechanism is a constant capture rate leading to a linear reduction in the probability of an individual spider being captured based on increasing population size, and a tendency for spiders at the periphery of a group to be more vulnerable to the predator. Contrary to this, the relationship between group size and probability of being killed by a predator was not linear for *M. incrassata* (Uetz and Hieber, 1994).

When web complexes of *M. incrassata* were large, an early-warning effect appeared to be more important than the selfish-herd effect. With many spiders present in their separate orb webs, the probability that at least one of these individuals would detect the predator's approach and take individual defensive measures was high. This, in turn, generated vibratory signals that alerted other members of the web complex to the presence of a predator (Uetz and Hieber, 1994, Uetz *et al.*, 2002). For example, a spider that detected an approaching predator might drop out of its web, setting off vibratory signals that, owing to webs being interconnected within the web complex, were transmitted efficiently to the rest of the colony.

For an example of social spiders mounting active communal defence against predators, we can turn to *Stegodyphus dumicola* (Eresidae). An important way in which this species differs from *M. incrassata* is that, instead of living in individual webs within a web complex, individuals of *S. dumicola* live together in a single communal web (Seibt and Wickler, 1988). In South Africa, *S. dumicola* is especially subject to predation by *Anoplolepis steingroeveri*, an ant species that is common in the same habitat. The spiders' defence against marauding bands of ants is to erect defensive barriers. These barriers are bands of silk on the branches under the web. By applying a covering of fine, sticky cribellate silk, these silk bands are made particularly difficult for ants to cross. Nonetheless, ants sometimes penetrate the barrier because ant bodies can accumulate on the silk and become bridges across which other ants can walk. The response of *S. dumicola* to these security breaches is to retreat to loosely woven silk tunnels below the nest, whereupon individual spiders take turns reinforcing the perimeter with cribellate silk. This defensive measure relies on working as a group, because an individual spider is unable to mobilise cribellate silk in the quantity needed for repelling the ants (Henschel, 1998).

Latrodectus hesperus (Theridiidae), a black widow spider, gives us an example of a non-social spider that uses flexibility in web-building behaviour in the context of anti-predator defence. These spiders build three-dimensional webs consisting of a sheet of silk and an embedded silk nest, with gumfooted threads (i.e. taut silk lines along the lower reaches of which there are droplets of sticky fluid; see Chapter 3) extending down from the sheet to the ground. The spider preys on ground-dwelling arthropods that blunder into, and adhere to, the gumfooted threads when passing under the web. The spider also surrounds its nest with a matrix of silk threads and these threads function in anti-predator defence by providing, via vibratory signals transmitted through the silk, early warning of impending attacks by predators (Blackledge and Zevenbergen, 2007). Flexibility is evident because sated spiders and spiders preparing to lay eggs shift to allocating more silk than usual to the matrix surrounding the nest and less to the gumfooted prey-capture threads. The subtlety in this example illustrates how flexibility works at many levels in spider anti-predator defences.

4.9   Predator-specific refinement of prey sensory ability

For prey, early detection and identification of predators can provide time to execute pre-emptive defence, and examples of specialised predator-specific detection and identification ability might be expected when a prey species is frequently targeted by particular predators. Here we will consider several examples in which both the predator and the prey are spiders.

A particularly clear example of a prey's ability to detect and modify its behaviour in response to cues from a major predator comes from two ground-dwelling lycosid species that are common in North America and which differ considerably in adult body size. *Pardosa milvina* is the smaller and *Hogna helluo* is the larger species. An individual of either species will prey on individuals of the other when size disparity favours it (Persons and Rypstra, 2001), but it is predation by *H. helluo* on *P. milvina* that we will consider here. Chemotactile traces from silk or excreta left by *H. helluo* when moving about on the substrate provide predator-identification cues for *P. milvina* (Persons *et al.* 2001), but only when the traces are recent (Barnes *et al.*, 2002) and only when the *H. helluo* individual that left the traces was at least as large as *P. milvina* (Persons and Rypstra, 2001). Instead of *P. milvina* distinguishing between large and small individuals of *H. helluo* on the basis of a qualitative difference in chemotactile cues, *P. milvina* seems to rely on the quantity of cues of silk or excreta, as its response to the cumulative chemotactile cues from a group of small *H. helluo* individuals is comparable to its response to a single large *H. helluo* individual (Persons and Rypstra, 2001). However, as *H. helluo* is not a social spider, a large quantity of fresh *H. helluo* silk is, in reality, more likely to be from a large individual of this species rather than a group of smaller individuals.

Hogna helluo uses prey movement as an especially important predation-eliciting cue (Uetz and Roberts, 2002). Upon detecting cues from *H. helluo*, *P. milvina* reduces its activity levels (Barnes *et al.*, 2002, Persons *et al.*, 2001) and tends to move into higher vegetation strata (Persons *et al.*, 2002). *Pardosa milvina* normally chooses complex substrates in preference to bare ground, and laboratory experiments show that on these substrates they are less likely to fall prey to *H. helluo* (Rypstra *et al.*, 2007). However, if cues from *H. helluo* are present in complex habitats and absent in the less preferred bare dirt habitat, *P. milvina*'s habitat preference is overridden (Rypstra *et al.*, 2007). Consequently, by being flexible in the ability to leave a habitat, *P. milvina* may lower its exposure to predators during especially dangerous periods. Indeed, it appears that individuals of *H. helluo* that have recently fed on *P. milvina* are especially dangerous (Persons and Rypstra, 2000) and *P. milvina* is strongly motivated to avoid substrates previously frequented by these individuals (Persons *et al.*, 2001).

There has been longstanding interest in the function of special silk decorations (sometimes called stabilimenta) that many spiders add to their webs (Chapter 3; Bruce, 2006, Herberstein *et al.*, 2000). Here we will consider a particularly well-studied example of flexibility in the use of web decorations. The decorations of *Argiope versicolor* (Araneidae) in Singapore are situated at the web hub and this spider usually rests on the decorations during the daytime. However, this makes *A. versicolor* especially conspicuous to a particular predator, *Portia labiata*, a spider with acute vision. In defence against *P. labiata*, *A. versicolor* has a predator-specific sensory ability in response to odour. Upon detecting specifically the odour of *P. labiata*, *A. versicolor* becomes less inclined to decorate webs (Li and Lee, 2004). Presumably this, in turn, translates into reduced predation, although this hypothesis has not yet been assessed.

Yet another spider has olfaction-based defence against *P. labiata*, but in this instance the effect is on the prey's eggs. The prey is *Scytodes pallida* (Scytodidae), a spitting spider. By spitting, a female of this species can readily defend herself against *P. labiata*, but spitting spiders carry their eggs in their mouths, blocking the source of the gummy spit and making the mother and her eggs especially vulnerable to *P. labiata* (Li and Jackson, 2003). Although the mechanism by which this is achieved is unknown, the eggs of *S. pallida* hatch more quickly when the odour of *P. labiata* is present (Li, 2002).

Predator-specific identification by prey based on vision can be found in another example from *Portia*, this time in a salticid–saliticid predator–prey system. In Queensland (Australia), *P. fimbriata* is a significant predator of an unusual salticid, *Euryattus* sp. Instead of spinning a cocoon-like nest, the type of nest typical of salticids (Richman and Jackson, 1992), *Euryattus* females find a rolled-up dead leaf and then, using silk guylines, suspend the leaf from vegetation, boulders, or tree trunks (Jackson, 1985). The female may perch on her leaf, using it as a base from which to leap on passing insects, but otherwise she shelters in the confines of the rolled-up leaf. A courting male visits the female's nest by moving slowly down a guyline, stepping out onto the leaf and then, by flexing his legs suddenly and forcefully, the male makes the leaf rock back and forth. The female responds to this courtship signal by coming out of her nest and either mating with the male on the leaf or chasing him away.

Upon finding one of these nests, *P. fimbriata* goes down a guyline onto the leaf and, after acquiring a position close to and facing an opening in the rolled-up leaf (i.e. a 'door'; Figure 4.1), suddenly and forcefully flexes its legs, making the leaf rock back and forth. The *Euryattus* female responds as though the signal came from a courting male, only to be attacked by the lurking predator as she emerges (Jackson and Wilcox, 1990). At least that is how it goes when *P. fimbriata* is successful, but sometimes things go wrong for *P. fimbriata* because *Euryattus* females have an uncanny ability to identify *P. fimbriata* by sight.

In Queensland, besides preying on *Euryattus*, *P. fimbriata* preys on many salticid species by stalking them across the ground, tree trunks or surfaces of boulders (Jackson and Blest, 1982). Owing to their exceptional eyesight, salticids might be difficult prey for *P. fimbriata* to approach. However, detritus mimicry, which we discussed earlier, functions for *P. fimbriata* as anti-predator defence and also provides a means of concealing its identity from keen-eyed salticid prey. When stalking a salticid, *P. fimbriata* moves especially slowly and tries to remain behind the salticid. *Portia fimbriata* also pulls its legs and palps in towards its body, obscuring the outlines of these appendages (Stevens and Merilaita, 2009) and thereby looking even less like an animal. This predatory tactic is known as cryptic stalking, and sometimes the salticid against which *P. fimbriata* is deploying cryptic stalking detects movement, pivots, and faces *P. fimbriata* head on. When this happens, *P. fimbriata* freezes until the prey salticid eventually turns away. One of the most striking aspects of these *Portia*–salticid prey-capture sequences is how prey salticids generally show little sign of having identified *Portia* as even an animal, let alone as a predator. At this stage, instead of attacking *Portia* or fleeing, the salticid typically turns away and resumes walking (Jackson and Pollard, 1996), unless the salticid is *Euryattus*.

Successful capture of *Euryattus* depends on *Portia* positioning itself at an opening in the leaf before having been seen by the *Euryattus* female inside (Jackson and Wilcox, 1990). When *Euryattus*, a stocky, powerful salticid, sees *Portia*, it clearly identifies it as a predator and actively defends itself. Occasionally *Euryattus* kills *Portia*, but attacks usually consist of *Euryattus* leaping on or head-butting *Portia*, sometimes knocking *Portia* off the leaf or guyline. The facility with which *Euryattus* identifies *Portia* is not specific to encounters at the leaf nest. *Portia* sometimes encounters *Euryattus* on the ground, or in other locations away from the nest. In these instances, although *Portia* adopts cryptic stalking, *Euryattus* still readily identifies and attacks *Portia*.

4.10   Ecotypic variation in predator-identification ability

The term 'ecotype' is used for populations within single species that are adapted to local conditions, with the adaptive differences between populations being genetically based (Leimu and Fischer, 2008, Turesson, 1922). Ecotypic variation in behaviour (Thompson 1999) may be a widespread phenomenon in spiders (e.g. Jackson, 1980, Jackson et al., 2006, Uetz and Cangialosi, 1986) and this includes behavioural ecotypes pertaining to anti-predator defence.

Agelenopsis aperta (Agelenidae), a North American spider, gives us an especially thoroughly studied example of ecotypic variation (Riechert, 1981, 1991, 1999, Riechert and Hedrick, 1990). These spiders build horizontal sheet webs for prey capture. Attached to the web there is a silk funnel that leads to a protected area in which the spider seeks shelter when it detects the approach of a predator.

When foraging, *A. aperta* sits with its legs outstretched at the border between the funnel and the sheet web surface, this being an optimal position from which to monitor vibratory signals from prey that land on the web. Riechert and co-workers have shown how variation in correlated behavioural traits (i.e. the expression of aggression towards conspecifics, predators and prey) can be explained as local adaptation to the conditions in local habitats. Populations from riparian sites are subject to heavy predation by birds and the spiders from these sites are less aggressive (i.e. more fearful) than spiders from desert grass-land habitats, which are depauperate in predators (Maupin and Riechert, 2001, Riechert and Hall, 2000, Riechert and Hedrick, 1993). When puffs of air are used to simulate the wingbeats of an approaching bird, the speed at which the spider retreats into the funnel depends on the population from which the spider originated, with spiders from riparian habitats responding more quickly. These differences are evident even for laboratory-reared spiders with no prior experience of the bird-related cues (Riechert and Hedrick, 1990).

Flexible anti-predator defences of spiders may have evolved especially when predator and prey have been linked in something like a coevolutionary arms race (Jackson and Pollard, 1996), the predator evolving prey-specific capture tactics while the prey evolves predator-specific defences against the predator's tactics. The arms race metaphor has been controversial (Abrams, 1986, Janzen, 1980), with hard evidence being elusive, and it may often be more realistic to consider more diffuse coevolution based on suites of predators and prey (Fox, 1988). Nonetheless, the way ecotypic variation is expressed in the aforemen-tioned example from *Euryattus* and *Portia* suggests coevolved specialised counter-adaptations of two species to each other.

The only locality in which *Euryattus* is known to be sympatric with *Portia* is in lowland Queensland rainforests. Laboratory experiments have shown that the specialised tactics by which the sympatric *Portia* targets *Euryattus* and the specialised *Portia*-identification ability of *Euryattus* are innate, neither requiring prior exposure to the respective prey or predator. Individuals of *Portia* from other localities in Australia and in Asia do not adopt the *Euryattus*-specific predatory tactics used by the Queensland *Portia* and they are decidedly ineffec-tive at capturing *Euryattus* (Jackson and Wilcox, 1990). Furthermore, some *Euryattus* populations in Queensland occur close by but at higher elevation, where *Portia* is absent. Experiments show that the Queensland *Portia*'s predatory success is significantly better when the *Euryattus* encountered is from an allopatric instead of a sympatric population. Concomitantly, allopatric *Euryattus* are noticeably inferior to sympatric *Euryattus* at identifying and then actively defending themselves against the Queensland *Portia* (Jackson and Wilcox, 1993).

4.11   Blurring the distinction between foraging and anti-predator defence

Among spiders, perhaps more than in other groups of animals, foraging behaviour and anti-predator defences often go hand in hand, as illustrated by the use of aggressive mimicry. Aggressive mimicry is a term widely used for foraging strategies based on predators resembling something that is attractive to their prey (Côté and Cheney, 2007, Vane-Wright, 1980), this being the type of mimicry for which *Portia* is best known. *Portia*'s prey is often the resident spider in the invaded web. When in another spider's web, *Portia* sometimes uses its appendages to mimic the web signals that would normally originate from a small ensnared insect (Tarsitano *et al.*, 2000) to lure the resident spider in close enough to be attacked and eaten (Chapter 2). This seems like straightforward aggressive mimicry, where a predator (*Portia*) deceives its prey (the resident spider) by resembling something that is salient to the prey (the resident spider's own prey). Yet, whenever we look closely at the biology of *Portia*, nothing seems to remain straightforward for long (Figure 4.3).

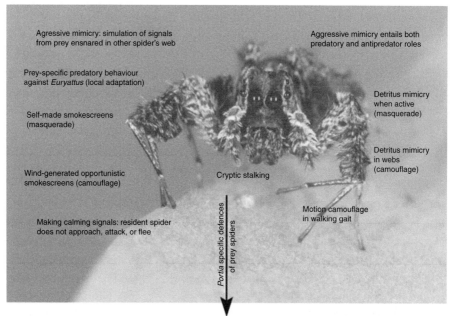

Agressive mimicry: simulation of signals from prey ensnared in other spider's web

Aggressive mimicry entails both predatory and antipredator roles

Prey-specific predatory behaviour against *Euryattus* (local adaptation)

Detritus mimicry when active (masquerade)

Self-made smokescreens (masquerade)

Detritus mimicry in webs (camouflage)

Wind-generated opportunistic smokescreens (camouflage)

Cryptic stalking

Making calming signals: resident spider does not approach, attack, or flee

Motion camouflage in walking gait

Portia specific defences of prey spiders

Reduced web-decorating behaviour in *Argiope* in response to chemical cues from *Portia*

Faster hatching of *Scytodes* eggs in response to chemical cues from *Portia*

Increase identification capacity and propensity to attack *Portia* by *Euryattus* (local adaptation)

Figure 4.3 *Portia* gives us an example of the variability and interconnected nature of foraging and anti-predator defences in spiders. See also colour plate.

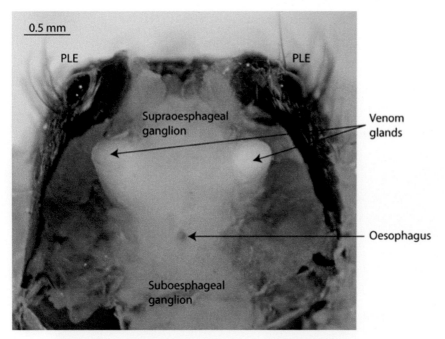

Figure 2.2 'Half frontal' view (posterior) of salticid (*Servaea* sp.) cephalothorax showing central nervous system (supraoesophageal and suboesophageal ganglia) and large venom glands. Supraoesophageal neuropil (fluffy white material) dominated by neurons used for processing input from eyes. Only PLE: (posterior lateral eyes) visible in this section through carapace.

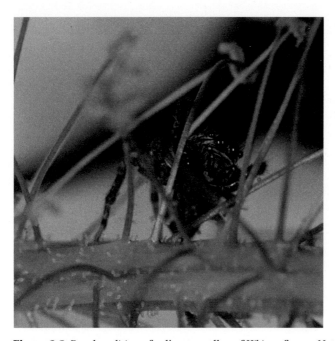

Figure 2.3 *Evarcha culicivora* feeding on pollen of *Hibiscus* flower. Note large anterior median eyes (characteristic of salticids).

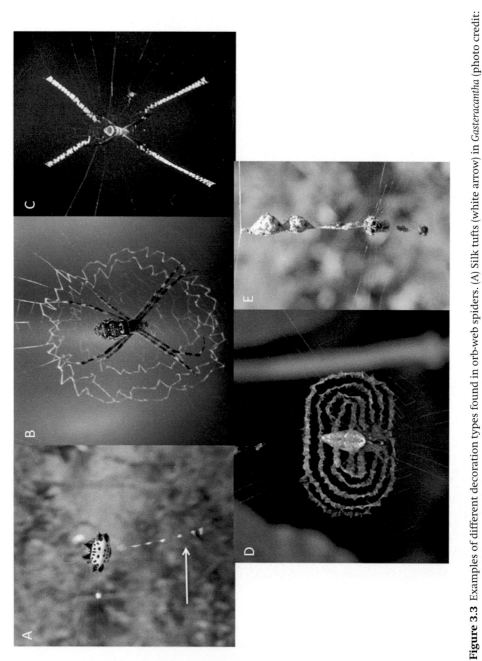

Figure 3.3 Examples of different decoration types found in orb-web spiders. (A) Silk tufts (white arrow) in *Gasteracantha* (photo credit: F. Gawryszewski). (B) Discoid decoration in *Argiope mascordi* (photo credit: G. Pappas). (C) Cruciate decorations in *Argiope keyserlingi* (photo credit: M. Herberstein). (D) Spiral decorations in *Cyclosa mulmeinensis* (photo credit: D. Li). (E) Egg-sac decoration in *Cyclosa* (photo credit: I. M. Tso).

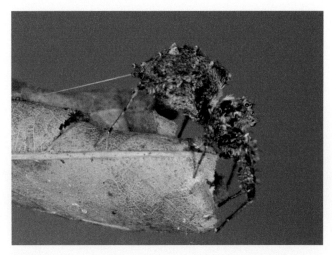

Figure 4.1 Detritus-like salticid *Portia fimbriata* standing at the door of the nest (rolled up dead leaf) of a female *Euryattus* sp.

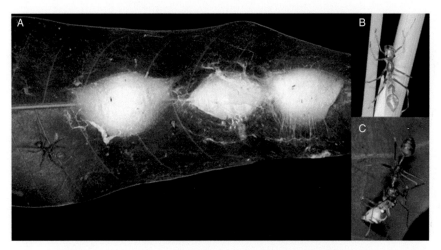

Figure 4.2 (A) Adult female ant-like *Myrmarachne assimilis* (body length, 7 mm) on mango leaf with crèche (three silk nests joined together) serving as defence against egg-eating ants. (B) Slim red body, modified to make the spider appear to have a head, thorax and abdomen, like an ant, instead of cephalothorax and abdomen, like a spider. Slender forelegs, held in characteristic posture, resemble ant's antennae. (C) *Oecophylla smaragdina*, ant model for *M. assimilis*, holding dead jumping spider in its jaws.

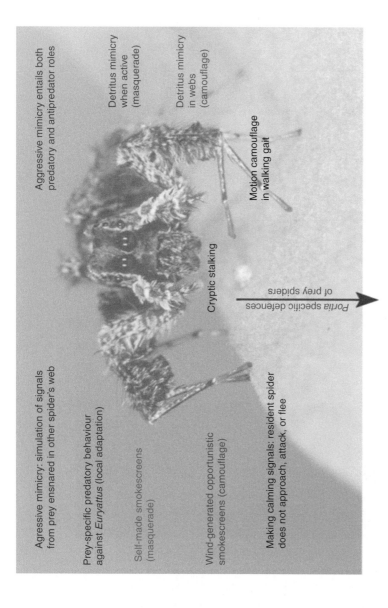

Aggressive mimicry: simulation of signals from prey ensnared in other spider's web

Prey-specific predatory behaviour against *Euryattus* (local adaptation)

Self-made smokescreens (masquerade)

Wind-generated opportunistic smokescreens (camouflage)

Making calming signals: resident spider does not approach, attack, or flee

Aggressive mimicry entails both predatory and antipredator roles

Detritus mimicry when active (masquerade)

Detritus mimicry in webs (camouflage)

Motion camouflage in walking gait

Cryptic stalking

Portia specific defences of prey spiders

Reduced web-decorating behaviour in *Argiope* in response to chemical cues from *Portia*

Faster hatching of *Scytodes* eggs in response to chemical cues from *Portia*

Increase identification capacity and propensity to attack *Portia* by *Euryattus* (local adaptation)

Figure 4.3 *Portia* gives us an example of the variability and interconnected nature of foraging and anti-predator defences in spiders. Blue font denotes *Portia* anti-predator adaptation, merging through to red font, which denotes *Portia* predatory behaviour. Green: defence behaviour of spiders commonly preyed on by *Portia*.

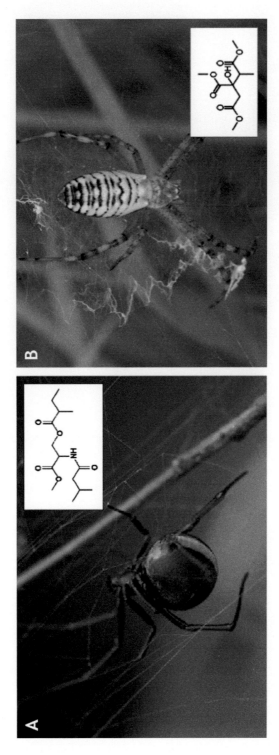

Figure 5.1 (A) Female *Latrodectus hasselti* (Theridiidae) with chemical structure of the amino-acid-derived pheromone (photo credit: M. B. C. Andrade). (B) Female *Argiope bruennichi* (Araneidae) with chemical structure of the citrate pheromone (photo credit: G. Uhl).

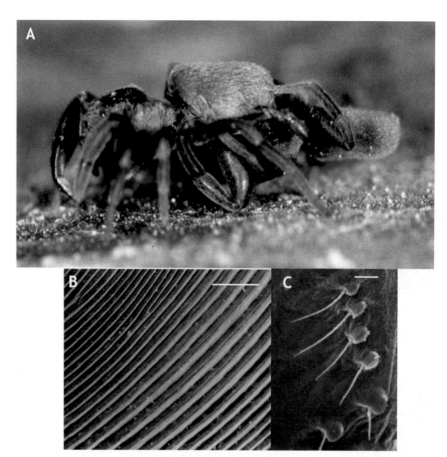

Figure 5.2 Stridulation in both sexes of *Palpimanus gibbulus* (Palpimanidae).
(A) Mating posture of *Palpimanus gibbulus*. Scale bar = 20 μm (photo credit: G. Uhl).
(B) SEM of the stridulatory ridges on the lateral side of both chelicerae (photo credit:
G. Uhl). (C) Pegs on the base of the pedipalpal femur. Scale bar = 20 μm.

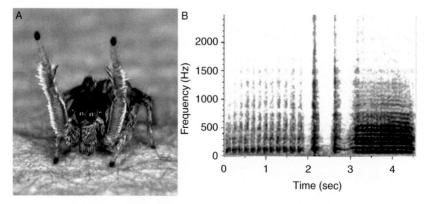

Figure 5.3 (A) Visual display of male *Habronattus dossenus* (Salticidae) (photo credit:
D. O. Elias). (B) Sonagram of male songs during courtship. Male acoustic display
including percussion, stridulation and tremulation mechanism was recorded using
laser Doppler vibrometry (photo credit: D. O. Elias).

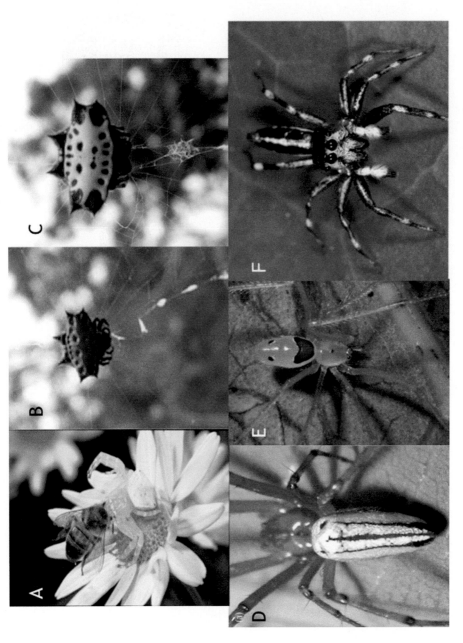

Figure 6.1 Examples of exuberantly coloured spiders. (A) Crab spider *Thomisus spectabilis* (photo credit: Ron Oldfield). (B and C) Different colour morphs of *Gasteracantha* (photo credit: F. Gawryszewski). (D) Orchid spider *Leucauge* (reprinted from Tso *et al.*, 2007, with kind permission from Elsevier). (E) Hawaiian happy face spider (photo credit: R. Gillespie). (F) *Cosmophasis* jumping spider from Singapore (photo credit: D. Li).

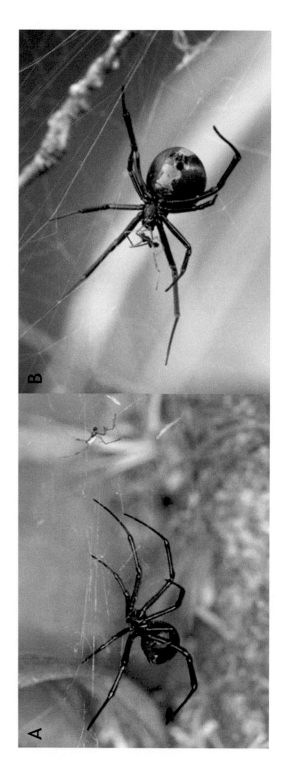

Figure 7.1 (A) Female redback spider (left) with much smaller, courting male (right) (photo credit: A. C. Mason). (B) Female redback spider with cannibalised male (photo credit: K. Jones).

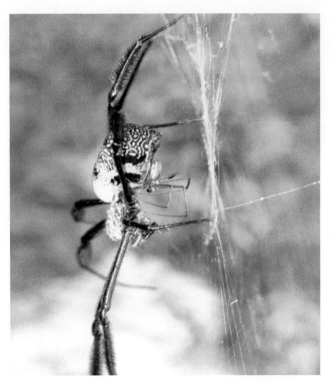

Figure 7.2 *Nephila fenestrata* during copulation. The small male inserts one of his pedipalps into one genital opening of the female. (Photo credit: J. M. Schneider.)

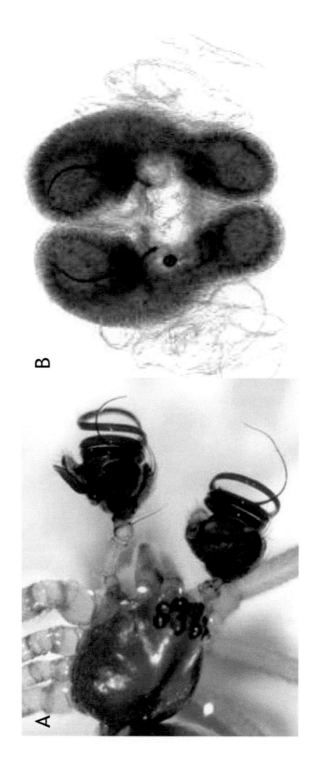

Figure 7.3 (A) Cephalothorax and pedipalps of male redback spider with both emboli partly uncoiled. The top pedipalp has been used in copulation and the apical sclerite has been broken off inside the female. The lower pedipalp has not yet been used and is intact. (B) Spermathecae and associated tubules of female redback spider (macerated with KOH to visualise the spermathecal contents). Two plugs are visible (dark curved lines), one in each spermatheca. Each is the apical sclerite of a male's pedipalp. (Photo credit: M. B. C. Andrade.

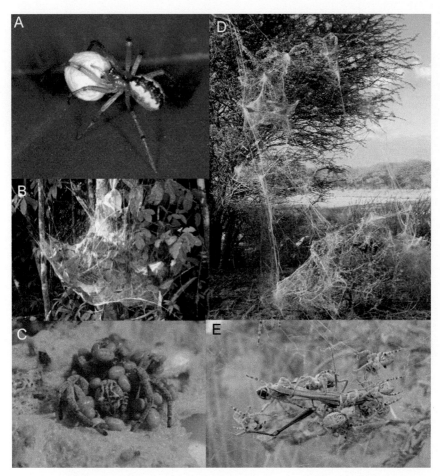

Figure 8.1 Subsocial and permanent social spiders. (A) Subsocial *Anelosimus akohi* female with egg sac. (B) Social *Anelosimus eximius* nest. (C) Subsocial *Stegodyphus lineatus* matriphagy; the young are feeding on the mother. (D) Social *Stegodyphus dumicola* nests with interconnected webs, on *Acacia* trees in Namibia. (E) Social *Stegodyphus dumicola* females capturing grasshopper in South Africa. (Photo credits: A and B: I. Agnarsson; C, D and E: T. Bilde.

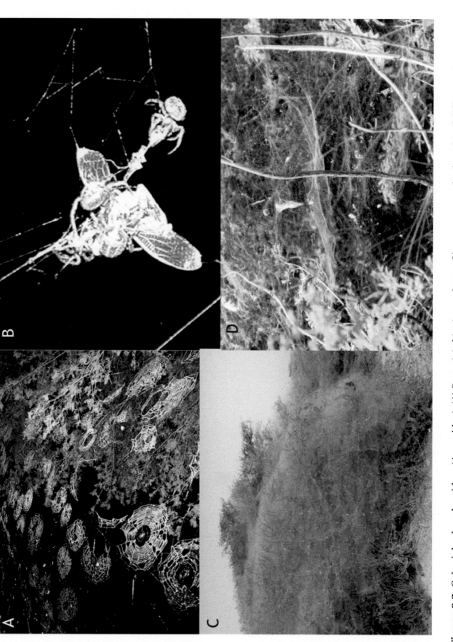

Figure 8.2 Colonial orb-web spiders (Araneidae). (A) *Parawixia bistriata* colony of interconnected orb webs of different sizes. The spiders are active at night and hide inside a communal retreat during the day. (B) *P. bistriata* individuals capturing a moth together. (C) Layered, interconnected, horizontal orb webs of *Cyrtophora citricola* in an *Acacia* tree. (D) A web of *C. citricola* with an egg-sac string above the drawn-up hub. (Photo credits: A and B: F. Fernández Campón; C and D: Y. Lubin.)

As *Portia* preys especially on other predators, with the predator targeted as prey often being quite capable of turning the tables and preying on *Portia* instead, the distinction between foraging and anti-predator defence becomes thoroughly intertwined (Figure 4.3). For example, *Portia*'s web signals often seem to function not simply as a mechanism for simulating the resident spider's prey, but instead as signals that keep the resident spider agitated and positioned out in the web while *Portia* moves in for the kill, all the while avoiding signals that might provoke a full-scale attack by the resident spider (Jackson *et al.*, 1998).

Portia also makes use of camouflage and masquerade in the sensory modality most relevant to the resident spider (Ruxton, 2009). Wind-derived web movement is noisy for web-building spiders, drowning out fainter signals such as *Portia*'s footsteps and, while in a web with the resident spider, *Portia* sometimes uses wind-derived noise as an opportunistic smokescreen. It does this by interrupting signalling when the wind blows, using this interval for stepping rapidly across the web towards the resident spider, then stopping in its tracks as soon as the wind dies down (Wilcox *et al.*, 1996). Wind is only one of the smokescreens behind which *Portia* hides (camouflages) its advancing steps towards the resident spider. For example, *Portia* also times its approaching steps so that they correspond to intervals during which the resident is wrapping its own prey (Jackson *et al.*, 2002). Additionally, in the absence of the wind offering an opportunistic smokescreen, *Portia* sometimes makes its own smokescreen (masquerade) by stepping towards the resident spider while simultaneously violently flexing all of its legs, thereby shaking the web much the same as during sudden gusts of wind (Tarsitano *et al.*, 2000). Flexibility is evident in the smokescreen strategy because *Portia* is selective, using opportunistic and self-made smokescreens when stalking spiders in webs but not when stalking relatively harmless prey such as insects ensnared in webs, and not when approaching to eat the egg sacs of the other spider.

4.12   Conclusions and outlook

If pressed for an overarching conclusion based on what we have discussed, it would be that, for spiders, flexibility in anti-predator defence is often mirrored by flexibility in the foraging strategies of the spider's predators, with the predators frequently being other spiders. In fact, predator–prey coevolution often seems to account for much of the complexity and flexibility in the strategies of the predator and the prey (Figure 4.3). Having taken Cloudsley-Thompson's (1995) warning to heart, we narrowed our focus to case studies that illustrate flexibility in how spiders defend themselves against predators and, accordingly, this conclusion is related specifically to the understanding of anti-predator flexibility. We end this chapter by offering two suggestions for future research.

The first recommendation is to 'wake up and look around'. Despite being acutely aware that we have reviewed only a fraction of a vast literature on spider anti-predator defences, we are now even more conscious of how much more research is needed. No one with an interest in spiders should ever despair of finding interesting topics to explore. A short stint outdoors demonstrates that there are seemingly endless examples of anti-predator defence awaiting closer examination.

Despite the wealth of potential, anti-predator defence as a topic for research seems to suffer from an interesting handicap. The temptation to let intuition substitute for data may be especially strong in the literature on anti-predator defence. Instead of letting intuition stand as foregone conclusions, we need well-formulated hypotheses that can be tested experimentally. Too often this may seem like an exercise in proving the obvious. Yet, in science, research on what at first may appear obvious has an uncanny way of uncovering unexpected, innovative discoveries.

Our second recommendation, based on the first, is simply to test ideas in the field. It is generally implicit that, when we use the term 'anti-predator defence', it is in the context of specific prey characteristics functioning as mechanisms that reduce predation in nature but, by and large, this critical type of data is lacking. There is no doubt that laboratory experiments have their place, as they can certainly influence our confidence in hypotheses about how anti-predator defences function in nature, especially if the design of experiments is based on a strong understanding of the natural history of the prey and the predator. Yet we should be ready to acknowledge that these experiments do not directly test the efficacy of anti-predator defences in nature. We should also do more than just accept this weakness, and rise to the challenge of finding ways to design and carry out experiments aimed more directly at determining how specific prey characteristics diminish predator-derived mortality in the field.

Acknowledgements

For financial support for much of the research reviewed in this manuscript, we gratefully acknowledge the Royal Society of New Zealand (Marsden Fund and James Cook Fellowship) and the National Geographic Society. We also acknowledge useful comments on the manuscript by John Prenter, Paul McDonald and Sara Kross.

References

Abrams, P. A. (1986). Is predator-prey coevolution an arms race? *Trends in Ecology and Evolution*, **1**, 108–110.

Amaya, C. C., Klawinski, P. D. and Formanowicz, D. R. (2001). The effects of leg autotomy on running speed and foraging ability in two species of wolf spider (Lycosidae). *American Midland Naturalist*, **145**, 201–205.

Andersson, M. (1994). *Sexual Selection*. Princeton, NJ: Princeton University Press.

Apontes, P. and Brown, C. A. (2005). Between-sex variation in running speed and a potential cost of leg autotomy in the wolf spider *Pirata sedentarius*. *American Midland Naturalist*, **154**, 115–125.

Barnes, M. C., Persons, M. H. and Rypstra, A. L. (2002). The effect of predator chemical cue age on antipredator behavior in the wolf spider *Pardosa milvina* (Araneae: Lycosidae). *Journal of Insect Behavior*, **15**, 269–281.

Blackledge, T. A. and Zevenbergen, J. M. (2007). Condition-dependent spider web architecture in the western black widow, *Latrodectus hesperus*. *Animal Behaviour*, **73**, 855–864.

Brautigam, M. and Persons, M. H. (2003). The effect of limb loss on the courtship and mating behaviour of the wolf spider *Pardosa milvina* (Araneae: Lycosidae). *Journal of Insect Behavior*, **16**, 571–587.

Briscoe, A. D. and Chittka, L. (2001). The evolution of colour vision in insects. *Annual Review of Entomology*, **46**, 471–510.

Bristowe, W. S. (1941). *The Comity of Spiders*. Publication 128. London: The Ray Society.

Bruce, M. J. (2006). Silk decorations: controversy and consensus. *Journal of Zoology*, **269**, 89–97.

Brueseke, M., Rypstra, A., Walker, S. and Persons, M. (2001). Leg autotomy in the wolf spider *Pardosa milvina*: a common phenomenon with few apparent costs. *American Midland Naturalist*, **146**, 153–160.

Cloudsley-Thompson, J. L. (1995). A review of the anti-predator devices of spiders. *Bulletin of the British Arachnological Society*, **10**, 81–96.

Côté, I. M. and Cheney, K. L. (2007). A protective function for aggressive mimicry? *Proceedings of the Royal Society of London, B*, **274**, 2445–2448.

Cott, H. B. (1940). *Adaptive Coloration in Animals*. London: Methuen.

Cushing, P. E. (1997). Myrmecomorphy and myrmecophily in spiders: a review. *Florida Entomologist*, **80**, 165–193.

Cuthill, I. C., Partridge, J. C., Bennett, A. T. D., *et al.* (2000). Ultraviolet vision in birds. *Advances in the Study of Behaviour*, **29**, 159–214.

Edmunds, M. (1974). *Defence in Animals: A Survey of Anti-Predator Defences*. London: Longman.

Fleming, P. A., Muller, D. and Bateman, P. W. (2007). Leave it all behind: a taxonomic perspective of autotomy in invertebrates. *Biological Reviews*, **82**, 481–510.

Foelix, R. F. (1996). *Biology of Spiders*, 2nd edn. Oxford, UK: Oxford University Press.

Formanowicz, D. R. (1990). The antipredator efficacy of spider leg autotomy. *Animal Behaviour*, **40**, 400–401.

Fox, L. R. (1988). Diffuse coevolution within complex communities. *Ecology*, **69**, 906–907.

Gabritchvesky, E. (1927). Experiments on the color changes and regeneration in the crab spider *Misumena vatia* (Cl.). *Journal of Experimental Zoology*, **47**, 251–267.

Garb, J. E., González, A. and Gillespie, R. G. (2004). The black widow spider genus *Latrodectus* (Araneae: Theridiidae): phylogeny, biogeography, and invasion history. *Molecular Phylogenetics and Evolution*, **31**, 1127–1142.

Gregory, R. L. (1998). *Eye and Brain: The Psychology of Seeing*, 5th edn. Oxford, UK: Oxford University Press.

Guffey, C. (1998). Leg autotomy and its potential fitness costs for two species of harvestmen (Arachnida, Opiliones). *Journal of Arachnology*, **26**, 296–302.

Guffey, C. (1999). Costs associated with leg autotomy in the harvestmen *Leiobunum nigripes* and *Leiobunum vittatum* (Arachnida: Opiliones). *Canadian Journal of Zoology*, **77**, 824–830.

Gullan, P. and Cranston, P. S. (2000). *The Insects: An Outline of Entomology*, 2nd edn. Oxford, UK: Blackwell.

Gunnarsson, B. (2007). Bird predation on spiders: ecological mechanisms and evolutionary consequences. *Journal of Arachnology*, **35**, 509–529.

Hamilton, W. D. (1971). Geometry for the selfish herd, *Journal of Theoretical Biology*, **31**, 295–311.

Hanlon, R. T., Chiao, C. C., Mäthger, L. M., *et al.* (2009). Cephalopod dynamic camouflage: bridging the continuum between background matching and disruptive coloration. *Philosophical Transactions of the Royal Society of London, B*, **364**, 429–437.

Harland, D. P. and Jackson, R. R. (2004). Portia perceptions: the *Umwelt* of an araneophagic jumping spider. In *Complex Worlds from Simpler Nervous Systems* (ed. F. R. Prete). Cambridge, MA: MIT Press, pp. 5–40.

Harland, D. P. and Jackson, R. R. (in press). How jumping spiders see the world. In *How Animals See the World: Behavior, Biology, and Evolution of Vision* (ed. O. Lazareva, T. Shimizu and E. Wasserman). New York: Oxford University Press.

Heiling, A. M., Herberstein, M. E. and Chittka, L. (2003). Pollinator attraction: crab spiders manipulate flower signals. *Nature*, **421**, 334.

Henschel, J. R. (1998). Predation on social and solitary individuals of the spider *Stegodyphus dumicola* (Araneae, Eresidae). *Journal of Arachnology*, **26**, 61–69.

Herberstein, M. E., Craig, C. L., Coddington, J. A. and Elgar, M. A. (2000). The functional significance of silk decorations of orb-web spiders: a critical review of the empirical evidence. *Biological Reviews*, **75**, 649–669.

Hölldobler, B. and Wilson, E. O. (1990). *The Ants*. Heidelberg, Germany: Springer Verlag.

Hurd, L. E. and Eisenberg, R. M. (1990). Arthropod community responses to manipulation of a biotrophic predator guild. *Ecology*, **71**, 2107–2114.

Jackson, R. R. (1980). The mating strategy of *Phidippus* (Araneae, Salticidae). IV. Interpopulational variation in courtship persistence. *Behavioral Ecology and Sociobiology*, **6**, 257–263.

Jackson, R. R. (1985). The biology of *Euryattus* sp. indet., a web-building jumping spider (Araneae, Salticidae) from Queensland: utilization of silk, predatory behaviour, and intraspecific interactions. *Journal of Zoology, London*, **B1**, 145–173.

Jackson, R. R. and Blest, A. D. (1982). The biology of *Portia fimbriata*, a web-building jumping spider (Araneae, Salticidae) from Queensland: utilization of webs and predatory versatility. *Journal of Zoology*, **196**, 255–293.

Jackson, R. R. and Pollard, S. D. (1996). Predatory behavior of jumping spiders. *Annual Review of Entomology*, **41**, 287–308.

Jackson, R. R. and Wilcox, R. S. (1990). Aggressive mimicry, prey-specific predatory behaviour and predator recognition in the predator-prey interactions of *Portia fimbriata* and *Euryattus* sp., jumping spiders from Queensland. *Behavioral Ecology and Sociobiology*, **26**, 111–119.

Jackson, R. R. and Wilcox, R. S. (1993). Predator-prey co-evolution of *Portia fimbriata* and *Euryattus* sp., jumping spiders from Queensland. *Memoirs of the Queensland Museum*, **33**, 557–560.

Jackson, R. R. and Pollard, S. D. (1997). Jumping spider mating strategies: sex among cannibals in and out of webs. In *The Evolution of Mating Systems in Insects and Arachnids* (ed. J. C. Choe and B. J. Crespi). Cambridge, UK: Cambridge University Press, pp.340–351.

Jackson, R. R., Cross, F. R. and Carter, C. M. (2006). Geographic variation in a spider's ability to solve a confinement problem by trial and error. *International Journal of Comparative Psychology*, **19**, 282–296.

Jackson, R. R., Li, D., Fijn, N. and Barrion, A. T. (1998). Predator-prey interactions between aggressive-mimic jumping spiders (Salticidae) and araeneophagic spitting spiders (Scytodidae) from the Philippines. *Journal of Insect Behavior*, **11**, 319–342.

Jackson, R. R., Pollard, S. D. and Cerveira, A. M. (2002). Opportunistic use of cognitive smokescreens by araneophagic jumping spiders. *Animal Cognition*, **5**, 147–157.

Janzen, D. H. (1980). When is it coevolution? *Evolution*, **34**, 611–612.

Jennions, M. D., Møller, A. P. and Petrie, M. (2001). Sexually selected traits and adult survival: a meta-analysis. *Quarterly Review of Biology*, **71**, 3–36.

Johnson, S. and Jakob, E. (1999). Leg autotomy in a spider has minimal costs in competitive ability and development. *Animal Behaviour*, **57**, 957–965.

Kaston, B. J. (1970). Comparative biology of American black widow spiders. *Transactions of the San Diego Society of Natural History*, **16**, 33–82.

Kelber, A., Vorobyev, M. and Osorio, D. (2003). Animal colour vision: behavioural tests and physiological concepts. *Biological Reviews*, **78**, 81–118.

Kiltie, R. A. (1988). Countershading: universally deceptive or deceptively universal. *Trends in Ecology and Evolution*, **3**, 21–23.

Kindlmann, P. and Houdková, K. (2006). Intraguild predation: fiction or reality? *Population Ecology*, **48**, 317–322.

Kotiaho, J. S. (2001). Costs of sexual traits: a mismatch between theoretical considerations and empirical evidence. *Biological Reviews*, **76**, 365–376.

Kotiaho, J. S., Alatalo, R. V., Mappes, J., Parri, S. and Rivero, A. (1998). Male mating success and risk of predation in a wolf spider: a balance between sexual and natural selection? *Journal of Animal Ecology*, **67**, 287–291.

Krafft, B. and Leborgne, R. (1979). Perception sensorielle et importance des phénomènes vibratoires chez les araignées. *Journal de Psychologie*, **3**, 299–334.

Land, M. F. and Nilsson, D. E. (2002). *Animal Eyes*. Oxford, UK: Oxford University Press.

Leimu, R. and Fischer, M. (2008). A meta-analysis of local adaptation in plants. *PLoS ONE*, **3**, e4010. doi:10.1371/journal.pone.0004010.

Li, D. (2002). Hatching responses of subsocial spitting spiders to predation risk. *Proceedings of the Royal Society of London, B*, **269**, 2155–2161.

Li, D. and Jackson, R. R. (2003). A predator's preference for egg-carrying prey: a novel cost of parental care. *Behavioral Ecology and Sociobiology*, **55**, 129–136.

Li, D. and Lee, W. S. (2004). Predator-induced plasticity in web-building behaviour. *Animal Behaviour*, **67**, 309–318.

Lim, M. L. M. and Li, D. (2006). Behavioural evidence of UV sensitivity in jumping spiders (Araneae: Salticidae). *Journal of Comparative Physiology, A*, **192**, 871–878.

Lima, S. L. and Dill, L. M. (1990). Behavioral decisions made under the risk of predation: a review and prospectus. *Canadian Journal of Zoology*, **68**, 619–640.

Lindström, L., Ahtiainen, J. J., Mappes, J., *et al.* (2006). Negatively condition dependent predation cost of positively condition dependent sexual signalling. *Journal of Evolutionary Biology*, **19**, 649–656.

Lohrey, A. K., Clark, D. L., Gordon, S. D. and Uetz, G. W. (2009). Antipredator responses of wolf spiders (Araneae: Lycosidae) to sensory cues representing an avian predator. *Animal Behaviour*, **77**, 813–821.

Lutzy, R. M. and Morse, D. H. (2008). Effects of leg loss on male crab spiders *Misumena vatia*. *Animal Behaviour*, **76**, 1519–1527.

Maupin, J. L. and Riechert, S. E. (2001). Superfluous killing in spiders: a consequence of adaptation to food-limited environments? *Behavioral Ecology*, **12**, 569–576.

Moya-Laraño, J. and Wise, D. H. (2007). Direct and indirect effects of ants on a forest-floor food web. *Ecology*, **88**, 1454–1465.

Nelson, X. J. and Jackson, R. R. (2006). Vision-based innate aversion to ants and ant mimics. *Behavioral Ecology*, **17**, 676–681.

Nelson, X. J. and Jackson, R. R. (2008). Anti-predator crèches and aggregations of ant-mimicking jumping spiders (Araneae: Salticidae). *Biological Journal of the Linnean Society*, **94**, 475–481.

Nelson, X. J. and Jackson, R. R. (2009). The influence of ants on the mating strategy of a myrmecophilic jumping spider (Araneae, Salticidae). *Journal of Natural History*, **43**, 713–735.

Nelson, X. J., Jackson, R. R., Edwards, G. B. and Barrion, A. T. (2004). Predation by ants on jumping spiders (Araneae: Salticidae) in the Philippines. *New Zealand Journal of Zoology*, **31**, 45–56.

Nelson, X. J., Jackson, R. R. and Li, D. (2006b). Conditional use of honest signaling by a Batesian mimic. *Behavioral Ecology*, **17**, 575–580.

Nelson, X. J., Li, D. and Jackson, R. R. (2006a). Out of the frying pan and into the fire: a novel trade-off for Batesian mimics. *Ethology*, **112**, 270–277.

Osorio, D. and Vorobyev, M. (2008). A review of the evolution of animal colour vision and visual communication signals. *Vision Research*, **48**, 2042–2051.

Oxford, G. S. and Gillespie, R. G. (1998). Evolution and ecology of spider coloration. *Annual Review of Entomology*, **43**, 619–643.

Persons, M. H. and Rypstra, A. L. (2000). Preference for chemical cues associated with recent prey in the wolf spider *Hogna helluo* (Araneae: Lycosidae). *Ethology*, **106**, 27–35.

Persons, M. H. and Rypstra, A. L. (2001). Wolf spiders show graded antipredator behavior in the presence of chemical cues from different sized predators. *Journal of Chemical Ecology*, **27**, 2493–2504.

Persons, M. H., Walker, S. E. and Rypstra, A. L. (2002). Fitness costs and benefits of antipredator behavior mediated by chemotactic cues in the wolf spider *Pardosa milvina* (Araneae: Lycosidae). *Behavioral Ecology*, **13**, 386–392.

Persons, M. H., Walker, S. E., Rypstra, A. L. and Marshall, S. D. (2001). Wolf spider predator avoidance tactics and survival in the presence of diet-associated predator cues (Araneae: Lycosidae). *Animal Behaviour*, **61**, 43–51.

Polis, G. A. and Strong, D. R. (1996). Food web complexity and community dynamics. *American Naturalist*, **147**, 813–842.

Poulton, E. B. (1890). *The Colours of Animals: Their Meaning and Use Especially Considered in the Case of Insects*. London: Kegan Paul, Trench, Truebner.

Pruden, A. J. and Uetz, G. W. (2004). Assessment of potential predation costs of male decoration and courtship display in wolf spiders using video digitization and playback. *Journal of Insect Behavior*, **17**, 67–80.

Rash, L. D. and Hodgson, W. C. (2002). Pharmacology and biochemistry of spider venoms. *Toxicon*, **40**, 225–254.

Rayor, L. S. and Uetz, G. W. (1990). Trade-offs in foraging success and predation risk with spatial position on colonial spiders. *Behavioral Ecology and Sociobiology*, **27**, 77–85.

Rayor, L. S. and Uetz, G. W. (1993). Ontogenic shifts within the selfish herd: predation risk and foraging trade-offs change with age in colonial web-building spiders. *Oecologia*, **95**, 1–8.

Richman, D. B. and Jackson, R. R. (1992). A review of the ethology of jumping spiders (Araneae, Salticidae). *Bulletin of the British Arachnological Society*, **9**, 33–37.

Riechert, S. E. (1981). The consequences of being territorial: spiders, a case study. *American Naturalist*, **117**, 871–892.

Riechert, S. E. (1988). The energetic cost of fighting. *American Zoologist*, **28**, 877–884.

Riechert, S. E. (1991). Prey abundance versus diet breadth in a spider test system. *Evolutionary Ecology*, **5**, 327–338.

Riechert, S. E. (1999). The use of behavioral ecotypes in the study of evolutionary processes. In *Geographic Variation in Behavior: Perspectives on Evolutionary Mechanisms* (ed. S. A. Foster and J. A. Endler). Oxford, UK: Oxford University Press, pp. 3–32.

Riechert, S. E. and Hall, R. F. (2000). Local population success in heterogeneous habitats: reciprocal transplant experiments completed on a desert spider. *Journal of Evolutionary Biology*, **13**, 541–550.

Riechert, S. E. and Hedrick, A. V. (1990). Levels of predation and genetically-based anti-predatory behaviour in the spider, *Agelenopsis aperta*. *Animal Behaviour*, **40**, 679–687.

Riechert, S. E. and Hedrick, A. V. (1993). A test for correlations among fitness-linked behavioral traits in the spider *Agelenopsis aperta* (Araneae, Agelenidae). *Animal Behaviour*, **46**, 669–675.

Roberts, J. A. and Uetz, G. W. (2008). Discrimination of variation in a male signaling trait affects optomotor response in visual predators. *Ethology*, **114**, 557–563.

Roberts, J. A., Taylor, P. W. and Uetz, G. W. (2006). Consequences of complex signalling: predator detection of multimodal cues. *Behavioral Ecology*, **18**, 236–240.

Roth, V. D. and Roth, B. M. (1984). A review of appendotomy in spiders and other arachnids. *Bulletin of the British Arachnological Society*, **6**, 137–146.

Ruxton, G. D. (2009). Non-visual crypsis: a review of the empirical evidence for camouflage to senses other than vision. *Philosophical Transactions of the Royal Society of London, B*, **364**, 549–557.

Ruxton, G., Sherratt, T. and Speed, M. (2004). *Avoiding Attack: The Evolutionary Ecology of Crypsis, Warning Signals and Mimicry*. Oxford, UK: Oxford University Press.

Rypstra, A. L., Schmidt, J. M., Reif, B. D., DeVito, J. and Persons, M. H. (2007). Tradeoffs involved in site selection and foraging in a wolf spider: effects of substrate structure and predation risk. *Oikos*, **116**, 853–863.

Scheffer, S. J., Uetz, G. W. and Stratton, G. E. (1996). Sexual selection, male morphology, and the efficacy of courtship signalling in two wolf spiders (Araneae: Lycosidae). *Behavioral Ecology and Sociobiology*, **38**, 17–23.

Seibt, U. and Wickler, W. (1988). Bionomics and social structure of 'family spiders' of the genus *Stegodyphus*, with special reference to the African species *Stegodyphus dumicola* and *Stegodyphus mimosarum* (Araneida, Eresidae). *Verhandlungen des Naturwissenschflichen Vereins in Hamburg*, **30**, 255–304.

Speed, M. P., Kelly, D. J., Davidson, A. M. and Ruxton, G. D. (2005). Countershading enhances crypsis with some bird species but not others. *Behavioral Ecology*, **16**, 327–334.

Spiller, D. A. and Schoener, T. W. (1998). Lizards reduce spider species richness by excluding rare species. *Ecology*, **79**, 503–516.

Spiller, D. A. and Schoener, T. W. (2001). An experimental test for predator-mediated interactions among spider species. *Ecology*, **82**, 1560–1570.

Stevens, M. (2007). Predator perception and the interrelation between different forms of protective coloration. *Proceedings of the Royal Society of London, B*, **274**, 1457–1464.

Stevens, M. and Merilaita, S. (2009). Defining disruptive coloration and distinguishing its functions. *Philosophical Transactions of the Royal Society of London, B*, **364**, 481–488.

Stuart-Fox, D. and Moussali, A. (2009). Camouflage, communication and thermoregulation: lessons from colour changing organisms. *Philosophical Transactions of the Royal Society of London, B*, **364**, 463–470.

Tarsitano, M. S., Jackson, R. R. and Kirchner, W. (2000). Signals and signal choices made by araneophagic jumping spiders while hunting the orb-weaving spiders *Zygiella x-notata* and *Zosis genicularis*. *Ethology*, **106**, 595–615.

Taylor, A. R., Persons, M. H. and Rypstra, A. L. (2005). The effect of perceived predation risk on male courtship and copulatory behaviour in the wolf spider *Pardosa milvina* (Araneae, Lycosidae). *Journal of Arachnology*, **33**, 76–81.

Taylor, P. W. and Jackson, R. R. (2003). Interacting effects of size and prior injury in jumping spider conflicts. *Animal Behaviour*, **65**, 787–794.

Théry, M. (2007). Colours of background reflected light and of the prey's eye affect adaptive coloration in female crab spiders. *Animal Behaviour*, **73**, 797–804.

Théry, M. and Casas, C. (2009). The multiple disguises of spiders: web colour and decorations, body colour and movement. *Philosophical Transactions of the Royal Society of London, B*, **364**, 471–480.

Thompson, D. B. (1999). Different spatial scales of natural selection and gene flow: the evolution of behavioral geographic variation and phenotypic plasticity. In *Geographic Variation in Behavior: Perspectives on Evolutionary Mechanisms* (ed. S. A. Foster and J. A. Endler). Oxford, UK: Oxford University Press, pp. 33–51.

Troscianko, T., Benton, C. P., Lovell, P. G., Tolhurst, D. J. and Pizlo, Z. (2009). Camouflage and visual perception. *Philosophical Transactions of the Royal Society of London, B*, **364**, 449–461.

Turesson, G. (1922). The species and the variety as ecological units. *Hereditas*, **3**, 100–113.

Uetz, G. W. and Cangialosi, K. R. (1986). Genetic differences in social behavior and spacing in populations of *Metepeira spinipes*, a communal-territorial orb weaver (Araneae, Araneidae). *Journal of Arachnology*, **14**, 159–173.

Uetz, G. W. and Hieber, C. S. (1994). Group size and predation risk in colonial web-building spiders: analysis of attack-abatement mechanisms. *Behavioral Ecology*, **5**, 326–333.

Uetz, G. W. and Roberts, J. A. (2002). Multi-sensory cues and multi-modal communication in spiders: insights from video/audio playback studies. *Brain, Behaviour and Evolution*, **59**, 222–230.

Uetz, G. W., Boyle, J., Hieber, C. S. and Wilcox, R. S. (2002). Anti-predator benefits of group living in colonial web-building spiders: the 'Early Warning' effect. *Animal Behaviour*, **63**, 445–452.

Uetz, G. W., McClintock, W. J., Miller, D., Smith, E. I. and Cook, K. K. (1996). Limb regeneration and subsequent asymmetry in a male secondary sexual character influences sexual selection in wolf spiders. *Behavioral Ecology and Sociobiology*, **38**, 253–257.

Vane-Wright, R. I. (1980). On the definition of mimicry. *Biological Journal of the Linnean Society*, **66**, 215–229.

Vetter, R. S. (1980). Defensive behavior of the black-widow spider *Latrodectus hesperus* (Araneae, Theridiidae). *Behavioral Ecology and Sociobiology*, **7**, 187–193.

Vetter, R. S. and Isbister G. K. (2008). Medical aspects of spider bites. *Annual Review of Entomology*, **53**, 409–429.

Vetter, R. S. and Visscher, P. K. (1998). Bites and stings of medically important venomous arthropods. *International Journal of Dermatology*, **37**, 481–496.

Wanless, F. R. (1978). A revision of the spider genus. I (Araneae: Salticidae). *Bulletin of the British Museum of Natural History*, **34**, 83–124.

Whitehouse, M. E. A. and Lubin, Y. (2005). The functions of societies and the evolution of group living: spider societies as a test case. *Biological Reviews*, **80**, 347–361.

Wickler, W. (1968). *Mimicry in Plants and Animals*. London: Weidenfeld and Nicholson.

Wilcox, R. S., Jackson, R. R. and Gentile, K. (1996). Spiderweb smokescreens: spider trickster uses background noise to mask stalking movements. *Animal Behaviour*, **51**, 313–326.

Wrinn, K. M. and Uetz, G. W. (2007). Impacts of leg loss and regeneration on body condition, growth, and development time in the wolf spider *Schizocosa ocreata*. *Canadian Journal of Zoology*, **85**, 823–831.

Zuk, M. and Kolluru, G. (1998). Exploitation of sexual signals by predators and parasitoids. *Quarterly Review of Biology*, **73**, 415–438.

Zylinski, S., Osorio, D. and Sholet, A. J. (2009). Perception of edges and visual texture in the camouflage of the common cuttlefish, *Sepia officianalis*. *Philosophical Transactions of the Royal Society of London, B*, **364**, 439–448.

5

Communication

GABRIELE UHL AND DAMIAN O. ELIAS

A spider's life is guided by sensory information completely alien to human observers unless specialised equipment is applied. Even in the case of spiders guided by vision, a sensory mode that humans can boast great acuity in, a large body of evidence suggests that spiders are most sensitive to ultraviolet light, light completely imperceptible to humans. The spider's world is thus unknown and only in the last two decades have researchers begun to make strides into understanding these fascinating creatures. Communication research has been a critical piece of the puzzle in our embryonic understanding of spiders. Although spiders generally live a solitary life, it has long been accepted that communication plays an important role throughout their lifetime. Spiders are now the subjects of intensive scientific research as it becomes more and more obvious that their communication systems are unique, highly complex, plastic and versatile.

5.1   Introduction

Generally, communication takes place when a signal is sent from one individual to another that alters the pattern of behaviour or the physiology in another organism (Wilson, 1975). Three processes are required for communication: the production of a signal or cue by a sender, its propagation through the environment via a transmission channel, and appropriate receptor sites to detect the signal by the receiver. The transmission channels used by spiders are chemical, tactile, acoustic and visual channels (Weygoldt, 1977, Witt and Rovner, 1982). Their use depends on the microhabitat in which the spider occurs and on its mode of living (Crane, 1949, Elias and Mason, in press, Tietjen and

Spider Behaviour: Flexibility and Versatility, ed. Marie Elisabeth Herberstein. Published by Cambridge University Press. © Cambridge University Press 2011.

Rovner, 1982). Even within species, the means of communication can be context specific where signal repertoires depend on where and when the signal is produced (e.g. Taylor and Jackson, 1999). The physical features of channels clearly limit the rate of transmission of signals and their susceptibility to background noise.

Chemical signals are very likely the oldest means of communication (Wyatt, 2003) but are especially understudied in spiders. Biofunctional molecules that spread information between individuals are called semiochemicals (from Greek *semeion* sign). In spiders, behavioural studies provide evidence for airborne and contact semiochemicals (Gaskett, 2007, Huber, 2005, Schulz, 2004). Airborne chemical communication can be active over long distances but has the disadvantage of being highly susceptible to air turbulence. Contact chemicals, by contrast, play an important role when draglines, webs or body surfaces of conspecifics are inspected. Assessment of potential mates or rivals is probably based on chemical as well as tactile signals, but the latter have been largely neglected. Acoustic, vibratory signals function mostly at short distances and have been investigated in much greater detail. Visual signals are the most derived means of communication in spiders; they occur in only a few spider families. In the last decade it became increasingly obvious that spiders rarely rely on one channel of communication. Even vision-based jumping spiders (Salticidae) communicate with chemical, tactile and acoustic signals (Elias *et al.*, 2005, Jackson and Pollard, 1997). Nevertheless, for ease of presentation we will describe the occurrence of various signals by different sensory channels and will come back to multimodal communication in the final part of the chapter.

Mainly due to a bias in research, this chapter will focus mainly on communication during male–female interactions. Male signalling is especially prominent because when a male encounters a conspecific female, he must communicate that he is a conspecific rather than the next meal. Selection due to species recognition, mate recognition, potential sexual cannibalism, male–male competition and finally female mate choice has strongly shaped male signalling behaviour. As a consequence, male spiders often show complex courtship displays in multiple sensory modes. However, the contexts in which spiders communicate are certainly not restricted to courtship and male agonistic encounters. Communication also plays a role in predation and predator avoidance and is suspected to be important in parent–offspring recognition and social dominance interactions. Generally, signals have the potential to contain information on an animal's identity (species, sex), developmental state (offspring, potential mate), behavioural state (level of aggression), relatedness (social groups) and health (condition, parasite load), and it is safe to assume that signals have evolved in all of these contexts in spiders.

5.2   Semiochemicals

5.2.1   *Introduction to semiochemicals*

Animals that are solitary, aggressive, widely dispersed or occurring at low densities, like the majority of spider species, need to communicate through remote chemoreception when they reach sexual maturity. Compared with vibratory or visual signals, chemical signals are advantageous as they are not limited by environmental barriers, are effective day or night, are needed in only small quantities, are relatively long lasting and are effective over long distances. Attracting or finding a mating partner using long-range signals is advantageous since the probability of small animals encountering each other by chance alone is negligibly small (Bristowe, 1939) and mortality during mate search is high (Andrade, 2003, Vollrath and Parker, 1992). Olfaction (i.e. remote chemoreception) relies on semiochemicals with low molecular weight that renders them volatile enough to become airborne, whereas taste (i.e. contact chemoreception or gustation) relies on substances that adhere to a substrate or to the animal's body surface.

Our understanding of the processes involved in olfaction and gustation in arthropods builds on extensive research on insects for which pheromones from over 3000 species have been identified (Blomqvist and Vogt, 2003). Studies on insects have advanced due to the readily identifiable response to pheromones by means of electroantennograms that allow electrophysiological investigations of responses to precise chemical mixtures. Only 1% of research effort on pheromones is dedicated to spider research (Symonds and Elgar, 2008), and methods involved are mainly limited to behavioural choice tests. Choice tests can be problematic since spiders often do not show any observable choice reaction under laboratory conditions, although they may well be able to perceive a given signal. Further, few semiochemicals have been identified to date and even fewer have been synthetically produced and tested under natural conditions. Surprisingly little is known about the location of the cells that produce the pheromones and the morphology and physiology of the chemoreceptors (Gaskett, 2007, Schulz, 2004).

Classically, semiochemicals that mediate interactions between individuals are divided into two groups, pheromones and allelochemicals, based on whether the participants involved in communication are from the same or different species. Pheromones comprise not only sex attractants but also trail, territorial marking and alarm substances. Pheromones can have immediate behavioural effects (releaser pheromones) or trigger physiological changes in the receiver that prime the animal for a different behavioural repertoire (primer pheromone; Wilson and Bossert, 1963). In spiders, releaser pheromones have been suggested for many species but reports on primer pheromones are rare (Gaskett, 2007). In *Latrodectus hasselti* (Theridiidae), exposure to female pheromones triggers fast development of males, resulting in small size, while no exposure leads to slow development and large males (Kasumovic and Andrade, 2006). Exposure of penultimate stage *Argiope bruennichi* (Araneidae) males to female pheromones leads to a higher probability of sexual cannibalism during mating (Nessler *et al.*, 2009). These findings suggest that the female signals act as primer pheromones: they serve as an estimate of the future competitive environment and cause changes in development trajectories and reproductive behaviour of males. The second group of semiochemicals encompasses allelochemicals that carry information from one animal to a member of a different species, as occurs with defensive signals and other substances that are involved in interspecific behaviours. In spiders, allelochemicals that benefit the sender (allomones) have received much attention since chemical aggressive mimicry has evolved in various intriguing ways. Kairomones, by contrast, are allelochemicals that benefit the receiver and are used to find prey or to avoid predators (see Section 5.2.4 and Chapters 2 and 6). Overall, semiochemicals are ubiquitous in spiders but notoriously understudied. Their versatile and flexible behaviour within and between species is only now starting to be explored.

5.2.2   *Chemicals in the context of mate attraction and mate choice*

Volatile substances

In web-building spiders, olfaction has long been suspected, since several males are often found at a single web in the field (Enders, 1975, Robinson and Robinson, 1980). Studies using females alone, females on webs, or webs alone report that they attract conspecific males (see references in Gaskett, 2007 as well as Andrade, 1996, Blanke, 1973, 1975, Jackson and Macnab, 1991, Olive, 1982). Females are generally highly attractive as virgins, either due to first male sperm priority or due to effective plugging of female genital openings (Uhl, 2000, Uhl *et al.*, 2010) but a specific time window within the virgin phase also seems to be important for mate attraction (Blanke, 1973, 1975, Miyashita and Hayashi, 1996). Once mated, females of many species cease to be attractive to males and stop pheromone production (e.g. Chinta *et al.*, 2010), but can readvertise receptivity months after mating (Perampaladas *et al.*, 2008). Choice studies should thus consider the effect of such time windows on strategic pheromone advertisement.

The spider species for which volatile pheromones have been identified are *Agelenopsis aperta* (Agelenidae: Papke *et al.*, 2001), *Argiope bruennichi* (Araneidae: Chinta *et al.*, 2010) and *Pholcus beijingensis* (Pholcidae: Xiao *et al.*, 2009). Rather than reiterating the extensive review by Anne Gaskett (2007) we will largely explore the recent developments in this field, focusing on the two last mentioned species.

The first pheromone recently identified from an orb-web spider is trimethyl methylcitrate from *Argiope bruennichi* (Chinta *et al.*, 2010). Methylcitric acid occurs naturally in many organisms but pheromones that are derivatives of the primary metabolite citric acid have not been reported from other animals. This substance, however, is closely related to the contact sex pheromone of *Cupiennius salei* (Table 5.1; Figure 5.1). Sampling of body and web extracts as well as headspace odours emitted by females of different reproductive states showed that only virgin adult females emitted the compound. The substance occurs in a diastereomeric ratio between 6:1 and 25:1 of (2*R*,3*S*)- and (2*S*,3*S*)-trimethyl methylcitrate in all extracts investigated. The effective stereochemistry, however, does not seem to be strongly fixed since synthesised substances with two different diastereomeric ratios (6:1 and 2:1) were equally attractive to males under natural conditions (Chinta *et al.*, 2010).

In *Pholcus beijingensis* (Xiao *et al.*, 2009), males are attracted by silk and extracts of receptive females in a two-choice arena system. Both virgin and mated females are receptive in this species, provided that the mated females do not carry an egg sac. Continuous receptivity and attractiveness corresponds with 50–90% last male fertilisation success found in all pholcid spiders investigated so far (Eberhard *et al.*, 1993, Schäfer and Uhl, 2002, Schäfer *et al.*, 2008). A blend of two acetates in a 2:1 ratio triggers male searching behaviour (Table 5.1). This is the first known case of a multicomponent pheromone in spiders. Both sex pheromones occur in various insects and rodent mammals, where blends of chemicals are common and function only when combined in a specific ratio (Wyatt, 2003). For spiders, it seems that multicomponent pheromones are rare but, considering the paucity in data, this can only be considered a preliminary statement.

It has long been suspected that it is not necessarily only the male who uses odour to find and assess a potential mating partner (Lopez, 1987, Richter *et al.*, 1971). Male signalling has recently been demonstrated in a number of species, among them jumping spiders (Salticidae), spitting spiders (Scytodidae) and wolf spiders (Lycosidae). In the sex role reversed burrowing wolf spiders *Allocosa brasiliensis* and *Allocosa alticeps*, females are the vagrant sex; they locate male burrows and initiate courtship when the burrows are inhabited by the male. Indeed, volatile substances that are emitted from the body surface of the male seem to trigger female courtship behaviour (Aisenberg *et al.*, 2010). Female preference for

Table 5.1 *Identified spider pheromones*

Spider taxa	Status of attractive individual	Test	Substance	Range	Effect	Reference
Agelenopsis aperta (Agelenidae)	older virgin females	laboratory study, 3-choice arena	8-methyl-2-nonanone	volatile	attracts males and elicits courtship	Papke et al., 2001
Pholcus beijingensis (Pholcidae)	silk and extracts of adult females without egg sacs	laboratory study 2-choice arena	2:1 ratio of (E,E)-farnesyl acetate and hexadecyl acetate	volatile	exploratory behaviour, no courtship	Xiao et al., 2009
Argiope bruennichi (Araneidae)	virgin females	field study, 2-choice test using synthetic substance	6:1–25:1 (2R,3S)- and (2S,3S)-trimethyl methylcitrate	volatile	attracts males and elicits courtship	Chinta et al., 2010
Linyphia triangularis (Linyphiidae)	virgin female webs	laboratory study, exposure to treated webs	(R,R)-3-(3-hydroxybutyryloxy)butyric acid, (R)-3-hydroxybutyric acid	contact, possibly volatile	induce web reduction behaviour in males, attract males to web	Schulz and Toft, 1993
Latrodectus hasselti (Theridiidae)	virgin female webs	laboratory study, exposure to treated filter paper	N-3-methyl-butyryl-O-(S)-2-methylbutyryl-L-serine methyl ester	contact, possibly volatile	elicits courtship, possibly attracts males	Jerhot et al., 2010
Cupiennius salei (Ctenidae)	dragline silk and extracts	laboratory study, exposure to treated dragline, electro-physiological response	(S)-enantiomer of asymmetric dimethyl citrate	contact	elicits courtship	Papke et al., 2000, Tichy et al. 2001
Tegenaria atrica (Agelenidae)	web and cuticular extracts	laboratory study, exposure tests	mixture of fatty acids and methyl stearate	contact	elicits courtship	Prouvost et al., 1999, Trabalon et al., 2005

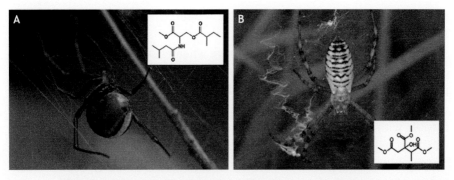

Figure 5.1 (A) Female *Latrodectus hasselti* (Theridiidae) with chemical structure of the amino-acid-derived pheromone (photo credit: M. B. C. Andrade). (B) Female *Argiope bruennichi* (Araneidae) with chemical structure of the citrate pheromone (photo credit: G. Uhl). See also colour plate.

male odour has recently been found in *Evarcha culicivora* (Salticidae; Cross *et al.*, 2009) in which both sexes engage in courtship and mate assessment. Males and females are able to discriminate between opposite-sex and same-sex conspecifics and developmental stages (juvenile–adult) on the basis of odour alone. Specific diet-related odours seem to have been incorporated into mate assessment since females prefer males that had a recent indirect blood meal – the spiders prefer to prey on blood-carrying mosquitoes, which they detect using olfaction (Jackson *et al.*, 2005). Possibly, diet odour and sex pheromone work in concert to stimulate mate attraction (Cross *et al.*, 2009). The compounds that are responsible for chemical discrimination in *E. culicivora* are not yet known.

An intriguing case of mate assessment on the basis of male volatile substances occurs in the spitting spider *Scytodes* sp. (Scytodidae; Koh *et al.*, 2009). Females that mated with the male whose dragline-borne odour they preferred during a choice trial produced more and larger eggs with higher hatching rate compared with those females that had to mate with the non-preferred male. It has been known for some time that mating with preferred mating partners can result in marked fitness consequences (Hettyey *et al.*, 2010, Sheldon, 2000). How the structure and composition of the chemical signal can reveal information on the genetic quality of the potential mating partner remains to be investigated.

Chemical contact communication

It is very likely that all solitary spider species use olfactory stimuli to detect and approach mating partners. Once in the vicinity of a female, males derive information from contact with female silk, female excreta or from pheromones deposited on the substratum by the female body (references in Gaskett, 2007, Tietjen and Rovner, 1982; also Fernández-Montraveta and

Ruano-Bellindo, 2000, Rypstra *et al.*, 2003, Schmitt *et al.*, 1992, Stoltz *et al.*, 2007, Trabalon and Assi-Bessekon, 2008).

A basic task that cursorial spiders have when encountering such cues is to determine the direction in which the spider went. A gradient of contact pheromones on the dragline silk has been suggested as the mechanism that would enable males to follow trails in the correct direction. However, this is only feasible with a pheromone that disintegrates extremely rapidly after release, which is atypical for chemical signals (Bossert and Wilson, 1963). It seems conceivable that dragline silk provides directional cues through a mechanical tactile component, such as position, angle and structure of the attachment disc that is produced to fix the dragline to the substratum as the spider moves (Tietjen, 1977). Specific chemical signals may thus be coupled with simple mechanical, tactile orientation signals that are used in concert to find potential mates.

A large number of behavioural studies indicate that chemical cues associated with female silk can convey information on the presence of a conspecific as well as on the reproductive status, age and receptivity of the sender (Gaskett, 2007). In *Phidippus johnsoni* (Salticidae), males cohabit in the nests of subadult females and the nest silk gradually becomes more effective in eliciting male courtship before the female's final moult (Jackson, 1986b). In *Metellina segmentata* (Tetragnathidae), males guard females often several days prior to courtship and mating and assess females solely on the presence of chemical cues/signals (Prenter *et al.*, 1994). When males are introduced to female webs, they enter an active process of information gathering and with significantly higher probability stay in the web of large, fecund females. Interestingly, male decision making in *M. segmentata* does not require the presence of the female, nor do males explore the web architecture but instead stay at the web periphery. Thus the only mechanism possible for mate choice is chemical communication through female silk. This was also shown for *Latrodectus hasselti* (Stoltz *et al.*, 2007). In both species females are sexually cannibalistic, and decision making on the web prior to body contact should be especially important for males considering the costs of sexual cannibalism.

The decision to stay or leave a female is probably the most important decision taken by male spiders. The closer a male approaches the female, the more information he should be able to receive through chemical signals. Indeed, courtship behaviour such as vibrating in the web, leg waving, lunging and retreating often require the physical presence and reciprocal activity of the female and are not released by silk alone (see references in Gaskett, 2007; also Cross *et al.*, 2007a, Rypstra *et al.*, 2003, Tietjen and Rovner, 1982, Xiao *et al.*, 2009). Once the potential partners come into body contact, close-range mate assessment on the tactile level is involved. Males drastically change courtship behaviour when in physical contact with a receptive female. Chemical signals contained in the web or dragline silk at this point probably become less important compared with chemical signals directly released from the female cuticle. In fact, chemical compounds found in the web and in the cuticle of females differ to a large extent in the agelenid *Tegenaria atrica*. Moreover, receptive and unreceptive females differ in the composition and quantity of chemical compounds present in their web and on their cuticle. These differences may contain information about potential mating partners that are used sequentially during the approach and contact phase (Prouvost *et al.*, 1999).

A contact pheromone was identified from the ctenid *Cupiennius salei* (Papke *et al.*, 2000; Table 5.1). The pheromone is a derivative of citric acid termed cupilure and is similar to the volatile pheromone from *Argiope bruennichi* (Chinta *et al.*, 2010). When male pedipalps contact the female dragline, males inspect the dragline and initiate courtship behaviour that results in reciprocal vibratory interactions when the female is close and receptive (Rovner and Barth, 1981; see Section 5.3.4). Thus in order for courtship to start, a female must be in the close vicinity and respond to male vibratory signals. The stereochemistry of the cupilure is crucial for eliciting a response in males. In the only electrophysiological study available to date, the neural response depended on which enantiomer of the synthetic cupilure was used for contact stimulation of a chemosensory sensillum (Tichy *et al.*, 2001).

Another set of pheromones was isolated from web silk of *Linyphia triangularis* and related linyphiid spiders (Schulz and Toft, 1993; Table 5.1). Spraying web extracts from virgin females onto inactive webs of mated females induced typical web reduction behaviour by the male (Schulz and Toft, 1993); that is, males that encounter the web of virgin females cut threads and pack the silk into a tight mass (Rovner, 1968). Interestingly, the contact pheromone that causes web reduction slowly degrades into two volatile substances that seem responsible for male attraction to the webs (Schulz, 2004, Watson, 1986). Using the decay process of a specific compound may be advantageous since it allows a constant rate of evaporation with relatively low production costs once a web is produced.

Degradation of contact pheromones can occur autocatalytically or by action of humidity. Generally, silk of various spiders remains attractive for several hours up to several weeks under laboratory conditions (Clark and Jackson, 1995a, Engelhardt, 1964, Jackson, 1987, Pollard *et al.*, 1987). Under natural conditions rain or dew may quickly render the contact pheromone inactive (Lycosidae and Theridiidae; Dondale and Hegdekar, 1973, Gwinner-Hanke, 1970, Roberts and Uetz, 2004a, Suter and Renkes, 1982, Tietjen, 1977). However, in the semi-aquatic hunting spider *Dolomedes triton* (Pisauridae) dragline signals elicit male responses even when deposited on the water surface. Interestingly, males show different response behaviour towards draglines found on land, demonstrating context-dependent behaviour (Roland and Rovner, 1983). Female draglines from tropical rainforest wolf spiders (Lycosidae) also showed no decrease in male response after they were subjected to water or were submerged (Lizotte and Rovner, 1989). Since the susceptibility of the signals to water is habitat and species dependent, structurally different chemicals can be suspected.

In the Australian redback spider *Latrodectus hasselti* (Theridiidae), volatile substances must be present in the webs of adult virgin females since males locate females from a distance, are able to discriminate conspecific female webs from those of heterospecific webs and even distinguish between conspecific webs from different geographical populations (Andrade and Kasumovic, 2005, Kasumovic and Andrade, 2004, Ross and Smith, 1979). Extracts of silk of virgin females contain two components that cannot be found in silk of mated females (Jerhot *et al.*, 2010). One of them was shown to be an amino acid derivative that evokes searching and courtship response when the male contacts treated filter paper. The other component was inactive under these conditions. It remains to be investigated whether one of these candidate substances is involved in mate attraction over longer distances or whether additional compounds are responsible for attraction. The contact pheromone is an unusual diacylated amino acid ester and its specific stereochemistry is highly important in eliciting a response by the male (Jerhot *et al.*, 2010; Table 5.1). Amino-acid-derived pheromones have not been reported from spiders but are found in *Phyllophaga* beetles, demonstrating their biochemical convergence (Robbins, 2009 and references therein). This type of pheromone may entail higher physiological costs compared with other known pheromone classes and may thus allow more detailed assessment of the female by the male. Why females should be selected to produce honest signals instead of signalling their mere presence to males remains to be investigated (see review by Johansson and Jones, 2007). It can be speculated, however, that the male self-sacrifice, which typically occurs in this species of widow spiders (Andrade, 2003, Forster, 1995), exerts strong selection pressure on male mate choice, possibly leading to partially reversed sex roles.

As with volatile pheromones, it would be misleading to assume that it is only the females who produce contact pheromones. In the lycosid *Trochosa*, females recognise conspecific males (Engelhardt, 1964), *Latrodectus hesperus* females (Theridiidae) show courtship behaviour in response to male silk (Ross and Smith, 1979) and females of *Tegenaria domestica* (Agelenidae) and *Coelotes terrestris* (Amaurobiidae) orient towards silk deposited by the male (Roland, 1984). In the linyphiid spider *Frontinella communis*, adult males also build webs that contain chemical signals (Suter and Hirscheimer, 1986). These long-established behavioural studies hint towards a more active role for males that has been neglected so far. Further, a common but largely unexplored phenomenon is silk deposition by males on the webs or on the bodies of the female before and during mating (e.g. araneid, thomisid and lycosid spiders; see references in Aisenberg *et al.*, 2008). Silk deposition on the female body as 'bridal veils' does not render the female physically less able to attack the male but may inhibit female aggression by transferring her into a state of quiescence. Since the silk lines deposited on the female inevitably come in contact with chemoreceptors on her legs (Aisenberg *et al.*, 2008), females may be able to receive information on male quality or may be subject to male neural manipulation (Ross and Smith, 1979). Male silk deposition on the female body or on her web may also have evolved in the context of male–male interactions as anti-aphrodisiacs or mating tags applied after mating.

5.2.3   *Male secretory head structures*

Chemical signals that play a role in species recognition or mate assessment have long been suspected to be produced in the bizarre head structures of male erigonines and some theridiids (e.g. *Argyrodes, Faiditus*; Lopez, 1987, *Diplocephalus,* Schaible and Gack, 1987). Males of these species have grooves, pits or turrets in the front part of the prosoma. In all species investigated so far, the male head structures are closely associated with pronounced glandular tissue (P. Michalik and G. Uhl, unpublished data). Contrary to previous suggestions, the secretory tissue does not seem to release a volatile substance that attracts females (G. Uhl and S. Schulz, unpublished data). Before and sometimes during mating, females contact the prosoma of the male with their mouthparts, release saliva and ingest the fluid. Delivery of gustatory rather than olfactory signals thus appears to be the function of these structures (Schlegelmilch, 1974, G. Uhl, personal observation). In fact, males of the erigonine *Oedothorax retusus* that offer accessible secretions have a higher mating probability compared with males that were experimentally hindered (K. Kunz and G. Uhl, unpublished data). In the erigonine *Diplocephalus permixtus*, a contact chemical or mechanical stimulus between male head structure and female mouthparts is required to trigger male pedipalp insertion (Uhl and Maelfait, 2008). Both findings suggest that the secretions facilitate mating. In the kleptoparasitic *Argyrodes elevatus* (Theridiidae), by contrast, males whose head structure was covered had similar mating probabilities but shorter copulation durations compared with non-covered males (G. Uhl, unpublished data; see Chapter 10 on kleptoparasites). The secretory head structures must have evolved several times independently in theridiids and erigonines and differ in their effects on the mating process.

5.2.4   Agonistic behaviour/predation and semiochemicals

Airborne as well as contact chemicals are used in agonistic encounters within and between species. Agonistic displays within species occur when rival males encounter conspecific female silk (e.g. Ayyagari and Tietjen, 1986, Schmitt et al., 1992). In *E. culicivora* (Salticidae) male odour leads to escalation in agonistic behaviour between females that actively court and assess males (Cross and Jackson, 2009a). When spiders encountered silk of conspecific same-sex individuals, they also reacted aggressively (Anava and Lubin, 1993, Clark and Jackson, 1994), suggesting that they are able to distinguish their own silk from that of other same-sex individuals. Moreover, females of *Portia labiata* (Salticidae) seem to recognise draglines from familiar same-sex conspecifics since they differ in residency time when given a choice between draglines of familiar and unfamiliar conspecifics (Clark and Jackson, 1995b). Consequently, there must be detectable variation between individual dragline silk and the ability to remember individual chemical cues.

Spiders as predators are prone to feed on other spiders or be fed on by other spiders (see Chapter 2). Chemical signals play a role in detecting and avoiding predators that occur in the same habitat (e.g. Persons et al., 2002, Schonewolf et al., 2006; Section 4.9 in this book). The salticid spider *Portia fimbriata* mainly feeds on the salticid *Jacksonoides queenslandicus*, the most abundant salticid in the natural habitat. Contact with draglines and odour of *J. queenslandicus*, and not the draglines of other salticids, heighten *P. fimbriata*'s attention to optical cues from *J. queenslandicus* (Jackson et al., 2002). Such attentional priming by kairomones does not appear to be based on prior experience but seems to be pre-programmed (see Section 2.4 in this book). Conversely, potential prey can derive information from volatile substances that are emitted by its predator. These kairomones can help to reveal detailed information about the presence, size and hunger level of the predator and thus lead to successful avoidance (see references in Bell et al., 2006). Lycosid spiderlings also reduce activity and show avoidance behaviour when encountering silk or excreta of other potentially predatory lycosids (Eiben and Persons, 2007). Although the spiderlings react innately to the kairomones, extended exposure enhances their anti-predator response (Eiben and Persons, 2007). Visual and vibratory cues seemed to be less effective in eliciting avoidance behaviour. Chemical cues help the linyphiid *Frontinella communis* to detect the presence of *Argyrodes trigonum* that inhabits its web, steals prey and also attacks the host (Suter et al., 1989). Anecdotal evidence further suggests that spiders sense volatile compounds from a pompilid wasp and try to escape as soon as the wasp appears (Bristowe, 1939). These kairomone-detecting sensory systems suggest that the species involved have interacted over relatively long periods of time (see Section 9.3.4).

Chemicals can also be used for prey attraction. Several genera of orb-web spiders (Araneidae) produce volatile substances that mimic the presence of female moths and function as a deadly attractant to males (Stowe *et al.*, 1987, Yeargan, 1994). Bolas spiders (*Mastophora*), for example, capture prey using a single silk line ending in a sticky ball (Eberhard, 1977) that contains substances that copy the odour of female moths not only in composition, but also in the ratio of the substances involved (Gemeno *et al.*, 2000). Using these allomones, only male moths are lured and captured by the bolas whirled by the spider (Eberhard, 1977). Interestingly, adult spiders attract moths whereas spiderlings attract nematocerus flies (Stowe *et al.*, 1995, Yeargan and Quate, 1996), suggesting that the chemical signals change during the lifetime of the spider (see Chapter 6 for more details).

An indirect use of volatile substances to attract prey has evolved in the colonial spider *Mallos gregalis*. The spiders accumulate organic matter in their webs that are decomposed by a yeast fungus. This fungus produces a strong smell, which attracts insects to the web (Tietjen *et al.*, 1987). Such indirect use of volatile substances may also play a role in other spider species that 'decorate' their webs with prey remains, as has recently been shown for *Nephila* and *Cyclosa* species (Bjorkman-Chiswell *et al.*, 2004).

Spiders also exploit chemical signals by eavesdropping on intraspecific signals of social insects, ant species (Stowe *et al.*, 1995) or termites (Eberhard, 1991). The spider *Habronestes bradleyi* (Zodariidae) is a highly specialised predator of the meat ant *Iridomyrmex purpureus* that it locates mainly by its alarm pheromone (Allan *et al.*, 1996). The salticid *Cosmophasis bitaeniata* even manages to reside in the nest of the green tree ant *Oecophylla smaragdina* even though the ant species is highly territorial and aggressive towards intruders, and has one of the most complex chemical communication systems known (Hölldobler and Wilson, 1990). *Cosmophasis bitaeniata* is an exploitative chemical mimic of its host and can enter nests unnoticed by major workers and can even take ant larvae from minor workers unharmed (Allan and Elgar, 2001). The hydrocarbon profiles of ants and salticids are strikingly similar and are acquired by the spider feeding on the ant larvae (Allan *et al.*, 2002, Elgar and Allan, 2004, 2006). Existing variation in the cuticular hydrocarbon profiles of the spiders can be explained by the variation of these profiles between ant colonies (Elgar and Allan, 2004).

5.2.5   *Species specificity of semiochemicals*

Accurate species recognition is an important component of mate identification, as it prevents hybridisation with genetically incompatible heterospecifics (Costa and Francescoli, 1991, Mayr, 1974, Wilson and Bossert, 1963). The risk of mortality during mate searching and approaching a predatory mate should further impose strong selection on males to use any available cue that facilitates rapid and accurate identification at a distance. Indeed, many studies on spiders report behavioural evidence for species discrimination through chemical cues transmitted via the silk, dragline or the air (e.g. Gaskett, 2007, Pollard et al., 1987). For example, male Latrodectus hesperus are able to discriminate conspecific female webs from those of L. hasselti females (Kasumovic and Andrade, 2004). Latrodectus hesperus males even discriminate against conspecific female silk from a different population (Kasumovic and Andrade, 2004). Tentatively it can be suggested that these populations are reproductively isolated and may be incipient biological species. Chemical extracts from the body surface of two sympatric Tegenaria species in fact show a large number of qualitative and quantitative differences. Females of the same species that were deodorised and subsequently treated with heterospecific extracts elicited little reaction in males and none of the males attempted courtship with these females (Trabalon et al., 1997). Both differences in the chemical composition or the specific stereochemistry of the compounds may be responsible for these strong discrimination effects.

Clearly, species-specific chemical communication can be part of a set of pre-mating isolation mechanisms. Nevertheless, chemical signals often seem to be conserved in congeners (Grasshoff, 1964 on Araneus, Roberts and Uetz, 2004a, 2004b on Schizocosa, Ross and Smith, 1979 on Latrodectus; Schulz, 1997 on liny-phiids as unpublished results, Tretzel, 1959 on Coelotes) and even across genera (Hegdekar and Dondale, 1969 on Pardosa and Schizocosa). The substances involved in mate attraction therefore seem to be less specific than assumed; however, as a critical test, sympatric species should be compared (see also Jackson, 1987). Pheromones attractive to congeners are abundant among insects, but in most cases the species are isolated by geographic range or, if sympatric, isolated by time of the day or reproductive season (Shorey, 1976). Likewise, sympatrically occurring A. trifasciata and A. aurantia are largely separated by different phenology (Olive, 1982). The fact that caged females of A. trifasciata were able to attract A. aurantia males in the field may be explained as an artefact of rearing the spiders in the laboratory and bringing them to the field much earlier than under natural phenology (Olive, 1982, but see Enders, 1975). Identification errors under laboratory conditions can also be explained by stimulus-deprived males reacting to subnormal stimuli. Engelhardt (1964) already reported that lycosid males courted only conspecific females when tested soon after having been captured in the field, whereas lab-reared males also courted heterospecific females. Detailed laboratory studies, however, can provide deeper insight into chemical recognition: males of the lycosid spider Schizocosa ocreata court in response to chemical cues of closely related species, but courtship behaviour towards heterospecific females is less intensive. Relative courtship intensity of males even varies significantly with phylogenetic distance (Roberts and Uetz, 2004b).

At the present state of knowledge, the specificity of signals seems to be extremely variable between spider taxa. However, in order to assess to what extent chemical signals are conserved or species specific, we need to investigate context-dependent response thresholds, compare response intensities, and consider if geographic range and mating seasons overlap. Species recognition via chemical signals certainly is complemented by vibratory and visual signals to reduce mistaken identity (see Sections 5.3.4 and 5.4.4).

5.2.6   *Production sites of chemical signals*

Hardly anything is known about the site of pheromone production in spiders. Behavioural studies in which spinnerets of female lycosid spiders were sealed resulted in little or no courtship response in males after the females had been removed from the testing chamber (Kaston, 1936, Lizotte and Rovner, 1989, Richter *et al.*, 1971, but see Bristowe and Locket, 1926). However, when females of the salticid *Phidippus audax* were prevented from depositing silk or faeces, males nevertheless spent more time at the site from which the female was removed (Oden cited in Pollard *et al.*, 1987). Consequently, candidate cells have been suspected in the ducts of the silk apparatus or in the integument (Kovoor, 1981, Kronestedt, 1986, Lopez, 1987, Suter *et al.*, 1987, Wanless, 1984). In the silk apparatus, peculiar gland cells were reported in the epithelium of ampullate excretory ducts (Lopez, 1987), but these glands as well as epithelial glands have not been sufficiently studied. In addition to female-produced pheromones, there is the possibility that males detect chemical substances emitted during the moulting process (Miyashita and Hayashi, 1996). The substance may therefore be a cue and not a signal specifically intended for information transfer (Maynard Smith and Harper, 2005).

The few known spider pheromones involved in the mating process are structurally very diverse (Table 5.1). It seems that pheromones can originate from various pathways; however, most of them are biosynthetically related to primary metabolites (volatile signal: Chinta *et al.*, 2010, Papke *et al.*, 2001; contact signal: Jerhot *et al.*, 2010, Papke *et al.*, 2000, Schulz and Toft, 1993), but there are also mixtures of fatty acids (Prouvost *et al.*, 1999, Trabalon *et al.*, 2005) and acetates (Xiao *et al.*, 2009). Whether pheromone synthesis in spiders is mostly linked with primary metabolism, in contrast to insects (Francke and Schulz, 2010), remains to be clarified.

5.2.7   *How are chemical signals perceived?*

Communication through sex pheromones requires both the capability for biosynthesis of the pheromone and appropriate receptor sites on chemosensory membranes. It is unclear how spiders perceive volatile substances. Hair sensilla responsible for olfaction similar to the typical wall pore sensilla of insects have rarely been found in spiders (Foelix, 1985) but are common in other arachnid orders, Amblypgi (Foelix *et al.*, 1975) and Acari (Foelix and Axtell, 1971). For a long time, the slit sensilla and tarsal organs were suspected to contain olfactory receptors (Dumpert, 1978, Keller, 1961). However, subsequent analyses supported vibration detection and proprioreception for slit sensilla and hygro- and thermoreception for tarsal organs (Barth, 2002, Ehn and Tichy, 1994, 1996a, 1996b). Possibly, all chemoreceptory sensilla are tip pore sensilla in spiders (Foelix and Chu-Wang, 1973). These sensilla can be distinguished from tactile sensilla by their steeper angle of insertion, a slight S-shape of the shaft and a blunt tip with a pore opening (Barth, 2002 and references therein, Foelix, 1985). The chemosensory cells respond to touching the sensillum tip with female silk (Tichy *et al.*, 2001). Probably, chemical stimuli dissolve in the fluid around the dendritic terminations that end close to the tip pore and interact with receptors in the membrane of the sensory cell (Foelix and Chu-Wang, 1973, Lindemann, 1996). Dendrites of up to 20 chemosensory cells were found innervating a single taste hair. In addition, two mechanosensitive dendritic endings attach to the socket of the hair and register any change in the position of the hair (Harris and Mill, 1973, Tichy *et al.*, 2001). Apparently, a single sensillum can respond to several sensory modalities. So far only in *C. salei* have the receptive sensory cells for contact pheromones been identified with electrophysiological methods and single cell recordings (Tichy *et al.*, 2001). Female silk or filter paper containing the synthetic pheromone elicited a neural response, whereas male silk did not. Contact with sodium chloride and saccharose, however, also resulted in a response (Tichy *et al.*, 2001). Different chemical compounds may thus cause different patterns of excitation across the set of sensory cells. Interestingly, chemosensitive sensilla on legs of *C. salei* have a broader reaction spectrum compared with sensilla on the palps and react towards various gustatory and olfactory stimuli (Gingl, 1998 cited in Barth, 2002, see also Holden, 1977 for *Araneus diadematus*). Recordings from single sensory cells are clearly needed in future studies in order to understand the neural processes of olfaction and gustation in spiders (Barth, 2002).

The distribution of putative chemosensitive hairs has been studied mostly in araneids and lycosids. In *Araneus* more than 1000 chemosensitive hairs have been counted on the legs of a single spider and most were concentrated on the tarsi and metatarsi (Foelix, 1970). There is also a marked age effect, with sub-adult individuals exhibiting fewer chemosensory hairs than adult spiders (Tietjen and Rovner, 1982). In adults, the number of hairs on the pedipalp is higher than on the walking legs. Both sexes show a similar distribution of mechanoreceptors on the palp, but males have more chemosensory hairs on the cymbium than the female (Kronestedt, 1979, Tietjen and Rovner, 1980). Considering that the need for chemical inspection of potential prey should be similar for both sexes, males invest more in sensory equipment than females. This may reflect stronger selection on fast and effective mate detection in males.

5.3   Acoustic signals

5.3.1   *Introduction to acoustic signalling*

Acoustics refers to particle motion in a fluid or elastic medium and thus includes a wide variety of animal signal types including airborne and water-borne 'sound' as well as seismic and other substrate-borne signals (reviewed in Hill, 2008, 2009). Acoustic communication signals can be defined either by the predominant medium that propagates particle motion (vibrations) or by the sensory receptors that detect said motion. Distinguishing between acoustic signal types is not a simple matter as the physics of propagating waves is complex and the interactions between waves propagating in different media are usually not independent. For example, airborne waves can excite substrate-borne waves and vice versa (Hill, 2001, 2008). In addition, it is important to distinguish whether it is the physical mode of propagation or the way in which receivers detect and process signal energy that determines signal type. In behavioural research it is usually preferable to take an organism-centric approach and define signal types by the way in which the receiver detects vibrations. Different receivers, however, may vary in the ways they detect acoustic signals. For example, vibrations that originate as an airborne signal can be detected via the air in one animal and via the substrate in another.

In a simplistic sense, there are three major types of acoustic signals in animals: water-borne, airborne and substrate-borne. To date little work has been conducted on water-borne signal communication with the exception of the mating behaviour of fishing spiders (Araneae: Pisauridae; Arnqvist, 1992; Bleckmann and Bender, 1987, Roland and Rovner, 1983). *Dolomedes triton* has the ability to detect differences between prey and predators based purely on water-borne cues (Barth *et al.*, 1988, Bleckmann, 1985, Bleckmann and Barth, 1984, Carico, 1973, Roland and Rovner, 1983). Male *D. triton* and *D. fimbriatus* both court females using a combination of visual (leg lifts) and percussive (leg and pedipalp drumming) displays (Arnqvist, 1992, Bleckmann and Bender, 1987,

Roland and Rovner, 1983). Percussive displays create low-frequency, long-lasting waves on the water that are distinct from prey cues (Bleckmann and Bender, 1987). It is yet unknown what, if any, information is carried in water-borne signals or if water-borne signals are used by females to select mates.

Airborne signals can be divided into two categories depending on whether local particle motion (near field sound) or the propagated pressure wave (far field sound) dominates airborne motion. Particle motion dominates only at extremely close distances to the vibrating object and evidence suggests that trichobothria receptors on spider legs are exquisitely sensitive at detecting this type of signal energy (reviewed in Barth, 2002, Fratzl and Barth, 2009). Although spiders presumably use near-field sound information (Frings and Frings, 1966) no explicit study has been conducted on near-field communication in spiders (but see Santer and Hebets, 2008). Near-field sound communication is potentially widespread and arachnids may be particularly well suited to study this virtually unknown phenomenon (Barth, 2002, Santer and Hebets, 2008, Rundus et al., 2010).

Far-field sound refers to vibrational energy dominated by a propagating pressure wave. Human ears are adept at detecting far-field sound and this has led to long-standing research biases on airborne components of signals in spiders. In spiders, however, no pressure detectors have been found. In the wandering spider *Cupiennius salei*, physiological recordings from one slit sensilla described sensitivity to far-field sound (Barth, 1967). The majority of physiological recordings from *C. salei*, however, have demonstrated that the vast majority of receptors respond to substrate-borne energy (reviewed in Barth, 2002). In one of the best-studied communication systems in spiders, in *Hygrolycosa rubrofasciata*, signalling rate was measured as far-field sound using microphones (Kotiaho et al., 1996, 1998, Lindstrom et al., 2006, Mappes et al., 1996, Parri et al., 1997, 2002, Rivero et al., 2000). Behavioural evidence, however, suggested that females responded faster to substrate-borne components and that signals were probably detected using substrate-vibration detectors (Parri et al., 2002). Substrate-borne vibrations in communication refer to any vibrations that are detected at the interface between different media (i.e. boundary waves; reviewed in Hill, 2008, 2009). Arrays of spider vibration receptors (slit and lyriform sensilla – see below) along a spider's leg are designed to detect strains in the cuticle caused by boundary waves propagated in the substrate (reviewed in Barth, 2002). Even with cues/signals that originate as far-field sounds (e.g. avian predator calls), spiders detect them as substrate vibrations (Lohrey et al., 2009). Most, if not all, spider communication thus occurs via vibrations in the substrate. A big exception to this, however, are spiders that communicate with non-spiders that do not have well-developed substrate-borne senses (e.g. vertebrates – see below).

5.3.2   Receptors for acoustic signals

To date, the majority of our knowledge on spider neurophysiology is due to the Herculean efforts of Friedrich Barth and colleagues (reviewed in Barth, 2002). For the purposes of this chapter we will only cover this topic briefly, but see excellent reviews by Barth (2002) and Fratzl and Barth (2009) for an in-depth coverage of spider physiology and mechanoreception.

Spiders detect vibrations through the use of slit sensilla that are unique to arachnids (Barth, 2002, Foelix, 1996). Slit sensilla occur on virtually every part of a spider's body and are particularly concentrated on the legs and pedipalps, close to joints in hard, sclerotised cuticle (Barth, 2002). *Cupiennius salei*, for example, are equipped with 3300 slit sense organs. Single slit sensilla are 8–200 μm long and 1–2 μm wide, and are covered by a thin epicuticular membrane to which a single dendrite is attached. Slit sensilla can also occur in groups of a few slits, or in larger conglomerations of up to 20 slits, called lyriform organs (Barth, 2002, Foelix, 1996). Stresses on the cuticle cause a compression of the slit, which in turn elicits a nerve signal response (action potential) at the dendritic ending of the sensory cell (Barth, 2002). Cuticular stresses can be caused by such things as muscular activity, changes in blood pressure, gravity, or substrate-borne vibrations (reviewed in Barth, 2002). Slit sensilla appear to serve different functions; for example, the metatarsal lyriform organ (see below) measures substrate-borne vibrations but also functions as a proprioceptor (Barth, 2002, Gingl *et al.*, 2006). Regardless of the source of cuticular stress, all mechanical information is encoded by slit sensilla, and the function of different slit sensilla and lyriform organs is usually due to its threshold activity, position and orientation on the body (Barth, 2002).

The metatarsal lyriform organ is the most sensitive substrate-borne vibration detector known in spiders (Barth, 2002, Gingl *et al.*, 2006 and references therein). It is located behind a cuticular ridge at the distal end of the metatarsus and consists of anywhere between 8 to 21 slits (reviewed in Barth, 2002). The meta-tarsal organ is capable of detecting a wide dynamic range of frequencies at very low thresholds (Barth and Geethabali, 1982). Virtually no frequency discrimination occurs at the receptor level and all biologically relevant frequencies elicit responses from the sensory receptors. While the overall activity of individual slits is similar, different slits have different thresholds and slightly different frequency properties. Frequency discrimination probably occurs by analysing slit ensemble changes in excitation at higher orders in the brain (Barth and Geethabali, 1982).

5.3.3   Acoustic signalling mechanisms

Acoustic signalling is common in spiders (reviewed in Elias and Mason, in press, Uetz and Stratton, 1982). Most of the behavioural descriptions available for spiders come from groups that produce signals with airborne components acquired using microphones (e.g. Maddison and Stratton, 1988b, Peretti *et al.*, 2006, Rovner, 1980). Microphone recordings of spider signals, however, will always be biased towards higher frequencies that are more likely to cause airborne vibrations (Elias and Mason, in press). Recordings directly off the substrate (e.g. piezo sensors, accelerometers, laser vibrometer devices) do not have these shortcomings and are becoming increasingly available (Elias *et al.*, 2005, 2006b, 2006d, Gibson and Uetz, 2008, Rovner and Barth, 1981, Uhl and Schmitt, 1996). These techniques have revealed that spider acoustic signals are ubiquitous and much more complex than once believed (reviewed in Elias and Mason, in press).

Acoustic signals have been described in 39 families of spiders (reviewed in Uetz and Stratton, 1982; Table 5.2) falling into three types of signal productions mechanisms: percussion, stridulation and tremulation (vibration in Uetz and Stratton, 1982; reviewed in Elias and Mason, in press, Uetz and Stratton, 1982). In modern studies that have used high-speed videography and laser vibrometry it is evident that spiders often use multiple mechanisms to produce acoustic signals (Dierkes and Barth, 1995, Elias *et al.*, 2003, 2006d). Spiders may use either independent mechanisms to produce different signals ('serial signal production' sensu Elias *et al.*, 2006d) or different mechanisms to produce a single multicomponent signal ('parallel signal production' sensu Elias *et al.*, 2006d). In addition, behavioural descriptions of spider displays often suggest the use of different mechanisms; for example combinations of 'body tremors' (tremulations) and 'leg tapping' (percussion) are exceedingly common (Lomborg and Toft, 2009, Lynam *et al.*, 2006).

Percussion

Percussion (described for 12 families of spiders; Table 5.2) occurs when animals produce substrate-borne vibrations using transient impacts of an appendage against another appendage or against the substratum (drumming), including 'web plucking' behaviour. Percussive impacts can sometimes be detected via microphone devices especially if appendages are drummed against certain substrates such as leaf litter (Kotiaho *et al.*, 2000).

Percussive signals potentially have many advantages. First, no specialised morphology is needed to produce signals, although many spiders have thickened plates in the areas that are used to drum against the substratum (e.g. Kronestedt, 1984). Secondly, as percussive signals contain broad frequencies, signal propagation is not necessarily limited to specific environments with particular transmission properties (Elias and Mason, in press, Hebets *et al.*, 2008). Hebets and colleagues (2008) proposed that by using percussive signals, *Schizocosa retrorsa*, a species of wolf spider that occupies several different

Table 5.2 *Acoustic signal production mechanisms in spiders*

Acoustic signal production mechanism	Spider families	References
Percussion	Anyphaenidae, Araneidae, Clubionidae, Ctenidae, Dipluridae, Lycosidae, Pisauridae, Salticidae, Sparassidae, Tetragnathidae, Theridiidae and Thomisidae	Albo *et al.*, 2007, Barth, 1982, Dierkes and Barth, 1995, Eberhard and Huber, 1998, Elias *et al.*, 2003, 2006d, Gibson and Uetz, 2008, Hebets *et al.*, 2008, Henschel, 2002, Krafft, 1978, Lim and Li, 2004, Lubin, 1986, Miller and Miller, 1987, Stratton and Uetz, 1983, Stropa, 2007, Uetz and Stratton, 1982 and references therein.
Stridulation	Agelenidae, Amaurobiidae, Anyphaenidae, Araneidae, Archaeidae, Austrochilidae, Barychelidae, Clubionidae, Corinnidae, Cyatholipidae, Diguetidae, Dipluridae, Erigonidae, Gnaphosidae, Hahniidae, Leptonetidae, Linyphiidae, Lycosidae, Mecysmaucheniidae, Mimetidae, Ochyroceratidae, Palpimanidae, Pholcidae, Phyxelididae, Salticidae, Scytodidae, Segestriidae, Sicariidae, Synotaxidae, Tetragnathidae, Theraphosidae, Theridiidae, Titanoecidae and Zodariidae	Agnarsson, 2004, 2006, Almeida-Silva *et al.* 2009, Arnedo *et al.* 2009, Bertani *et al.*, 2008, Bristowe, 1929, Eberhard, 1994, Eberhard *et al.*, 1993, Elias *et al.*, 2003, 2006d, Fernández-Montraveta *et al.*, 2000, Fischer *et al.*, 2009, Forster and Platnick, 1984, Gertsch, 1979, Grismado and Lopardo 2003, Griswold *et al.*, 2005, Gwinner-Hanke 1970, Hebets, 2008, Jocqué, 2005, Legendre, 1963, Lomborg and Toft, 2009, Lynam *et al.*, 2006, Maddison and Stratton, 1988a, 1988b, Peretti *et al.*, 2006, Pérez-Miles *et al.*, 1996, 2005, Ramírez *et al.*, 2001, Singer *et al.*, 2000, Stratton, 1991, 2005, Stratton and Uetz, 1983, Uetz and Stratton, 1982 and references therein, Uhl and Schmitt, 1996, Charles Griswold, personal communication
Tremulation (Vibration in Uetz and Stratton, 1982)	Agelenidae, Amaurobiidae, Ctenidae, Linyphiidae, Lycosidae, Pholcidae, Salticidae, Sparassidae and Tetragnathidae	Aisenberg, 2009, Barth, 1982, 1993, Dierkes and Barth, 1995, Elias *et al.*, 2003, 2006a, 2006d, 2008, Krafft, 1978, Huber and Eberhard, 1997, Rovner, 1980, Rovner and Barth, 1981, Schuch and Barth, 1985, 1990, Singer *et al.*, 2000, Suter and Keiley, 1984, Suter and Renkes, 1984

microhabitats, compensates for variation in habitat-dependent transmission, allowing for successful mating in a variety of habitats. Most percussive signal characters are unlikely targets of mate choice as they have a limited range of reliable characters (e.g. rate), compared with other potential signal characters (e.g. frequency, amplitude modulation, syllable structure, etc.) (Elias and Mason, in press). One potential function of percussive signals may be to signal distance information. Higher frequencies tend to attenuate rapidly, relative to lower frequencies (Dierkes and Barth, 1995, Michelsen *et al.*, 1982). Assessing the relative contributions of low versus high frequencies in percussive signals could be used to assess how close receivers are to the senders. This has been suggested in a variety of spiders that signal via percussion, although this function has not been empirically demonstrated (Barth and Schmitt, 1991, Elias *et al.*, 2003, 2006d, Schuch and Barth, 1985).

Stridulation

Stridulation is a signal production mechanism by which an animal rubs two rigid body parts (usually a 'pick' and 'file') against each other (Dumortier, 1963). Stridulation often transfers vibrations simultaneously to both the air and substrate (Hill, 2008). In spiders, stridulatory structures are usually single or paired (reviewed in Jocqué, 2005, Uetz and Stratton, 1982). Single stridulatory structures consist of files made of pegs, stiff setae, or ridged structures on the back of the cephalothorax that are rubbed against 'picks' or 'plectrums' on the front of the abdomen (reviewed in Jocqué, 2005, Uetz and Stratton, 1982; see Figure 5.2). Paired stridulatory structures are more common and consist of files found on bilateral appendages such as the palps (e.g. Elias *et al.*, 2006d, Rovner, 1975), chelicerae (e.g. Agnarsson, 2004, Forster *et al.*, 1990) and legs (reviewed in Jocqué, 2005, Uetz and Stratton, 1982). Stridulatory structures have been identified on several body parts including abdomen–prosoma, appendage–appendage, appendage–abdomen, appendage–book lung and adjacent joints on a single appendage (Jocqué, 2005, Uetz and Stratton, 1982). In the genus *Mallinella* (Zodariidae), six different stridulatory structures have been described in a single male (Jocqué, 2005). Putative stridulatory structures have attracted the attention of arachnologists for a century, especially in instances where spiders produce airborne sound (Pocock, 1895a, 1895b, 1899, Wood-Mason, 1876). In fact, stridulatory structures have been used widely in systematics in many spider families, especially the Linyphiidae, Theraphosidae and Theridiidae (Agnarsson, 2006, Arnedo 2009, Pérez-Miles *et al.*, 1996). To date, stridulatory structures have been found in 34 spider families (Table 5.2). Stridulatory mechanisms potentially play a major role in mating behaviour because they often occur only in the male sex or are sexually dimorphic

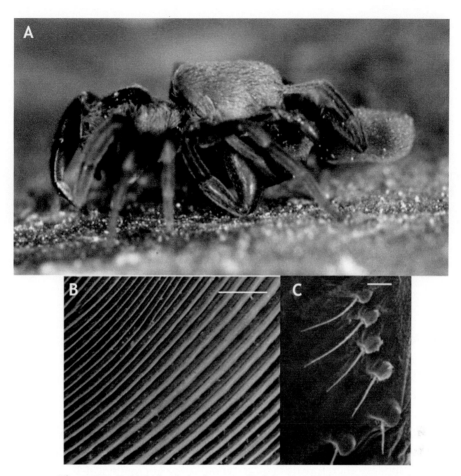

Figure 5.2 Stridulation in both sexes of *Palpimanus gibbulus* (Palpimanidae).
(A) Mating posture of *Palpimanus gibbulus*. Scale bar = 20 μm (photo credit: G. Uhl).
(B) SEM of the stridulatory ridges on the lateral side of both chelicerae (photo credit:
G. Uhl). See also colour plate. (C) Pegs on the base of the pedipalpal femur.
Scale bar = 20 μm.

(Knoflach and Pfaller, 2004, Maddison and Stratton, 1988a). In some cases,
stridulatory structures are found in both sexes (Figure 5.2) and are thought to
serve a defensive function against vertebrate predators (see below) (Hrušková-
Martišová *et al.*, 2008, Marshall *et al.*, 1995, Uhl and Schmitt, 1996). Currently, the
number of putative stridulatory structures in spiders is vastly greater than the
number of matching signal recordings, and future research is needed to examine acoustic signals produced by spiders.

   Stridulatory structures function as frequency multipliers, producing high-
frequency signals with low-frequency body movements (Dumortier, 1963). The
signal frequencies emitted during stridulation are a function of the file structure

as well as the velocity of pick movement across the file. Stridulatory signals can be used to concentrate vibrational energy to particular frequency bands and if the transmission properties of a spider's environment are predictable, stridulatory signals could potentially transmit signals for long distances and contain a variety of potential information such as rate, frequency and amplitude (Elias and Mason, in press). Another advantage of stridulatory structures is their ability to excite airborne vibrations (Hill, 2008, 2009). High-frequency airborne signals may enable spiders to signal defensively against potential vertebrate predators that can only detect airborne 'sound' (Hrušková-Martišová et al., 2008, Marshall et al., 1995). For example, *Theraphosa blondi* (Theraphosidae) use defensive hissing sounds produced by stridulations (Marshall et al., 1995) coupled with defensive urticating hairs. This broadband hissing is similar to other defensive sounds made by other theraphosids, suggesting acoustic aposematism for vertebrate predators (Marshall et al., 1995).

Tremulation

A tremulation mechanism (Morris, 1980) occurs when an animal oscillates its body or appendage and the energy from these oscillations is transferred directly into the substrata through one or more of the animal's legs (Elias et al., 2003, 2006d, Rovner, 1980, Uetz and Stratton, 1982). Vibration, body tremors/shakes/quivers, and opisthosomal signals are all examples of tremulations (Barth, 2002, Hoefler et al., 2009a, Jackson, 1977). Tremulation signals require no specialised morphology and are low in frequency since they are limited by how fast an animal can oscillate its body (reviewed in Elias and Mason, in press). Tremulations are therefore difficult to record using microphone devices and to date most of our knowledge about tremulation signals involves the observation that spiders frequently oscillate their legs or abdomens during mating interactions (Aisenberg, 2009, Eberhard and Huber, 1998, Suter and Renkes, 1984). These movements, however, may serve other functions, and combinations of signal recordings and behavioural experiments are needed to verify that these movements are communication signals.

Rovner (1967) in pioneering studies on wolf spider signalling behaviour successfully recorded stridulatory signals using microphones but obvious abdominal oscillations were undetectable. In species that use different mechanisms to produce different acoustic signals, tremulation signals are often the highest intensity when recorded in the substrate (Elias et al., 2003) due to the fact that these lower frequencies propagate through substrates with relatively little attenuation (Dierkes and Barth, 1995). To date tremulation signals have been recorded and/or verified as important in mating behaviour in nine families (Table 5.2). Tremulation signals are, by virtue of the way they are produced, relatively tonal in structure and thus extremely sensitive to environment-dependent signal propagation as well as any perturbations in that environment (Elias and Mason, in press). The tonal structure of the signal, however, can potentially carry a large array of information (rate, frequency, amplitude, modulations, etc.) if propagated in a predictable environment.

5.3.4   Substrate-borne communication

Substrate-borne signals are thought to function in several non-mutually exclusive contexts in spiders: (1) for species recognition, (2) to signal quality for use in mate choice, (3) to signal competitive ability, and (4) to stimulate female mating behaviour and to suppress female aggressiveness.

Species recognition signals

One of the best-studied spider species is the wandering spider *Cupiennius salei* (reviewed in Barth, 2002). *Cupiennius salei* is found on banana plants in the New World tropics (Rovner and Barth, 1981). Males begin producing substrate-borne signals when they encounter female silk containing pheromonal signals (Barth, 1993). Males produce a series of courtship vibrations consisting of abdominal tremulations (oscillations) and pedipalpal drumming (Barth, 2002). If females are sexually receptive, females answer back with a female-specific tremulation signal, which is then used as a location signal for males (Barth, 2002, Dierkes and Barth, 1995). Females tend to respond more strongly to species-specific signalling patterns when co-occurring with another *Cupiennius* species (Barth and Schmitt, 1991). In experiments with *C. salei* using live female responses to synthetic male signals, females were tolerant to a limited amount of variation in certain male traits, specifically spectral frequency, duration, and temporal pattern of abdominal tremulations (Schuch and Barth, 1990). Other parameters such as signal shape and amplitude were less important (Schuch and Barth, 1990).

Wolf spiders from the genus *Schizocosa* inhabit numerous leaf litter habitats and have been the focus of many studies (reviewed in Stratton, 2005, Uetz and Roberts, 2002). *Schizocosa* is a genus that consists of 23 species in North America (Stratton, 2005). While some species include visual signals, all described *Schizocosa* species use substrate-borne signals in communication (Stratton, 2005). Species recognition in two species, *S. ocreata* and *S. rovneri*, appears to be based on substrate-borne signalling (Stratton, 1983, Stratton and Uetz, 1981, 1983, 1986). *Schizocosa rovneri* males produce signals using a combination of palpal stridulations and body percussion (Stratton and Uetz, 1986, Uetz and Denterlein, 1979). *Schizocosa ocreata*, by contrast, produce signals using a complex series of motions that include a variety of signal production mechanisms including abdominal tremulations, palpal stridulations, and leg percussion ('jerky tapping'; Gibson and Uetz, 2008, Stratton and Uetz, 1986). The percussive displays of *S. rovneri* appear well suited to propagate in their microhabitat of compressed floodplain leaf litter, while the complex displays of *S. ocreata* may function to overcome the heterogeneity of upland leaf litter habitats (Stratton and Uetz, 1983, 1986). Males of both species court females indiscriminately and hybrids between *S. ocreata* and *S. rovneri* are viable in the laboratory (Stratton, 1983, Stratton and Uetz, 1981, 1983). No hybrids have been reported in the field, however, and females only respond to conspecific signals, leading to the conclusion that courtship displays in *Schizocosa* function as species recognition signals (Stratton and Uetz, 1983, 1986).

Mate quality signals

Many species of spiders are cursorial and live in leaf litter habitats on forest floors. Leaf litter habitats are complex and spiders that live in these habitats often court over long distances (Elias and Mason, in press, Hebets *et al.*, 2008, Uetz and Stratton, 1982). One well-studied spider mating system is the wolf spider *Hygrolycosa rubrofasciata* from the work of Kotiaho and colleagues. *Hygrolycosa rubrofasciata* are found in moist meadow and bog habitats consisting of moss, hay, sedge and leaf litter of willow and birch leaves. Male distribution is highly patchy in these habitats and males prefer elevated habitats with abundant dry leaf litter cover (Kotiaho *et al.*, 2000). In the mating season, *H. rubrofasciata* males court females using percussive displays where males drum their abdomens against the leaf litter substrate (Kronestedt, 1996). Male drumming is intense and comes with significant metabolic costs and is considered an honest indicator of quality as drum rate is condition dependent (Kotiaho *et al.*, 1998, 2000, Mappes *et al.*, 1996, Rivero *et al.*, 2000). In addition, signalling comes with significant immunological (Ahtiainen *et al.*, 2005, 2006) and viability costs (Kotiaho *et al.*, 1998, 1999). Females signal willingness to mate by tremulation ('body shakes' in Kronestedt, 1996) and choose males based on drumming rate which is highly repeatable within males but highly variable between males (Kotiaho *et al.*, 1996, Parri *et al.*, 1997, Rivero *et al.*, 2000). Signal frequency, however, is highly variable within and between males (Kotiaho *et al.*, 1999, Rivero *et al.*, 2000). By choosing males with high drumming rates, females ensure offspring with higher survival and better immune systems (Ahtiainen *et al.*, 2004, 2005, 2006, Alatalo *et al.* 1998).

Work on the wolf spider *Schizocosa ocreata* also suggests that substrate-borne signals may function as mate quality signals (Gibson and Uetz, 2008). Although *S. ocreata* signals contain strong visual components (Hebets and Vink, 2007,

McClintock and Uetz, 1996), mating can occur in the absence of any visual cues (Taylor *et al.*, 2006). A variety of acoustic signal traits are correlated with female receptivity including signal amplitude, peak frequency, stridulatory pulse duration and percussive strike rate (Gibson and Uetz, 2008). Successful males were also in overall better condition, suggesting that substrate-borne signals transmit information about male quality (Gibson and Uetz, 2008). Courtship rate in another wolf spider species, *Pardosa milvina*, also suggests that acoustic signals function as mate quality signals (Hoefler *et al.*, 2008, 2009a). Male *P. milvina* court females using a combination of visual (leg raise) and tremulation (body shake) signals (Hoefler *et al.*, 2008, Rypstra *et al.*, 2003). Females preferred males that engaged in more vigorous courtship (Rypstra *et al.*, 2003) and males that had more vigorous courtship were of generally higher quality, produced more offspring, had offspring that developed faster, and survived longer than offspring from less vigorously courting males (Hoefler *et al.*, 2008, 2009). Similar results are also found in the congener *P. prativaga* where diet manipulations enhanced male courtship displays (Lomborg and Toft, 2009). In this species, males that courted at higher rates also experienced greater mating success (Lomborg and Toft, 2009).

Female choice on courtship length has also been implicated in several widow species. In redbacks (*Latrodectus hasselti*) and white widows (*L. pallidus*), males perform vibratory courtship on the female web consisting of abdominal tremulations and web plucking over several hours (Andrade, 1996, Andrade and Banta, 2002, Forster, 1995, Harari *et al.*, 2009, Stoltz *et al.*, 2008, 2009). In *Latrodectus hasselti* females punish short courtship by cannibalising males and selection on displays appears to be on duration of the entire display and not on individual vibratory components (Snow and Andrade, 2004, Stoltz *et al.*, 2008, 2009). Similar results were found in *L. pallidus* as virgin females prevented males that had not performed long displays from entering nests and mounting (Harari *et al.*, 2009, Segoli *et al.*, 2006).

Signals in some web-building spiders are also thought to function as mate quality indicators. Male funnel-web spiders *Agelenopsis aperta* court females on webs using a combination of abdominal ('waggle') and web ('flex') tremulations as well as web drumming (Singer *et al.*, 2000). After a period of web courtship, a male will approach the female and mount her, after which the male continues tactile courtship by stroking the sides of her abdomen with his legs (Becker *et al.*, 2005, Singer *et al.*, 2000). This usually is followed by female catalepsy where females become immobile and unresponsive even to prodding and manipulation (Pruitt and Riechert, 2009). Male web courtship both precedes and follows female catalepsy and males will often abandon the immobile female to once again resume courtship on the web (Pruitt and Riechert, 2009, Singer and

Riechert, 1995). Females are more likely to mate with larger males (Riechert and Singer, 1995, Singer and Riechert, 1994, Singer et al., 2000) and males that produce higher frequency tremulation signals (Singer et al., 2000). Singer and colleagues proposed that female funnel-web spiders select males based on information in vibratory signals (Singer and Riechert, 1995, Singer et al., 2000). Similar results were found in the orb-web spider *Leucauge mariana* (Aisenberg, 2009). *Leucauge mariana* males that performed more abdominal tremulations ('bobbing') and leg tapping behaviours were more likely to mate with already mated females (Aisenberg, 2009). Females were also more likely to mate a second time if initial matings were short, suggesting that females use information from vibratory signals to determine paternity patterns (Aisenberg, 2009). In the Sierra Dome spider *Neriene litigiosa*, females prefer larger males that perform more vigorous courtship (Watson, 1998). Offspring of larger, more vigorously courting males grew faster and achieved larger size, suggesting higher reproductive fitness for females that preferred males that courted at higher rates (Watson, 1998).

Competition and aggressive signals

Male–male competition for access to females may play an important role in many spider systems (Cross et al., 2007b, Elias et al., 2008, Riechert, 1988, Taylor et al., 2001). Animal contests in most instances are settled on the basis of resource holding potential (RHP) and RHP assessment can occur based on characters correlated with fighting ability including acoustic signals (reviewed in Hsu et al., 2006).

In ground-breaking studies of contest behaviour in animals, Riechert (reviewed in Riechert, 1988) investigated competition in the funnel-web spider *Agelenopsis aperta*. Male *A. aperta* defend web sites against any intruding spiders (Riechert, 1978, 1979). Contestants display behavioural strategies relative to their RHP, showing increased willingness to escalate contests if they are residents, and if they are larger than their opponents (Reichert, 1988). RHP assessment is predicted to be based on the assessment of vibratory signals (Riechert, 1978). Vibratory signalling behaviours are common in early phases of contests and usually, in instances with size disparities, lead to the retreat of the smaller individuals. As RHP disparities decrease, signalling increases and often leads to direct confrontations and significant risks of damage. In other scenarios, males continue to display after winning contests potentially signalling the winner's intent to escalate to potentially damaging behaviours (Riechert, 1978).

During the breeding season adult male jumping spiders *Phidippus clarus* visit and guard immature female nests over a period of several weeks (Elias et al., 2008, Hoefler, 2007, Kasumovic et al., 2009a, 2009b). During this period of time males engage in repeated contests for access to female nests. Male contests begin with an assessment period where males display to each other using a combination of visual and acoustic signals (Elias *et al.*, 2008). Males produce short bursts of abdominal tremulations at opponents, and signal number is correlated with both size and contest success (Elias *et al.*, 2008). Males produce vibratory signals only as they approach opponents and small differences in vibratory signals usually rapidly escalate to direct fights (Elias *et al.*, 2008). Elias and colleagues (2008) suggested that vibratory signals function to inform opponents of their willingness to escalate contests in a similar way to *Agelenopsis aperta* (see above). This was further supported by the observation that males that had lost contests avoided further interactions and dramatically reduced their signalling behaviour, while the winners' signalling was unchanged (Elias *et al.*, 2008). Male bowl and doily spiders *Linyphia triangularis* and *Frontinella communis* also fight for access to females (Suter and Keiley, 1984). In the initial phase of contests, males display at each other using visual leg waves and abdominal tremulations. Mismatches between the relative sizes of opponents usually lead to the smaller male retreating, while size-matched pairings usually lead to escalation in aggression, suggesting that vibratory displays are used to assess size and competitive ability in contestants.

Female sexual stimulation and aggression deterrent signals

Female spiders are often aggressive and sexual cannibalism is common in many species (reviewed in Elgar, 1992). Males that do not perform the proper mating displays are often at risk of becoming a female's meal (Elias *et al.*, 2005, Stoltz *et al.*, 2008, 2009). Females in the species *Stegodyphus lineatus* are sedentary and build conical web nests with a large capture area. After their last moult, males wander in search of females and upon encountering female webs, begin courtship displays consisting of leg and abdominal vibrations on the capture portion of the female web (Maklakov *et al.*, 2003). Male acoustic signals propagate towards the female nests and males repeatedly enter the female nest, contact the female, and return to courtship displays. Males that produced courtship vibrations were more likely to mate with virgin females within three hours, but within these three hours measures such as vibration rate did not predict mating success. Maklakov and colleagues (2003) suggested that this pattern was consistent with the hypothesis that vibratory displays functioned to stimulate receptive females rather than as mate assessment and mate choice. Experiments with mated females supported this hypothesis as males were less likely to perform vibratory displays to unreceptive mated females (Maklakov *et al.*, 2003). Experiments with the bowl and doily spider *Frontinella communis* suggested that signals function to decrease female aggression (Suter and

Hirscheimer, 1986). Upon arrival at female webs, males start long courtship displays consisting of different abdominal tremulations (Suter and Renkes, 1984). The frequency characteristics of male signals are stereotyped and female aggression only occurs at the beginning of courtship, leading to the conclusion that male signals curtail female aggression (Suter and Renkes, 1984). While stimulating females' receptivity and decreasing aggression seem to be a critical part of all spider displays, it remains to be investigated to what extent this role may be independent from species recognition and mate choice.

In the pholcid *Physocyclus globosus*, males perform courtship displays consisting of abdominal tremulations ('abdomen bobbing') and stridulation (Huber and Eberhard, 1997). Male abdominal tremulations are correlated with mating success as males that perform more signals are more likely to sire offspring and females are less likely to dump their sperm after copulation (Peretti and Eberhard, 2010). Once males begin to copulate, females and not males stridulate (Peretti *et al.*, 2006). Females stridulate during male copulatory squeezes, usually resulting in males relaxing the intensity of the 'squeeze'. Peretti and colleagues (2006) suggested that female signals ensure that male movements do not damage female genitalia. This tactile, stridulatory dialogue is important in paternity as males that responded to female stridulations were more likely to father offspring than males that did not (Peretti *et al.*, 2006). Tactile, copulatory communication may be a common phenomenon in spiders but has thus far been overlooked in the literature (Eberhard, 1994, 2004).

5.4   Visual signals

5.4.1   *Introduction to visual signalling*

As a general rule, spiders have poor vision and are only able to form low resolution images on their principal image-forming eyes (Land, 1985, Land and Nilsson, 2002). Eyes of many web spiders are also not suitable for assessing visual signals and are probably used for coarse navigation purposes only (Land and Nilsson, 2002). Several spider families, however, are exceptions to this rule. In particular, cursorial spiders from the families Salticidae, Lycosidae, Sparassidae, Thomisidae, Oxyopidae and Deinopidae have relatively well developed vision (reviewed in Foelix, 1996, Land, 1985, Land and Nilsson, 2002).

Animals are capable of measuring many properties of emitted or reflected light including intensity (luminance, radiance), contrast (differences in luminance between two adjacent areas), wavelength (hue, colour), and/or polarisation. By integrating these measurements with spatial and temporal information, animals also have the ability to process the size and shape of objects as well as motion (reviewed in Land and Nilsson, 2002). Work on visual communication in other animal groups suggests that relative contrast, colour and size/shape/timing of visual signals are important in mate choice (Andersson, 1994, Maynard Smith and Harper, 2005). In spiders, work on visual communication has mainly focused on the wavelengths and size of visual ornaments as well as motion (Clark and Biesiadecki, 2002, Cross *et al.*, 2007b, Elias *et al.*, 2006c, Hebets *et al.*, 2006, Lim *et al.*, 2008, Persons and Uetz, 2005).

The ability for animals to detect luminance, contrast, size and shape of images depends on the optical performance of the eyes. Generally there are two components of optical performance in eyes, spatial resolution and sensitivity (Land, 1985, Land and Nilsson, 2002). Colour has also been implicated in many animal mating systems including spiders. Perception of colour is dependent on the number and types of photo pigments present in the retina (reviewed in Land and Nilsson, 2002). Multiple photoreceptor types have been found in several spider species (Koyanagi *et al.*, 2008, Tiedemann *et al.*, 1986, Walla *et al.*, 1996, Yamashita, 1985) and behavioural discrimination of colours has been demonstrated for jumping and crab spiders (Bhaskara *et al.*, 2009, Heiling *et al.*, 2005a, 2005b, Nakamura and Yamashita, 2000, VanderSal and Hebets, 2007).

5.4.2   *Receptors for visual signals*

Spiders typically have eight eyes arranged in two or three rows. Spiders are the only major terrestrial invertebrate group that uses cornea-lens combination eyes, similar to those used by mammals (Land and Nilsson, 2002). Of all the spider visual systems studied, however, jumping spiders (Salticidae) alone exploit the full optical resolving power of a corneal lens system through the use of many unique adaptations in their principal eyes, including a tiered retina (reviewed in Forster, 1982a, 1982b, Land, 1985, Land and Nilsson, 2002). Functionally spider eyes are divided into two groups, the principal eyes (anterior median eyes) and the secondary eyes (anterior lateral, posterior median and posterior lateral eyes) (Foelix, 1996). In general, secondary eyes are thought to be better suited to detecting motion while primary eyes are better suited for fine-scale discrimination of objects. While spider vision has been demonstrated to function in predation (Bhaskara *et al.*, 2009, Harland and Jackson, 2002, Neuhofer *et al.*, 2009, Théry and Casas, 2009), navigation (Nørgaard *et al.*, 2008, Reyes-Alcubilla *et al.*, 2009, Schmid, 1998) and predator avoidance (Neuhofer *et al.*, 2009), only jumping (Salticidae) and wolf (Lycosidae) spiders have been shown to use visual signals in communication (reviewed in Forster, 1982b, Framenau and Hebets, 2007, Stratton, 2005).

Jumping and wolf spider eyes are very different. Jumping spiders have enlarged primary eyes, giving them remarkable spatial discrimination abilities. For example, the spatial resolution of the jumping spider *Portia* principal eye is more than 175 times greater than the wolf spider *Lycosa* principal eye (data from Land, 1985). Not surprisingly, jumping spiders use vision as the dominant sense in predation (Harland and Jackson, 2001, Jackson, 1982, Jakob *et al.*, 2007, Nelson and Jackson, 2009), navigation (Hill, 1979, Hoefler and Jakob, 2006), courtship (Clark and Biesiadecki, 2002, Cross *et al.*, 2008, Maddison and McMahon, 2000, Masta and Maddison, 2002) and competition behaviours (Chan *et al.*, 2008, Cross *et al.*, 2007b, Faber and Baylis, 1993, Taylor *et al.*, 2001, Wells, 1988). In contrast, wolf spiders have enlarged secondary eyes and a reflecting tapetum, imparting high visual sensitivity. For example, the sensitivity of the wolf spider *Lycosa* secondary eyes is 90 times that of the jumping spider *Portia* principal eyes (data from Land, 1985).

Jumping spider eyes are well suited for colour vision (Forster, 1982a, 1982b, Koyanagi *et al.*, 2008, Land, 1985). Behavioural experiments have demonstrated their ability to distinguish between different colours (Hoefler and Jakob, 2006, Jakob *et al.*, 2007, Peaslee and Wilson, 1989, VanderSal and Hebets, 2007) and anatomical experiments have demonstrated dichromatic (Blest *et al.*, 1981), trichromatic (DeVoe, 1975, Koyanagi *et al.*, 2008) and tetrachromatic vision (Yamashita and Tateda, 1976). It is yet unknown whether the discrepancies between studies represent species-specific differences in colour vision or differences in experimental methodologies. Wolf spiders may also have some ability to discriminate colour. DeVoe (1972) found that in the principal eyes of *Lycosa*, photoreceptors contained photo pigments sensitive to both UV and green wavelengths. In the wolf spider species studied, however, spatial resolution of principal eyes is much lower than the secondary eyes, which only contain green sensitive photoreceptors (DeVoe, 1972).

5.4.3   *Visual signalling mechanisms*

Spider visual ornaments are composed of scales, flattened setae overlying the surface of the cuticle (Townsend and Felgenhauer, 1999). There are three different acknowledged scale types, lanceolate, spatulate, and plumose scales, each with divergent shape and structure (Townsend and Felgenhauer, 1998). Spider scales sometimes have embedded pigment, structural or florescent coloration (Andrews *et al.*, 2007, Oxford and Gillespie, 1998, Taylor and McGraw, 2007). Ommochrome pigments are usually used in yellow, orange, red, brown and black coloration (Oxford and Gillespie, 1998) while white is generated by reflections from guanine crystals (Foelix, 1996).

Some spiders, notably jumping spiders, use structural colour for green, white, orange and UV coloration (Parker and Hegedus, 2003). Structural colours are produced through reflections off alternating layers of low (air) and high (chitin) refractive index material, and through a constructive interference process are usually very bright (reviewed in Land, 1972). Varying the thickness between chitin and air layers leads to a shift in reflected colour (Land, 1972, Land *et al.*, 2007, Parker and Hegedus, 2003, Taylor and McGraw, 2007). The iridescent scales from the jumping spider *Cosmophasis umbratica*, for example, reflect UV and green-orange light (Land *et al.*, 2007). The coloration is a result of a highly organised nanostructure wherein scales are made up of an alternating chitin–air–chitin sandwich, the chitin layers of which are precisely three quarters of a wavelength thick while the air gap is a quarter wavelength thick; other scales without the air gap produce a dull purple reflection (Land *et al.*, 2007). Females use information from these scales in mate choice (Lim *et al.*, 2007, 2008). Some spiders also sequester fluorophores, molecules that absorb energy of a specific wavelength and re-emit energy at a different wavelength in their scales (Andrews *et al.*, 2007).

5.4.4   *Visual communication*

Species recognition signals

Evidence that females discriminate between males of sympatric species on the basis of visual signals alone is scarce (Jackson, 1982). Many of the species studied produce visual signals in combination with other signals in different modalities (Elias *et al.*, 2003, 2006c, Jackson, 1977, Uetz and Roberts, 2002). Male jumping spider displays are often stereotyped to such an extent that they are useful as taxonomic characters (Richman, 1982) suggesting a role in species recognition, although many spiders have context-dependent displays (Cross *et al.*, 2008, Jackson and Pollard, 1997, Nelson and Jackson, 2007). In one species, females in some populations even preferred mating with males that included novel display elements (Elias *et al.*, 2006a, Hebets and Maddison, 2005). For *Cosmophasis umbratica*, however, females produce a sex- and species-specific fluorescent signal using their pedipalps (Lim *et al.*, 2007). In experiments where fluorescence signals were blocked, Lim and colleagues (2007) demonstrated that males become unresponsive, suggesting that fluorescent signals are used by males to identify conspecifics. The extent that visual signals are used as recognition signals in other species remains an open question.

Mate quality signals

One well-studied visual communication system is that of the wolf spider *Schizocosa ocreata* (Delaney *et al.*, 2007, Hebets and Vink, 2007, McClintock and Uetz, 1996, Uetz *et al.*, 2009a). The tibiae of *S. ocreata* forelegs have black pigmentation and associated tufts of bristles ('brushes'; Stratton, 2005, Stratton and Uetz, 1981). Pigmentation and the presence of brushes are associated with motion displays of those appendages (Hebets and Uetz, 2000). During mate choice trials on field-collected substrates, tuft size (relative to body size) was the only trait associated with mating success, with males with larger tufts being more likely to mate with females (Persons and Uetz, 2005). In addition, the probability of attempted sexual cannibalism varied with tuft size (Persons and Uetz, 2005). Tuft asymmetry also appears to be important for mate choice (Uetz and Smith, 1999, Uetz et al., 1996). Decreased mating success is associated with asymmetric tufts if asymmetry results from previously lost legs or if symmetry is experimentally manipulated by shaving the tufts on one side (Uetz et al., 1996). In the field, male body condition and size is negatively correlated with tuft asymmetry (Uetz and Smith, 1999) and increased tuft asymmetry is associated with periods of environmental stress (Uetz et al., 2009b). Female receptivity displays are more likely to occur for males with symmetric tufts, even when the effects of male size, condition and behaviour are held constant (Uetz and Smith, 1999). Schizocosa ocreata displays, however, have strong substrate-borne components and females have been shown to mate in the absence of visual signals (Taylor et al., 2006). Also, during experiments in open arenas with no natural substrates, experimental manipulations of tufts had no effect on mating behaviour (Scheffer et al., 1996). These diverging results suggest that tufts are used for mate choice in certain conditions when the propagation of substrate-borne signals is unpredictable (Uetz and Smith, 1999).

In another species of Schizocosa, S. uetzi, the tibia on the forelegs have associated black pigmentation (Hebets et al., 2006). Black pigmentation is variable within populations and the proportion of black pigmentation is correlated with male weight, suggesting that coloration may be used by females to assess quality (Hebets et al., 2006, Shamble et al., 2009). In video playback experiments, females were more receptive to males with ornamented forelegs in the presence of substrate-borne signals. However, this preference was only seen when male ornamentation was greater than that observed in natural populations (Hebets, 2005, Shamble et al., 2009). In experiments with live males and females, the degree of black ornamentation did not influence mate choice; instead, courtship rate was the only significant predictor of copulation success (Shamble et al., 2009). Interestingly though, females that had experienced courtship from males with black pigmentation as subadults preferred pigmented males as adults (Hebets, 2003) suggesting preferences for visual ornamentation is dependent on experience (Shamble et al., 2009).

Cosmophasis umbratica jumping spider males perform complex visual courtship displays consisting of a variety of behaviours including skittering (rapid stop and go stepping behaviour), leg and abdominal arching and waving, and palpal vibration (Lim and Li, 2004). The male appendages used during courtship dances also have associated bright coloration (Lim and Li, 2004). All male sex-specific ornaments shown to females during displays reflect highly in the UV range (300–400 nm; Lim and Li, 2006a). Females preferred viewing males that reflected UV light, and when UV was absent they essentially ignored male displays (Lim and Li, 2006a, 2006b, 2007). Ultraviolet ornamentation is condition dependent, with poorly fed males reflecting less UV light than well fed males, and young males reflecting longer UV wavelengths relative to older males (Lim *et al.*, 2007). These data suggest that UV ornaments are quality signals (reviewed in Taylor and McGraw, 2007). *Phintella vittata* males also use UV ornaments, but in this case male ornaments reflect in the UV-B range (280–315 nm; Li *et al.*, 2008a). This type of reflection is not strongly represented in natural light and no other animals have been shown to use UV-B ornaments in communication (Li *et al.*, 2008a). Females prefer males that reflect UV-B, once again suggesting a role in female mate choice and possibly species recognition (Li *et al.*, 2008b).

Male competition signals

Many jumping spiders use foreleg waving in male–male aggressive displays where higher rate signalling is associated with fighting success (Cross *et al.*, 2007b, Jackson *et al.*, 2006, Taylor *et al.*, 2001). For example, males in the species *Plexippus paykulli* display at each other by raising their bodies off the ground, pointing the abdomen downward, and waving their forelegs (Taylor *et al.*, 2000). Abdomen size is a potential visual signal reflecting overall body size and fighting ability, while ornaments on the abdomen serve as amplifiers, making assessments of abdominal size easier for opponents (Taylor *et al.*, 2001). In addition to visual signals of opponents, jumping spider males also use visual information from nearby females when deciding whether or not to escalate to potentially costly interactions (Cross *et al.*, 2006, 2007b, Jackson *et al.*, 2006, Wells, 1988).

Attention primer signals

Attracting a female's attention is also critical in mate choice. *Maevia inclemens* is a jumping spider that is found in the eastern and mid-western United States. Male *M. inclemens* have two distinct morphs, a tufted and a grey morph. Tufted morph males are black in body coloration, have white legs and have three tufts of setae on their anterior cephalothorax. Grey morph males are black and white striped, and have orange pedipalps and no tufts (Clark and Uetz, 1990). Tufted morph displays consist of the male 'standing up' and waving the forelegs while swinging the abdomen side to side, usually at a distance of 9 cm from the female (Clark, 1994, Clark and Uetz, 1993). Grey morph courtship is very different and consists of males lowering their body to the substrate and sidling back and forth with the legs outstretched forward in a triangular configuration. This display usually occurs at a distance of 3 cm from the female (Clark, 1994, Clark and Uetz, 1993). Females choose males that they see move first, independent of morphotype, and different morphs are more likely to draw a female's attention at different distances (Clark, 1992, Clark and Biesiadecki, 2002, Clark and Morjan, 2001).

5.5   Multimodal signals

Spiders have long been considered sensory specialists par excellence. Web-building spiders and wandering spiders are models in studying substrate-borne vibration physiology and behaviour while jumping spiders are models in studying visual optics and behaviour (reviewed in Barth, 2002, Forster, 1982a, Land, 1985). Many animals, however, communicate using multiple signals across more than one sensory modality (Candolin, 2003, Hebets and Papaj, 2005, Partan and Marler, 2005, Rowe, 1999). The function of multimodal signals and the conditions leading to the evolution of multimodal communication is under considerable debate (Hebets and Papaj, 2005, Iwasa and Pomiankowski, 1994, Pomiankowski and Iwasa, 1993) and spiders have been at the forefront of this research (Elias *et al.*, 2003, Hebets and Uetz, 1999, Uetz and Roberts, 2002).

In multimodal signals, separate components can relay either redundant or non-redundant information (Partan and Marler, 2005). Multimodal signals that relay redundant information are also known as 'back up signals' (Johnstone, 1996). Empirically, redundant signal components will have equivalent effects when presented independently, and identical or enhanced responses when presented together (Hebets and Papaj, 2005, Partan and Marler, 2005). Multimodal signals that relay non-redundant information are also known as 'multiple messages' (Johnstone, 1996, Møller and Pomiankowski, 1993). Empirically, non-redundant signal components will have different effects when presented independently, and when presented together can have a variety of complex effects including dominance or enhancement of one sensory com-ponent, or entirely new responses resulting from emergent properties of the multimodal signal (Hebets and Papaj, 2005, Partan and Marler, 2005). Wolf spider male *Pardosa milvina*, for example, use chemical signals from silk to find females and visual cues to focus their attention on the location of nearby females (Hoefler *et al.*, 2008, 2009b, Rypstra *et al.*, 2003, 2009). Both signals provide redundant information on female location but when males detect mated female silk and the visual presence of any female their courtship activity and aggressive behaviours dramatically increase (Rypstra *et al.*, 2009).

Spider mating behaviour often involves multiple sensory systems at different stages of mating behaviour. For example, the wandering spider *Cupiennius salei* uses different sensory systems in each of three phases. The first, chemical, phase ensures that males are sexually stimulated and is driven by pheromones in female silk; the second, vibratory, phase ensures species isolation and high-quality mates; and the third, tactile, phase ensures that male and female reproduction is coordinated and is the final stage for mate assessment (Barth and Schmitt, 1991, Schmitt *et al.*, 1993). The use of multiple modalities at different stages prevents costly mistakes, may compensate for errors in signal propagation, and may serve to avoid cannibalism. Information from multiple modalities may also serve to modulate preferences and mating behaviour. For example, in the blood-feeding jumping spider *Evarcha culicivora*, both males and females use visual signals for mate choice decisions (Cross and Jackson, 2009b, Cross *et al.*, 2007a, 2008, 2009); individuals choose larger mates on the basis of visual signals (Cross *et al.*, 2007a) but more frequently approach odours from opposite-sex individuals that recently fed on blood (Cross and Jackson, 2009b). Other spider species emphasise either visual signals or substrate-borne signals depending on context. For example, *Phidippus johnsoni* jumping spider males court females by using visual signals if they find them away from nests or by using substrate-borne signals if they find them in nests (Jackson, 1982). This courtship versatility has also been found in other jumping spiders (Cross *et al.*, 2008, Jackson, 1983, 1986a, Jackson and Pollard, 1997). Multimodal signals are often emitted together. Jumping spiders from the genus *Habronattus* (Figure 5.3), for example, precisely coordinate visual displays with substrate-borne signals (Elias *et al.*, 2003, 2006c). Distinct visual displays are produced with different substrate-borne signals, suggesting that each component contributes to an overall integrative signal (Elias *et al.*, 2006c).

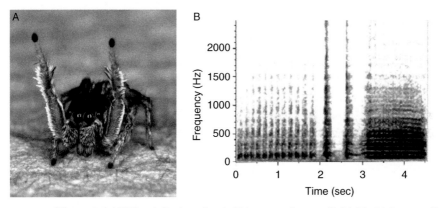

Figure 5.3 (A) Visual display of male *Habronattus dossenus* (Salticidae) (photo credit: D. O. Elias). (B) Sonagram of male songs during courtship. Male acoustic display including percussion, stridulation and tremulation mechanism was recorded using laser Doppler vibrometry (photo credit: D. O. Elias). See also colour plate.

In a comparative study on wolf spiders in the genus *Schizocosa*, it was found that in female receptivity responses to visual and substrate-borne signals in isolation, only species with strong visual ornamentation (tufts) responded to visual signals alone while all species studied responded to conspecific substrate-borne signals (Hebets and Uetz, 1999, Scheffer *et al.*, 1996, Uetz and Roberts, 2002). In addition, for species that produced multimodal signals, variation was observed between responses to isolated and combined signals, suggesting that in some species different signals served as back-ups, while in others multimodal signals provide non-redundant information and may interact (Hebets and Papaj, 2005, Roberts *et al.*, 2007). In one species with foreleg ornamentation, *Schizocosa uetzi*, no effect was observed if visual signals were removed (Hebets, 2005). When visual and substrate-borne signals were presented together, however, female preferences to visual signals dramatically increased, suggesting intersignal interactions where signals in one modality (substrate-borne vibrations) alter attention to another (visual) (Hebets, 2005). These data suggest that assessment of traits important to mate choice may occur only in situations where the correct combination of multisensory information is available (Hebets, 2008, Rundus *et al.*, 2010).

5.6   Social interactions

Tolerance and cooperation is necessary within groups of subsocial and social spiders and is also required to some extent in spiders that form aggregations under specific conditions (Krafft, 1982, Lubin and Bilde, 2007, Whitehouse and Lubin, 2005; see Chapter 8 in this book). However, spider communication in this context is little investigated.

Many spiders show maternal care of their young. Egg-sac-carrying female wolf spiders detect vibrations from the egg sac that indicate that the young are about to hatch and, as a consequence, they tear open the egg sacs (Uetz and Stratton, 1983). Complex interactions between parent and hatched offspring occur in species where mothers catch prey for their offspring or feed them by regurgitation (Lubin and Bilde, 2007). In colonial spiders, mainly vibratory communication signals are considered to be used as warning signals, to mediate spacing and web construction, and are involved in cooperative foraging decisions (Burgess and Uetz, 1982, Vakanas and Krafft, 2004).

In social spiders, the potential for aggressive interactions between group members is higher compared with eusocial insects as there is no division of labour (Lubin and Bilde, 2007). Vibratory signals transmitted in competition over preferred feeding positions probably lead to competitive advantages (Buskirk, 1975, Whitehouse and Lubin, 1999). Chemical signals seem to play a crucial role for colony adhesion in social spiders (Krafft, 1982, Krafft and Roland,

1980). Anaesthetised conspecifics of *Stegodyphus sarasinorum* are recognised and tolerated, whereas other immobile spider species are accepted as prey (Kullmann and Zimmermann, 1972). Further, in *S. sarasinorum* (Eresidae) and *Agelena consociata* (Agelenidae) the silk provides a cue that mediates orientation and aggregation of conspecifics (Roland, 1984). In *Anelosimus studiosus*, in which social behaviour differs along a latitudinal gradient, females from social nests (same and foreign) were attracted to one another in contrast to females from solitary female nests (Riechert and Jones, 2008). How social spiders recognise individuals with whom to cooperate is only starting to be investigated. Indications for kin recognition have been found in the subsocial *Stegodyphus lineatus* and in the social *Diaea ergandros* (Bilde and Lubin 2001, Evans, 1999). Cuticular hydrocarbons were investigated in spiderlings of *S. lineatus* that stay in their mother's nest for about two weeks where they are fed by regurgitation and prey provisioning (L. Grinsted, T. Bilde and P. d'Ettore, unpublished data). The chemical profiles are sibling-group specific and point towards branched alkanes as signals for kin recognition, similar to what is known for insects. Further, the composition of cuticular compounds changes during the spiderlings' development in *S. lineatus* and in another subsocial spider, *Tegenaria atrica* (Agelenidae) (L. Grinsted, unpublished data, Pourié *et al.*, 2005 and references therein). In the subsocial *Coelotes terrestris* (Amaurobiidae), the female's web changes in chemistry from the pre- to the post-dispersal phase of her young (Trabalon and Assi-Bessekon, 2008). The social and non-social phase is therefore accompanied by qualitative and quantitative changes in cuticular or web-based chemicals, which strongly suggests that chemicals are involved in regulating the degree of tolerance and aggression in different phases.

5.7   Conclusion and outlook

We are beginning to understand the sensory world of spiders through work on different communication modalities: olfactory, visual and acoustic. Communication in spiders encompasses all aspects of a spider's life: food acquisition, predator avoidance, agonistic encounters, identification of conspecifics, mate assessment as well as social interactions. Several key areas are neglected, however. Firstly, we know very little about the role and function of chemicals in communication. Secondly, we still need to identify the mechanisms responsible for the production, detection and processing of chemical, acoustic and visual signals in spiders. Work on chemical communication, the biomechanics of signal production, and physiology of signal processing is sorely needed. Thirdly, we need to adopt integrative approaches to study spider communication as spider signals are, as a general rule, multicomponent and multimodal. Although there is still a need to explore the specific role of individual signals in isolation, we need to pay tribute to the true complexity of spider communication by investigating the interactions of the many sensory modalities used by spiders to process and navigate their environment. Experimental approaches are required that investigate receiver responses to isolated and combined signals (Hebets and Papaj, 2005, Partan and Marler 2005). In theory, redundant multicomponent signals provide flexibility to different environmental conditions as well as enhance the behavioural responses of the receiver. Non-redundant signals, by contrast, can prime attentional or behavioural changes when used sequentially or can provide enhanced responses when used simultaneously (Partan and Marler, 1999, 2005). The theoretical framework for complex signals is growing and investigations on spiders are playing a key role in this process.

References

Agnarsson, I. (2004). Morphological phylogeny of cobweb spiders and their relatives (Araneae, Araneoidea, Theridiidae). *Zoological Journal of the Linnean Society*, **141**, 447–626.

Agnarsson, I. (2006). Asymmetric female genitalia and other remarkable morphology in a new genus of cobweb spiders (Theridiidae, Araneae) from Madagascar. *Biological Journal of the Linnean Society*, **87**, 211–232.

Ahtiainen, J. J., Alatalo, R. V., Kortet, R. and Rantala, M. J. (2005). A trade-off between sexual signalling and immune function in a natural population of the drumming wolf spider *Hygrolycosa rubrofasciata*. *Journal of Evolutionary Biology*, **18**, 985–991.

Ahtiainen, J. J., Alatalo, R. V., Kortet, R. and Rantala, M. J. (2006). Immune function, dominance and mating success in drumming male wolf spiders *Hygrolycosa rubrofasciata*. *Behavioral Ecology and Sociobiology*, **60**, 826–832.

Ahtiainen, J. J., Alatalo, R. V., Mappes, J. and Vertainen, L. (2004). Decreased sexual signalling reveals reduced viability in small populations of the drumming wolf spider *Hygrolycosa rubrofasciata*. *Proceedings of the Royal Society of London, B*, **271**, 1839–1845.

Aisenberg, A. (2009). Male performance and body size affect female re-mating occurrence in the orb-web spider *Leucauge mariana* (Araneae, Tetragnathidae). *Ethology*, **115**, 1127–1136.

Aisenberg, A., Baruffaldi, L. and González, M. (2010). Behavioural evidence of male volatile pheromones in the sex-role reversed wolf spiders *Allocosa brasiliensis* and *Allocosa alticeps*. *Naturwissenschaften*, **97**, 63–70.

Aisenberg, A., Estramil, N., González, M., Toscano-Gadea, C. A. and Costa, F. G. (2008). Silk release by copulating *Schizocosa malitiosa* males (Araneae, Lycosidae): a bridal veil? *Journal of Arachnology*, **36**, 204–206.

Alatalo, R. V., Kotiaho, J., Mappes, J. and Parri, S. (1998). Mate choice for offspring performance: major benefits or minor costs? *Proceedings of the Royal Society of London, B*, **265**, 2297–2301.

Albo, M. J., Viera, C. and Costa, F. G. (2007). Pseudocopulation and male-male conflict elicited by subadult females of the subsocial spider *Anelosimus* cf. *studiosus*. (Theridiidae). *Behaviour*, **144**, 1217–1234.

Allan, R. A. and Elgar, M. A. (2001). Exploitation of the green tree ant, *Oecophylla smaragdina*, by the salticid spider *Cosmophasis bitaeniata*. *Australian Journal of Zoology*, **49**, 129–137.

Allan, R. A., Capon, R. J., Brown, W. V. and Elgar, M. A. (2002). Mimicry of host cuticular hydrocarbons by salticid spider *Cosmophasis bitaeniata* that preys on larvae of tree ants *Oecophylla smaragdina*. *Journal of Chemical Ecology*, **28**, 835–848.

Allan, R. A., Elgar, M. A. and Capon, R. J. (1996). Exploitation of an ant chemical alarm signal by the zodariid spider *Habronestes bradleyi* Walckenaer. *Proceedings of the Royal Society of London, B*, **263**, 69–73.

Almeida-Silva, L., Brescovit, A. and Griswold, C. E. (2009). On the poorly known genus *Anuvinda* Lehtinen, 1967 (Araneae, Titanoecidae). *Zootaxa*, **2266**, 61–68.

Anava, A. and Lubin, Y. (1993). Presence of gender cues in the web of a widow spider, *Latrodectus revivensis*, and a description of courtship behaviour. *Bulletin of the British Arachnological Society*, **9**, 119–122.

Andersson, M. (1994). *Sexual Selection*. Princeton, NJ: Princeton University Press.

Andrade, M. C. B. (1996). Sexual selection for male sacrifice in the Australian redback spider. *Science*, **271**, 70–72.

Andrade, M. C. B. (2003). Risky mate search and male self-sacrifice in redback spiders. *Behavioral Ecology*, **14**, 531–538.

Andrade, M. C. B. and Banta, E. M. (2002). Value of male remating and functional sterility in redback spiders. *Animal Behaviour*, **63**, 857–870.

Andrade, M. C. B. and Kasumovic, M. M. (2005). Terminal investment strategies and male mate choice: extreme tests of Bateman. *Integrative and Comparative Biology*, **45**, 838–847.

Andrews, K., Reed, S. M. and Masta, S. E. (2007). Spiders fluoresce variably across many taxa. *Biology Letters*, **3**, 265–267.

Arnedo, M. A., Hormiga, G. and Scharff, N. (2009). Higher-level phylognetics of linyphiid spiders (Araneae, Linyphiidae) based on morphological and molecular evidence. *Cladistics*, **25**, 1–32.

Arnqvist, G. (1992). Courtship behavior and sexual cannibalism in the semi-aquatic fishing spider, *Dolomedes fimbriatus* (Clerck) (Araneae: Pisauridae). *Journal of Arachnology*, **20**, 222–226.

Ayyagari, L. R. and Tietjen, W. J. (1986). Preliminary isolation of male-inhibitory pheromone of the spider *Schizocosa ocreata* (Araneae, Lycosidae). *Journal of Chemical Ecology*, **13**, 237–244.

Barth, F. G. (1967). Ein einzelnes Spaltsinnesorgan auf dem Spinnentarsus: seine Erregung in Abhängigkeit von den Parametern des Lustschallreizes. *Zeitschrift für vergleichende Physiologie*, **55**, 407–499.

Barth, F. G. (1982). Spiders and vibratory signals: sensory reception and behavioral significance. In *Spider Communication: Mechanism and Ecological Significance* (ed. P. N. Witt and J. S. Rovner). Princeton, NJ: Princeton University Press, pp. 67–122.

Barth, F. G. (1993). Sensory guidance in spider pre-copulatory behavior. *Comparative Biochemistry and Physiology, A*, **104**, 717–733.

Barth, F. G. (2002). *A Spider's World: Senses and Behavior.* Berlin: Springer Verlag.

Barth, F. G. and Geethabali (1982). Spider vibration receptors: threshold curves of individual slits in the metatarsal lyriform organ. *Journal of Comparative Physiology*, **148**, 175–185.

Barth, F. G. and Schmitt, A. (1991). Species recognition and species isolation in wandering spiders (*Cupiennius* spp.; Ctenidae). *Behavioral Ecology and Sociobiology*, **29**, 333–339.

Barth, F. G., Bleckmann, H., Bohnenberger, J. and Seyfarth, E.-A. (1988). Spiders of the genus *Cupiennius* Simon 1891 (Araneae, Ctenidae). II. On the vibratory environment of a wandering spider. *Oecologia*, **77**, 194–201.

Becker, E., Riechert, S. and Singer, F. (2005). Male induction of female quiescence/catalepsis during courtship in the spider *Agelenopsis aperta. Behaviour*, **142**, 57–70.

Bell, R. D., Rypstra, A. L. and Persons, M. H. (2006). The effect of predator hunger on chemically mediated antipredator responses and survival in the wolf spider *Pardosa milvina* (Araneae: Lycosidae). *Ethology*, **112**, 903–910.

Bertani, R., Fukushima, C. S. and da Silva, Jr., P. I. (2008). Mating behavior of *Sickius longibulbi* (Araneae, Theraphosidae, Ischnocolinae), a spider that lacks spermathecae. *Journal of Arachnology*, **36**, 331–335.

Bhaskara, R. M., Brijesh, C. M., Ahmed, S. and Borges, R. M. (2009). Perception of ultraviolet light by crab spiders and its role in selection of hunting sites. *Journal of Comparative Physiology, A*, **195**, 409–417.

Bilde, T. and Lubin, Y. (2001). Kin recognition and cannibalism in a subsocial spider. *Journal of Evolutionary Biology*, **14**, 959–966.

Bjorkman-Chiswell, B. T., Kulinski, M. M., Muscat, R. L., *et al.* (2004). Web-building spiders attract prey by storing decaying matter. *Naturwissenschaften*, **91**, 245–248.

Blanke, R. (1973). Nachweis von Pheromonen bei Netzspinnen. *Naturwissenschaften*, **60**, 481.

Blanke, R. (1975). Untersuchungen zum Sexualverhalten von *Cyrtophora cicatrosa* (Stoliczka) (Araneae, Araneidae). *Zeitschrift für Tierpsychologie*, **37**, 62–74.

Bleckmann, H. (1985). Discrimination between prey and non-prey wave signals in the fishing spider *Dolomedes triton* (Pisauridae). In *Acoustic and Vibrational Communication in Insects* (ed. K. Kalmring and N. Elsner). Berlin: Verlag Paul Parey, pp. 215–222.

Bleckmann, H. and Barth, F. G. (1984). Sensory ecology of a semi-aquatic spider (*Dolomedes triton*). II. The release of predatory behavior by water surface waves. *Behavioral Ecology and Sociobiology*, **14**, 303–312.

Bleckmann, H. and Bender, M. (1987). Water surface waves generated by the male pisaurid spider *Dolomedes triton* (Walckenaer) during courtship behaviour. *Journal of Arachnology*, **15**, 363–369.

Blest, A. D., Hardie, R. C., McIntyre, P. and Williams, D. S. (1981). The spectral sensitivities of identified receptors and the function of retinal tiering in the principal eyes of a jumping spider. *Journal of Comparative Physiology*, **145**, 227–239.

Blomquist, G. J. and Vogt, R. G. (2003). *Insect Pheromone Biochemistry and Molecular Biology: The Biosynthesis and Detection of Pheromones and Plant Volatiles*. Amsterdam, the Netherlands: Elsevier Academic Press.

Bossert, W. H. and Wilson, E. O. (1963). The analysis of olfactory communication among animals. *Journal of Theoretical Biology*, **5**, 443–469.

Bristowe, W. S. (1929). The mating habits of spiders, with special reference to the problems surrounding sex dimorphism. *Proceedings of the Zoological Society of London*, **1929**, 309–358.

Bristowe, W. S. (1939). *The Comity of Spiders*. London: The Ray Society.

Bristowe, W. S. and Locket, G. H. (1926). The courtship of British lycosid spiders, and its probable significance. *Proceedings of the Zoological Society of London*, **22**, 317–147.

Burgess, J. W. and Uetz, G. W. (1982). Social spacing strategies in spiders. In *Spider Communication: Mechanism and Ecological Significance* (ed. P. N. Witt and J. S. Rovner). Princeton, NJ: Princeton University Press, pp. 317–351.

Buskirk, R. (1975). Aggressive display and orb defense in a colonial spider, *Metabus gravidus*. *Animal Behaviour*, **23**, 560–567.

Candolin, U. (2003). The use of multiple cues in mate choice. *Biological Reviews*, **78**, 575–595.

Carico, J. E. (1973). The nearctic species of the genus *Dolomedes* (Araneae: Pisauridae). *Bulletin of the Museum of Comparative Zoology*, **144**, 435–488.

Chan, J. P. Y., Lau, P. R., Tham, A. J. and Li, D. Q. (2008). The effects of male-male contests and female eavesdropping on female mate choice and male mating success in the jumping spider, *Thiania bhamoensis* (Araneae: Salticidae). *Behavioral Ecology and Sociobiology*, **62**, 639–646.

Chinta, S. P., Goller, S., Lux, J., *et al.* (2010). The sex pheromone of the wasp spider *Argiope bruennichi*. *Angewandte Chemie International Edition*, **49**, 2033–2036.

Clark, D. L. (1992). Male dimorphism and species recognition in the jumping spider *Maevia inclemens* (Araneae: Salticidae). Cincinnati, OH: University of Cincinnati.

Clark, D. L. (1994). Sequence analysis of courtship behavior in the dimorphic jumping spider *Maevia inclemens* (Araneae, Salticidae). *Journal of Arachnology*, **22**, 94–107.

Clark, D. L. and Biesiadecki, B. (2002). Mating success and alternative reproductive strategies of the dimorphic jumping spider, *Maevia inclemens* (Araneae, Salticidae). *Journal of Arachnology*, **30**, 511–518.

Clark, D. L. and Morjan, C. L. (2001). Attracting female attention: the evolution of dimorphic courtship displays in the jumping spider *Maevia inclemens* (Araneae: Salticidae). *Proceedings of the Royal Society of London, B*, **268**, 2461–2465.

Clark, D. L. and Uetz, G. W. (1990). Video image recognition by the jumping spider, *Maevia inclemens* (Araneae: Salticidae). *Animal Behaviour*, **40**, 884–890.

Clark, D. L. and Uetz, G. W. (1993). Signal efficacy and the evolution of male dimorphism in the jumping spider, *Maevia inclemens*. *Proceedings of the National Academy of Sciences of the USA*, **90**, 11 954–11 957.

Clark, R. J. and Jackson, R. R. (1994). Self recognition in a jumping spider: *Portia labiata* females discriminate between their own draglines and those of conspecifics. *Ethology, Ecology and Evolution*, **6**, 371–375.

Clark, R. J. and Jackson, R. R. (1995a). Dragline-mediated sex recognition in two species of jumping spiders (Araneae, Salticidae), *Portia labiata* and *P. fimbriata*. *Ethology, Ecology and Evolution*, **7**, 73–77.

Clark, R. J. and Jackson, R. R. (1995b). Araneophagic spiders discriminate between the draglines of familiar and unfamiliar conspecifics. *Ethology, Ecology and Evolution*, **7**, 185–190.

Costa, F. G. and Francescoli, G. (1991). Analyse espérimentale de l'isolement reproductive entre deux espèces jumelles et sympatriques d'araignées: le *Lycosa thorelli* (Keyserling) et le *Lycosa carbonelli* Costa et Capocasale. *Canadian Journal of Zoology*, **69**, 1768–1776.

Crane, J. (1949). Comparative biology of salticid spiders at Rancho Grande, Venezuela. IV. An analysis of display. *Zoologica (Scientific Contributions to the New York Zoological Society)*, **34**, 159–214.

Cross, F. R. and Jackson, R. R. (2009a). How cross-modality effects during intraspecific interactions of jumping spiders differ depending on whether a female-choice or mutual-choice mating system is adopted. *Behavioural Processes*, **80**, 162–168.

Cross, F. R. and Jackson, R. R. (2009b). Mate-odour identification by both sexes of *Evarcha culicivora*, an East African jumping spider. *Behavioural Processes*, **81**, 74–79.

Cross, F. R., Jackson, R. R. and Pollard, S. D. (2007a). Male and female mate-choice decisions by *Evarcha culicivora*, an East African jumping spider. *Ethology*, **113**, 901–908.

Cross, F. R., Jackson, R. R. and Pollard, S. D. (2008). Complex display behaviour of *Evarcha culicivora*, an East African mosquito-eating jumping spider. *New Zealand Journal of Zoology*, **35**, 151–187.

Cross, F. R., Jackson, R. R. and Pollard, S. D. (2009). How blood-derived odor influences mate-choice decisions by a mosquito-eating predator. *Proceedings of the National Academy of Sciences of the USA*, **106**, 19 416–19 419.

Cross, F. R., Jackson, R. R., Pollard, S. D. and Walker, M. W. (2006). Influence of optical cues from conspecific females on escalation decisions during male-male interactions of jumping spiders. *Behavioural Processes*, **73**, 136–141.

Cross, F. R., Jackson, R. R., Pollard, S. D. and Walker, M. W. (2007b). Cross-modality effects during male-male interactions of jumping spiders. *Behavioural Processes*, **75**, 290–296.

Delaney, K. J., Roberts, J. A. and Uetz, G. W. (2007). Male signaling behavior and sexual selection in a wolf spider (Araneae: Lycosidae): a test for dual functions. *Behavioral Ecology and Sociobiology*, **62**, 67–75.

DeVoe, R. D. (1972). Dual sensitivities of cells in wolf spider eyes at ultraviolet and visible wavelengths of light. *Journal of General Physiology*, **59**, 247.

DeVoe, R. D. (1975). Ultraviolet and green receptors in principal eyes of jumping spiders. *Journal of General Physiology*, **66**, 193–207.

Dierkes, S. and Barth, F. G. (1995). Mechanism of signal production in the vibratory communication of the wandering spider *Cupiennius getazi* (Arachnida, Araneae). *Journal of Comparative Physiology, A*, **176**, 31–44.

Dondale, C. D. and Hegdekar, B. M. (1973). The contact sex pheromone of *Pardosa lapidicina* Emerton (Araneida: Lycosidae). *Canadian Journal of Zoology*, **52**, 400–401.

Dumortier, B. (1963). Sound emissions in Arthropoda. In *Acoustic Behavior of Animals* (ed. R. G. Busnel). Amsterdam, the Netherlands: Elsevier, 277–338.

Dumpert, K. (1978). Spider odor receptor: electrophysiological proof. *Experientia*, **34**, 754–756.

Eberhard, W. G. (1977). Aggressive chemical mimicry by a bolas spider. *Science*, **198**, 1173–1175.

Eberhard, W. G. (1991). *Chrosiothes tonala* (Araneae, Theridiidae): a web-building spider specializing on termites. *Psyche*, **98**, 7–20.

Eberhard, W. G. (1994). Evidence for widespread courtship during copulation in 131 species of insects and spiders, and implications for cryptic female choice. *Evolution*, **48**, 711–733.

Eberhard, W. G. (2004). Why study spider sex: special traits of spiders facilitate studies of sperm competition and cryptic female choice. *Journal of Arachnology*, **32**, 545–556.

Eberhard, W. G. and Huber, B. A. (1998). Courtship, copulation, and sperm transfer in *Leucauge mariana* (Araneae, Tetragnathidae) with implications for higher classification. *Journal of Arachnology*, **26**, 342–368.

Eberhard, W. G., Guzman Gomez, S. and Catley, K. M. (1993). Correlation between spermathecal morphology and mating systems in spiders. *Biological Journal of the Linnean Society*, **50**, 197–209.

Ehn, R. and Tichy, H. (1994). Hygro- and thermoreceptive tarsal organ in the spider *Cupiennius salei*. *Journal of Comparative Physiology, A*, **174**, 345–350.

Ehn, R. and Tichy, H. (1996a). Response characteristics of a spider warm cell: temperature sensitivities and structural properties. *Journal of Comparative Physiology, A*, **178**, 537–542.

Ehn, R. and Tichy, H. (1996b). Threshold for detecting temperature changes in a spider thermoreceptor. *Journal of Neurophysiology*, **76**, 2608–2613.

Eiben, B. and Persons, M. (2007). The effect of prior exposure to predator cues on chemically-mediated defensive behavior and survival in the wolf spider *Rabidosa rabida* (Araneae: Lycosidae). *Behaviour*, **144**, 889–906.

Elgar, M. A. (1992). Sexual cannibalism in spiders and other invertebrates. In *Cannibalism: Ecology and Evolution Among Diverse Taxa* (ed. M. A. Elgar and B. J. Crespi). Oxford, UK: Oxford University Press, pp. 128–155.

Elgar, M. A. and Allan, R. A. (2004). Predatory spider mimics aquire colony-specific cuticular hydrocarbons from their ant model prey. *Naturwissenschaften*, **91**, 143–147.

Elgar, M. A. and Allan, R. A. (2006). Chemical mimicry of the ant *Oecophylla smaragdina* by the myrmecophilous spider *Cosmophasis bitaeniata*: is it colony-specific? *Journal of Ethology*, **24**, 239–246.

Elias, D. O. and Mason, A. C. (in press). Signaling in variable environments: substrate-borne signaling mechanisms and communication behavior in spiders. In *The Use of Vibrations in Communication: Properties, Mechanisms and Function Across Taxa* (ed. C. O'Connell-Rodwell). Kerala, India: Research Signpost.

Elias, D. O., Hebets, E. A. and Hoy, R. R. (2006a). Female preference for complex/novel signals in a spider. *Behavioral Ecology*, **17**, 765–771.

Elias, D. O., Hebets, E. A., Hoy, R. R., Maddison, W. P. and Mason, A. C. (2006b). Regional seismic song differences in sky island populations of the jumping spider *Habronattus pugillis* Griswold (Araneae, Salticidae). *Journal of Arachnology*, **34**, 545–556.

Elias, D. O., Hebets, E. A., Hoy, R. R. and Mason, A. C. (2005). Seismic signals are crucial for male mating success in a visual specialist jumping spider (Araneae: Salticidae). *Animal Behaviour*, **69**, 931–938.

Elias, D. O., Kasumovic, M. M., Punzalan, D., Andrade, M. C. B. and Mason, A. C. (2008). Assessment during aggressive contests between male jumping spiders. *Animal Behaviour*, **76**, 901–910.

Elias, D. O., Land, B. R., Mason, A. C. and Hoy, R. R. (2006c). Measuring and quantifying dynamic visual signals in jumping spiders. *Journal of Comparative Physiology, A*, **192**, 785–797.

Elias, D. O., Lee, N., Hebets, E. A. and Mason, A. C. (2006d). Seismic signal production in a wolf spider: parallel versus serial multi-component signals. *Journal of Experimental Biology*, **209**, 1074–1084.

Elias, D. O., Mason, A. C., Maddison, W. P. and Hoy, R. R. (2003). Seismic signals in a courting male jumping spider (Araneae: Salticidae). *Journal of Experimental Biology*, **206**, 4029–4039.

Enders, F. (1975). Airborne pheromone probable in orb webs spider *Argiope aurantia* (Araneidae). *British Arachnological Society Newsletter*, **13**, 5–6.

Engelhardt, W. (1964). Die Mitteleuropäischen Arten der Gattung Trochosa C. L. Koch, 1848 (Araneae, Lycosidae). Morphologie, Chemotaxonomie, Biologie, Autökologie. *Zeitschrift für Morphologie und Ökologie der Tiere*, **54**, 219–392.

Evans, T. A. (1999). Kin recognition in a social spider. *Proceedings of the Royal Society of London, B*, **266**, 287–292.

Faber, D. B. and Baylis, J. R. (1993). Effects of body size on agonistic encounters between male jumping spiders (Araneae: Salticidae). *Animal Behaviour*, **45**, 289–299.

Fernández-Montraveta, C. and Ruano-Bellido, J. (2000). Female silk and mate attraction in a burrowing wolf-spider (Araneae, Lycosidae). *Bulletin of the British Arachnological Society*, **11**, 361–366.

Fernández-Montraveta, C., Moya-Laraño, J. and Orta-Ocaña, M. (2000). An SEM study on pedipalpal stridulation in Iberian lycosids (genera *Lycosa* and *Hogna*; Araneae, Lycosidae). *Bulletin of the British Arachnological Society*, **11**, 289–292.

Fischer, M. L., Cokl, A., Ramires, E. N., *et al.* (2009). Sound is involved in multimodal communication of *Loxosceles intermedia* Mell-Leitão, 1934 (Araneae; Sicariidae). *Behavioural Processes*, **82**, 236–243.

Foelix, R. F. (1970). Chemosensitive hairs in spiders. *Journal of Morphology*, **132**, 313–334.

Foelix, R. F. (1985). Mechano- and chemoreceptive sensilla. In *Neurobiology of Arachnids* (ed. F. G. Barth). Berlin: Springer Verlag, pp. 118–137.

Foelix, R. F. (1996). *The Biology of Spiders*, 2nd edn. New York: Oxford University Press.

Foelix, R. F. and Axtell, R. C. (1971). Fine structure of tarsal sensilla in the tick *Amblyomma americanum* (L.). *Zeitschrift für Zellforschung*, **114**, 22–37.

Foelix, R. F. and Chu-Wang, I.-W. (1973). The morphology of spider sensilla. II. Chemoreceptors. *Tissue and Cell*, **5**, 461–478.

Foelix, R. F., Chu-Wang, I.-W. and Beck, L. (1975). Fine structure of tarsal sensory organs in the whip spider *Admetus pumilo* (Amblypygi, Arachnida). *Tissue and Cell*, **7**, 331–346.

Forster, L. (1982a). Vision and prey-catching strategies in jumping spiders. *American Scientist*, **70**, 165–175.

Forster, L. (1982b). Visual communication in jumping spiders (Salticidae). In *Spider Communication: Mechanism and Ecological Significance* (ed. P. N. Witt and J. S. Rovner). Princeton, NJ: Princeton University Press, pp. 161–212.

Forster, L. (1995). The behavioural ecology of *Latrodectus hasselti* (Thorell), the Australian redback spider (Araneae: Theridiidae): a review. *Records of the Australian Museum, Supplement*, **52**, 13–24.

Forster, R. R. and Platnick, N. I. (1984). A review of the archaeid spiders and their relatives, with notes on the limits of the superfamily Palpimanoidea. *Bulletin of the American Museum of Natural History*, **178**, 1–106.

Forster, R., Platnick, N. and Coddington, J. (1990). A proposal and review of the spider family Synotaxidae (Araneae, Araneoidea), with notes on theridiid interrelationships. *Bulletin of the American Museum of Natural History*, **193**, 1–116.

Framenau, V. W. and Hebets, E. A. (2007). A review of leg ornamentation in male wolf spiders, with the description of a new species from Australia, *Artoria schizocoides* (Araneae, Lycosidae). *Journal of Arachnology*, **35**, 89–101.

Francke, W. and Schulz, S. (2010). Pheromones of terrestrial invertebrates. In *Comprehensive Natural Products Chemistry*, vol. 4, 2nd edn. (ed. K. Mori, L. Mander and H.-W.O. Liu). Amsterdam, the Netherlands: Elsevier, pp. 153–223.

Fratzl, P. and Barth, F. G. (2009). Biomaterial systems for mechanosensing and actuation. *Nature*, **462**, 442–448.

Frings, H. and Frings, M. (1966). Reactions of orb-weaving spiders (Argiopidae) to airborne sounds. *Ecology*, **47**, 578–588.

Gaskett, A. C. (2007). Spider sex pheromones: emission, reception, structures, and function. *Biological Reviews*, **82**, 27–48.

Gemeno, C., Yeargan, K. V. and Haynes, K. F. (2000). Aggressive chemical mimicry by the bolas spider *Mastophora hutchinsoni*: identification and quantification of a major prey's sex pheromone components in the spider's volatile emissions. *Journal of Chemical Ecology*, **26**, 1235–1243.

Gertsch, W. J. (1979). *American Spiders*. New York: Van Nostrand.

Gibson, J. S. and Uetz, G. W. (2008). Seismic communication and mate choice in wolf spiders: components of male seismic signals and mating success. *Animal Behaviour*, **75**, 1253–1262.

Gingl, E., Burger, A. M. and Barth, F. G. (2006). Intracellular recording from a spider vibration receptor. *Journal of Comparative Physiology, A*, **192**, 551–558.

Grasshoff, M. (1964). Die Kreuzspinne *Araneus pallidus*: ihr Netzbau und ihre Paarungsbiologie. *Natur und Museum*, **94**, 305–314.

Grismado, C. J. and Lopardo, L. (2003). Nuevos datos sobre la distribución geográfica de las familias australes de aranas Malkaridae y Mecysmaucheniidae (Arachnida: Araneae), con la descripción de la hembra de *Mecysmaucheniius thayerae* Forster and Platnick. *Revista Ibérica de Aracnología*, **8**, 37–43.

Griswold, C. E., Ramírez, M. J., Coddington, J. and Platnick, N. (2005). Atlas of phylogenetic data for entelegyne spiders (Araneae: Araneomorphae: Entelegynae) with comments on their phylogeny. *Proceedings of the California Academy of Sciences, 4th Series*, **56**, Supplement II, 1–324.

Gwinner-Hanke, H. (1970). Zum Verhalten zweier stridulierender Spinnen, *Steatoda bipunctata* Linné und *Teutana grossa* Koch (Theridiidae, Araneae), unter besonderer Berücksichtigung des Fortpflanzungsverhaltens. *Zeitschrift für Tierpsychologie*, **27**, 649–678.

Harari, A. R., Ziv, M. and Lubin, Y. (2009). Conflict or cooperation in the courtship display of the white widow spider, *Latrodectus pallidus*. *Journal of Arachnology*, **37**, 254–260.

Harland, D. P. and Jackson, R. R. (2001). Prey classification by *Portia fimbriata*, a salticid spider that specializes at preying on other salticids: species that elicit cryptic stalking. *Journal of Zoology*, **255**, 445–460.

Harland, D. P. and Jackson, R. R. (2002). Influence of cues from the anterior medial eyes of virtual prey on *Portia fimbriata*, an araneophagic jumping spider. *Journal of Experimental Biology*, **205**, 1861–1868.

Harris, D. J. and Mill, P. J. (1973). The ultrastructure of chemoreceptor sensilla in *Ciniflo* (Araneida, Arachnida). *Tissue and Cell*, **5**, 679.

Hebets, E. A. (2003). Subadult experience influences adult mate choice in an arthropod: exposed female wolf spiders prefer males of a familiar phenotype. *Proceedings of the National Academy of Sciences of the USA*, **100**, 13 390–13 395.

Hebets, E. A. (2005). Attention-altering signal interactions in the multimodal courtship display of the wolf spider *Schizocosa uetzi*. *Behavioral Ecology*, **16**, 75–82.

Hebets, E. A. (2008). Seismic signal dominance in the multimodal display of the wolf spider *Schizocosa stridulans*. Stratton 1991. *Behavioral Ecology*, **19**, 1250–1257.

Hebets, E. A. and Maddison, W. P. (2005). Xenophilic mating preferences among populations of the jumping spider *Habronattus pugillis* Griswold. *Behavioral Ecology*, **16**, 981–988.

Hebets, E. A. and Papaj, D. R. (2005). Complex signal function: developing a framework of testable hypotheses. *Behavioral Ecology and Sociobiology*, **57**, 197–214.

Hebets, E. A. and Uetz, G. W. (1999). Female responses to isolated signals from multimodal male courtship displays in the wolf spider genus *Schizocosa* (Aranerae: Lycosidae). *Animal Behaviour*, **57**, 865–872.

Hebets, E. A. and Uetz, G. W. (2000). Leg ornamentation and the efficacy of courtship display in four species of wolf spider (Araneae: Lycosidae). *Behavioral Ecology and Sociobiology*, **47**, 280–286.

Hebets, E. A. and Vink, C. J. (2007). Experience leads to preference: experienced females prefer brush-legged males in a population of syntopic wolf spiders. *Behavioral Ecology*, **18**, 1010–1020.

Hebets, E. A., Cuasay, K. and Rivlin, P. K. (2006). The role of visual ornamentation in female choice of a multimodal male courtship display. *Ethology*, **112**, 1062–1070.

Hebets, E. A., Elias, D. O., Mason, A. C., Miller, G. L. and Stratton, G. E. (2008). Substrate-dependent signalling success in the wolf spider, *Schizocosa retrorsa*. *Animal Behaviour*, **75**, 605–615.

Hegdekar, B. M. and Dondale, C. (1969). A contact sex pheromone and some response parameters in lycosid spiders. *Canadian Journal of Zoology*, **47**, 1–4.

Heiling, A. M., Cheng, K., Chittka, L., Goeth, A. and Herberstein, M. E. (2005a). The role of UV in crab spider signals: effects on perception by prey and predators. *Journal of Experimental Biology*, **208**, 3925–3931.

Heiling, A. M., Chittka, L., Cheng, K. and Herberstein, M. E. (2005b). Colouration in crab spiders: substrate choice and prey attraction. *Journal of Experimental Biology*, **208**, 1785–1792.

Henschel, J. R. (2002). Long-distance wandering and mating by the dancing white lady spider (*Leucorchestris arenicola*) (Araneae, Sparassidae) across Namib dunes. *Journal of Arachnology*, **30**, 321–330.

Hettyey, A., Hegyi, G., Puurtinen, M., *et al.* (2010). Mate choice for genetic benefits: time to put the pieces together. *Ethology*, **116**, 1–9.

Hill, D. E. (1979). Orientation by jumping spiders of the genus *Phidippus* (Araneae: Salticidae) during the pursuit of prey. *Behavioral Ecology and Sociobiology*, **5**, 301–322.

Hill, P. S. M. (2001). Vibration as a communication channel: a review. *American Zoologist*, **41**, 1135–1142.

Hill, P. S. M. (2008). *Vibrational Communication in Animals*. Cambridge, MA: Harvard University Press.

Hill, P. S. M. (2009). How do animals use substrate-borne vibrations as an information source? *Naturwissenschaften*, **96**, 1355–1371.

Hoefler, C. D. (2007). Male mate choice and size-assortative pairing in a jumping spider, *Phidippus clarus*. *Animal Behaviour*, **73**, 943–954.

Hoefler, C. D. and Jakob, E. M. (2006). Jumping spiders in space: movement patterns, nest site fidelity and the use of beacons. *Animal Behaviour*, **71**, 109–116.

Hoefler, C. D., Carlascio, A. L., Persons, M. H. and Rypstra, A. L. (2009a). Male courtship repeatability and potential indirect genetic benefits in a wolf spider. *Animal Behaviour*, **78**, 183–188.

Hoefler, C. D., Guhanarayan, G., Persons, M. H. and Rypstra, A. L. (2009b). The interaction of female condition and mating status on male-male aggression in a wolf spider. *Ethology*, **115**, 331–338.

Hoefler, C. D., Persons, M. H. and Rypstra, A. L. (2008). Evolutionarily costly courtship displays in a wolf spider: a test of viability indicator theory. *Behavioral Ecology*, **19**, 974–979.

Holden, W. (1977). Behavioral evidence of chemoreception on the legs of the spider *Araneus diadematus* Cl. *Journal of Arachnology*, **3**, 207–210.

Hölldobler, B. and Wilson, E. O. (1990). *The Ants*. Berlin: Springer.

Hrušková-Martišová, M., Pekár, S. and Gromov, A. (2008). Analysis of the stridulation in solifuges (Arachnida: Solifugae). *Journal of Insect Behaviour*, **21**, 440–449.

Hsu, Y. Y., Earley, R. L. and Wolf, L. L. (2006). Modulation of aggressive behaviour by fighting experience: mechanisms and contest outcomes. *Biological Review*, **81**, 33–74.

Huber, B. A. (2005). Sexual selection research on spiders: progress and biases. *Biological Reviews*, **80**, 363–385.

Huber, B. A. and Eberhard, W. G. (1997). Courtship, genitalia and genital mechanics in *Physocyclus globosus* (Araneae, Pholcidae). *Canadian Journal of Zoology*, **74**, 905–918.

Iwasa, Y. and Pomiankowski, A. (1994). The evolution of mate preferences for multiple sexual ornaments. *Evolution*, **48**, 853–867.

Jackson, R. R. (1977). Courtship versitility in the jumping spider, *Phidippus johnsoni* (Araneae: Salticidae). *Animal Behaviour*, **25**, 953–957.

Jackson, R. R. (1982). The behavior of communicating in jumping spiders (Salticidae). In *Spider Communication: Mechanism and Ecological Significance* (ed. P. N. Witt and J. S. Rovner). Princeton, NJ: Princeton University Press, pp. 213–247.

Jackson, R. R. (1983). The biology of *Mopsus mormon*, a jumping spider (Araneae, Salticidae) from Queensland: intraspecific interactions. *Australian Journal of Zoology*, **31**, 39–53.

Jackson, R. R. (1986a). Interspecific interactions of communal jumping spiders (Araneae, Salticidae) from Kenya: mechanisms of sex- and species-recognition. *Behaviour*, **97**, 297–307.

Jackson, R. R. (1986b). Use of pheromones by males of *Phidippus johnsoni* (Araneae, Salticidae) to detect subadult females that are about to molt. *Journal of Arachnology*, **14**, 137–139.

Jackson, R. R. (1987). Comparative study of releaser pheromones associated with the silk of jumping spiders (Araneae, Salticidae). *New Zealand Journal of Zoology*, **14**, 1–10.

Jackson, R. R. and Macnab, A. M. (1991). Comparative study of the display and mating behavior of lyssomanine jumping spiders (Araneae: Salticidae), especially *Asemonea tenuipes*, *Goleba puella*, and *Lyssomanes viridis*. *New Zealand Journal of Zoology*, **18**, 1–23.

Jackson, R. R. and Pollard, S. D. (1997). Jumping spider mating strategies: sex among cannibals in and out of webs. In *Mating Systems in Insects and Arachnids* (ed. J. Choe and B. Crespi). Cambridge, UK: Cambridge University Press, pp. 340–351.

Jackson, R. R., Clark, R. J. and Harland, D. P. (2002). Behavioural and cognitive influences of kairomones on an araneophagic jumping spider. *Behaviour*, **139**, 749–775.

Jackson, R. R., Nelson, X. J. and Sune, G. O. (2005). A spider that feeds indirectly on vertebrate blood by choosing female mosquitoes as prey. *Proceedings of the National Academy of Sciences of the USA*, **102**, 15 155–15 160.

Jackson, R. R., Walker, M. W., Pollard, S. D. and Cross, F. R. (2006). Influence of seeing a female on the male-male interactions of a jumping spider, *Hypoblemum albovittatum*. *Journal of Ethology*, **24**, 231–238.

Jakob, E. M., Skow, C. D., Haberman, M. P. and Plourde, A. (2007). Jumping spiders associate food with color cues in a T-maze. *Journal of Arachnology*, **35**, 487–492.

Jerhot, E., Stoltz, J. A., Andrade, M. C. B. and Schulz, S. (2010). Acylated serine derivative: a new class of arthropod pheromones of the Australian redback spider, *Latrodectus hasselti*. *Angewandte Chemie International Edition*, **49**, 1–5.

Jocqué, R. (2005). Six stridulating organs on one spider (Araneae, Zodariidae): is this the limit? *Journal of Arachnology*, **33**, 597–603.

Johansson, B. G. and Jones, T. M. (2007). The role of chemical communication in mate choice. *Biological Reviews*, **82**, 265–289.

Johnstone, R. A. (1996). Multiple displays in animal communication: 'Backup signals' and 'multiple messages'. *Philosophical Transactions of the Royal Society of London, B*, **351**, 329–338.

Kaston, B. J. (1936). The senses involved in the courtship of some vagabond spiders. *Entomologica Americana*, **16**, 97–167.

Kasumovic, M. M. and Andrade, M. C. B. (2004). Discrimination of airborne pheromones by mate-searching male western black widow spiders (*Latrodectus hesperus*): species- and population-specific responses. *Canadian Journal of Zoology*, **82**, 1027–1034.

Kasumovic, M. M. and Andrade, M. C. B. (2006). Male development tracks rapidly shifting sexual versus natural selection pressures. *Current Biology*, **16**, R242.

Kasumovic, M. M., Elias, D. O., Punzalan, D., Mason, A. C. and Andrade, M. C. B. (2009a). Experience affects the outcome of agonistic contests without affecting the selective advantage of size. *Animal Behaviour*, **77**, 1533–1538.

Kasumovic, M. M., Elias, D. O., Punzalan, D., Mason, A. C. and Andrade, M. C. B. (2009b). The role of multiple experiences on contest outcome and patterns of selection in a jumping spider. *Animal Behaviour*, **77**, 1533–1538.

Keller, L. R. (1961). Untersuchungen über den Geruchssinn der Spinnenart *Cupiennius salei* Keyserling. *Zeitschrift für Vergleichende Physiologie*, **44**, 576–612.

Knoflach, B. and Pfaller, K. (2004). Comb-footed spiders: an introduction (Araneae, Theridiidae). *Denisia*, 111–160.

Koh, T. H., Seah, W. K., Yap, L.-M. Y. L. and Li, D. (2009). Pheromone-bases female mate choice and its effect on reproductive investment in a spitting spider. *Behavioral Ecology and Sociobiology*, **63**, 923–930.

Kotiaho, J. S., Alatalo, R. V., Mappes, J., *et al.* (1998). Energetic costs of size and sexual signalling in a wolf spider. *Proceedings of the Royal Society of London, B*, **265**, 2203–2209.

Kotiaho, J. S., Alatalo, R. V., Mappes, J. and Parri, S. (1996). Sexual selection in a wolf spider: male drumming activity, body size and viability. *Evolution*, **50**, 1977–1981.

Kotiaho, J. S., Alatalo, R. V., Mappes, J. and Parri, S. (1999). Sexual signalling and viability in a wolf spider (*Hygrolycosa rubrofasciata*): measurements under laboratory and field conditions. *Behavioral Ecology and Sociobiology*, **46**, 123–128.

Kotiaho, J. S., Alatalo, R. V., Mappes, J. and Parri, S. (2000). Microhabitat selection and audible sexual signalling in the wolf spider *Hygrolycosa rubrofasciata* (Araneae, Lycosidae). *Acta Ethologica*, **2**, 123–128.

Kovoor, J. (1981). Une source probable de phéromones sexuelles: les glandes tégumentaires de la région génitale des femelles d'araignées. *Atti della Società Toscana di Scienze Naturali, Memorie, B, Suppl.*, **88**, 1–15.

Koyanagi, M., Nagata, T., Katoh, K., Yamashita, S. and Tokunaga, F. (2008). Molecular evolution of arthropod color vision deduced from multiple opsin genes of jumping spiders. *Journal of Molecular Evolution*, **66**, 130–137.

Krafft, B. (1978). The recording of vibratory signals performed by spiders during courtship. *Symposia of the Zoological Society of London*, **42**, 59–67.

Krafft, B. (1982). The significance and complexity of communication in spiders. In *Spider Communication: Mechanism and Ecological Significance* (ed. P. N. Witt and J. S. Rovner). Princeton, NJ: Princeton University Press, pp. 15–65.

Krafft, B. and Roland, C. (1980). Quelques remarques au sujet de communication chimique chez les araignées. *Comptes Rendus du Colloque Arachnologique IX*. Barcelona, Spain: University of Barcelona, pp. 129–135.

Kronestedt, T. (1979). Study on chemosensitive hairs in wolf spiders (Araneae, Lycosidae) by scanning electron microscopy. *Zoologica Scripta*, **8**, 279–285.

Kronestedt, T. (1984). Ljudalstring hos vargspindeln *Hygrolycosa rubrofasciata*. *Fauna Flora (Stockholm)*, **79**, 97–107.

Kronestedt, T. (1986). A presumptive pheromone-emitting structure in wolf spiders (Araneae, Lycosidae). *Psyche*, **93**, 127–131.

Kronestedt, T. (1996). Vibratory communication in the wolf spider *Hygrolycosa rubrofasciata*. *Revue Suisse de Zoologie*, 341–354.

Kullmann, E. and Zimmermann, W. (1972). Versuche zur Toleranz bei der permanent sozialen Spinnenart *Stegodyphus sarasinorum* Karsch (Fam. Eresidae). In *Proceedings of 5th International Congress of Arachnology, Brno, 1971*. Berlin: International Society of Arachnology, pp. 175–182.

Land, M. F. (1972). The physics and biology of animal reflectors. *Progress in Biophysics and Molecular Biology*, **24**, 75–106.

Land, M. F. (1985). The morphology and optics of spider eyes. In *Neurobiology of Arachnids* (ed. F. G. Barth). Berlin: Springer Verlag, pp. 53–78.

Land, M. F. and Nilsson, D. E. (2002). *Animal Eyes*. Oxford, UK: Oxford University Press.

Land, M. F., Lim, M. L. M. and Li, D. (2007). Optics of the ultra-violet reflecting scales of a jumping spider. *Proceedings of the Royal Society of London, B*, **274**, 1583–1589.

Legendre, R. (1963). L'audition et l'émission de sons chez les aranéides. *Annales Biologiques*, **2**, 371–390.

Li, J. J., Lim, M. L. M, Zhang, Z. T., *et al.* (2008a). Sexual dichromatism and male colour morph in ultraviolet-B reflectance in two populations of the jumping spider

Phintella vittata (Araneae: Salticidae) from tropical China. *Biological Journal of the Linnean Society*, **94**, 7–20.

Li, J. J., Zhang, Z. T., Liu, F. X., *et al.* (2008b). UVB-based mate-choice cues used by females of the jumping spider *Phintella vittata. Current Biology*, **18**, 699–703.

Lim, M. L. M. and Li, D. (2004). Courtship and male–male agonistic behaviour of *Cosmophasis umbratica* Simon, an ornate jumping spider (Araneae: Salticidae) from Singapore. *Raffles Bulletin of Zoology*, **52**, 435–448.

Lim, M. L. M. and Li, D. (2006a). Extreme ultraviolet sexual dimorphism in jumping spiders (Araneae: Salticidae). *Biological Journal of the Linnean Society*, **89**, 397–406.

Lim, M. L. M. and Li, D. Q. (2006b). Behavioural evidence of UV sensitivity in jumping spiders (Araneae: Salticidae). *Journal of Comparative Physiology, A*, **192**, 871–878.

Lim, M. L. M. and Li, D. Q. (2007). Effects of age and feeding history on structure-based UV ornaments of a jumping spider (Araneae: Salticidae). *Proceedings of the Royal Society of London, B*, **274**, 569–575.

Lim, M. L. M., Land, M. F. and Li, D. Q. (2007). Sex-specific UV and fluorescence signals in jumping spiders. *Science*, **315**, 481.

Lim, M. L. M., Li, J. and Li, D. (2008). Effect of UV-reflecting markings on female mate-choice decisions in *Cosmophasis umbratica*, a jumping spider from Singapore. *Behavioral Ecology*, **19**, 61–66.

Lindemann, B. (1996). Taste reception. *Physiological Reviews*, **76**, 719–766.

Lindstrom, L., Ahtiainen, J. J., Mappes, J., *et al.* (2006). Negatively condition dependent predation cost of a positively condition dependent sexual signalling. *Journal of Evolutionary Biology*, **19**, 649–656.

Lizotte, R. and Rovner, J. S. (1989). Water-resistant sex pheromones in lycosid spiders from a tropical wet forest. *Journal of Arachnology*, **17**, 122–125.

Lohrey, A. K., Clark, D. L., Gordon, S. D. and Uetz, G. W. (2009). Antipredator responses of wolf spiders (Araneae: Lycosidae) to sensory cues representing an avian predator. *Animal Behaviour*, **77**, 813–821.

Lomborg, J. P. and Toft, S. (2009). Nutritional enrichment increases courtship intensity and improves mating success in male spiders. *Behavioral Ecology*, **20**, 700–708.

Lopez, A. (1987). Glandular aspects of sexual biology. In *Ecophysiology of Spiders* (ed. W. Nentwig). Heidelberg, Germany: Springer, pp. 121–141.

Lubin, Y. (1986). Courtship and alternative mating tactics in a social spider. *Journal of Arachnology*, **14**, 239–257.

Lubin, Y. and Bilde, T. (2007). The evolution of sociality in spiders. *Advances in the Study of Behavior*, **37**, 83–145.

Lynam, E. C., Owens, J. C. and Persons, M. H. (2006). The influence of pedipalp autotomy on the courtship and mating behavior of *Pardosa milvina* (Araneae: Lycosidae). *Journal of Insect Behaviour*, **19**, 63–75.

Maddison, W. and McMahon, M. (2000). Divergence and reticulation among montane populations of a jumping spider (*Habronattus pugillis* Griswold). *Systematic Biology*, **49**, 400–421.

Maddison, W. P. and Stratton, G. E. (1988a). A common method of sound production by courting male jumping spiders (Araneae, Salticidae). *Journal of Arachnology*, **16**, 267–269.

Maddison, W. P. and Stratton, G. E. (1988b). Sound production and associated morphology in male jumping spiders of the *Habronattus agilis* species group (Araneae, Salticidae). *Journal of Arachnology*, **16**, 199–211.

Maklakov, A. A., Bilde, T. and Lubin, Y. (2003). Vibratory courtship in a web-building spider: signalling quality or stimulating the female? *Animal Behaviour*, **66**, 623–630.

Mappes, J., Alatalo, R. V., Kotiaho, J. and Parri, S. (1996). Viability costs of condition-dependent sexual male display in a drumming wolf spider. *Proceedings of the Royal Society of London, B*, **263**, 785–789.

Marshall, S. D., Thoms, E. M. and Uetz, G. W. (1995). Setal entanglement: an undescribed method of stridulation by a neotropical tarantula (Araneae, Theraphosidae). *Journal of Zoology*, **235**, 587–595.

Masta, S. E. and Maddison, W. P. (2002). Sexual selection driving diversification in jumping spiders. *Proceedings of the National Academy of Sciences of the USA*, **99**, 4442–4447.

Maynard Smith, J. and Harper, D. (2005). *Animal Signals*. New York: Oxford University Press.

Mayr, E. (1974). *Populations, Species, and Evolution*. Cambridge, MA: Harvard University Press.

McClintock, W. J. and Uetz, G. W. (1996). Female choice and pre-existing bias: visual cues during courtship in two *Schizocosa* wolf spiders (Araneae: Lycosidae). *Animal Behaviour*, **52**, 67–181.

Michelsen, A., Fink, F., Gogala, M. and Traue, D. (1982). Plants as transmission channels for insect vibrational songs. *Behavioural Ecology and Sociobiology*, **11**, 269–281.

Miller, G. L. and Miller, P. R. (1987). Life cycle and courtship behavior of the burrowing wolf spider *Geolycosa turricola* (Treat) (Araneae, Lycosidae). *Journal of Arachnology*, **15**, 385–394.

Miyashita, T. and Hayashi, H. (1996). Volatile chemical cue elicits mating behavior of cohabiting males of *Nephila clavata* (Araneae, Tetragnathidae). *Journal of Arachnology*, **24**, 9–15.

Møller, A. P. and Pomiankowski, A. (1993). Why have birds got multiple sexual ornaments? *Behavioral Ecology and Sociobiology*, **32**, 167–176.

Morris, G. K. (1980). Calling display and mating behavior of *Copiphora rhinoceros pictet* (Orthoptera, Tettigoniidae). *Animal Behaviour*, **28**, 42–51.

Nakamura, T. and Yamashita, S. (2000). Learning and discrimination of colored papers in jumping spiders (Araneae, Salticidae). *Journal of Comparative Physiology, A*, **186**, 897–901.

Nelson, X. J. and Jackson, R. R. (2007). Complex display behaviour during the intraspecific interactions of myrmecomorphic jumping spiders (Araneae, Salticidae). *Journal of Natural History*, **41**, 1659–1678.

Nelson, X. J. and Jackson, R. R. (2009). Prey classification by an araneophagic ant-like jumping spider (Araneae: Salticidae). *Journal of Zoology*, **279**, 173–179.

Nessler, S. H., Uhl, G. and Schneider, J. M. (2009). Scent of a woman: the effect of female presence on sexual cannibalism in an orb-weaving spider (Araneae: Araneidae). *Ethology*, **115**, 633–640.

Neuhofer, D., Machan, R. and Schmid, A. (2009). Visual perception of motion in a hunting spider. *Journal of Experimental Biology*, **212**, 2819–2823.

Nørgaard, T., Nilsson, D. E., Henschel, J. R., Garm, A. and Wehner, R. (2008). Vision in the nocturnal wandering spider *Leucorchestris arenicola* (Araneae: Sparassidae). *Journal of Experimental Biology*, **211**, 816–823.

Olive, C. W. (1982). Sex pheromones in two orbweaving spiders (Araneae, Araneidae): an experimental field study. *Journal of Arachnology*, **10**, 241–245.

Oxford, G. S. and Gillespie, R. G. (1998). Evolution and ecology of spider coloration. *Annual Review of Entomology*, **43**, 619–643.

Papke, M., Schulz, S., Tichy, H., Gingl, H. and Ehn, R. (2000). Identification of a new sex pheromone from the silk dragline of the tropical wandering spider *Cupiennius salei*. *Angewandte Chemie International Edition*, **39**, 4339–4341.

Papke, M. D., Riechert, S. E. and Schulz, S. (2001). An airborne female pheromone associated with male attraction and courtship in a desert spider. *Animal Behaviour*, **61**, 877–886.

Parker, A. R. and Hegedus, Z. (2003). Diffractive optics in spiders. *Journal of Optics, A*, **5**, S111–S116.

Parri, S., Alatalo, R. V., Kotiaho, J. and Mappes, J. (1997). Female choice for male drumming in the wolf spider *Hygrolycosa rubrofasciata*. *Animal Behaviour*, **53**, 305–312.

Parri, S., Alatalo, R. V., Kotiaho, J. S., Mappes, J. and Rivero, A. (2002). Sexual selection in the wolf spider *Hygrolycosa rubrofasciata*: female preference for drum duration and pulse rate. *Behavioral Ecology*, **13**, 615–621.

Partan, S. R. and Marler, P. (1999). Communication goes multimodal. *Science*, **283**, 1272–1273.

Partan, S. R. and Marler, P. (2005). Issues in the classification of multimodal communication signals. *American Naturalist*, **166**, 231–245.

Peaslee, A. G. and Wilson, G. (1989). Spectral sensitivity in jumping spiders (Araneae, Salticidae). *Journal of Comparative Physiology, A*, **164**, 359–363.

Perampaladas, K., Stoltz, J. A. and Andrade, M. C. B. (2008). Mated redback spider females re-advertise receptivity months after mating. *Ethology*, **114**, 589–598.

Peretti, A. V. and Eberhard, W. G. (2010). Cryptic female choice via sperm dumping favours male copulatory courtship in a spider. *Journal of Evolutionary Biology*, **23**, 271–281.

Peretti, A., Eberhard, W. G. and Briceno, R. D. (2006). Copulatory dialogue: female spiders sing during copulation to influence male genitalic movements. *Animal Behaviour*, **72**, 413–421.

Pérez-Miles, F., de Oca, L. M., Postigliioni, R. and Costa, F. G. (2005). The stridulatory setae of *Acanthoscurria suina* (Araneae, Theraphosidae) and their possible role in sexual communication: an experimental approach. *Iheringia, Série Zoologia*, **95**, 365–371.

Pérez-Miles, F., Lucas, S. M., da Silva Junior, P. I. and Bertani, R. (1996). Systematic revision and cladistic analysis of Theraphosinae (Araneae: Theraphosidae). *Mygalomorph*, **1**, 33–68.

Persons, M. H. and Uetz, G. W. (2005). Sexual cannibalism and mate choice decisions in wolf spiders: influence of male size and secondary sexual characters. *Animal Behaviour*, **69**, 83–94.

Persons, M. H., Walker, S. E. and Rypsta, A. L. (2002). Fitness costs and benefits of antipredator behavior mediated by chemotactic cues in the wolf spider *Pardosa milvina* (Araneae: Lycosidae). *Behavioral Ecology*, **13**, 386–392.

Pocock, R. I. (1895a). Musical boxes in spiders. *Natural Science, London*, **6**, 44–50.

Pocock, R. I. (1895b). On a new sound-producing organ in a spider. *Annals and Magazine of Natural History*, **16**, 230–233.

Pocock, R. I. (1899). A new stridulating theraphosid spider from South America. *Annals and Magazine of Natural History*, **3**, 347–349.

Pollard, S. D., Macnab, A. M. and Jackson, R. R. (1987). Communication with chemicals: pheromones and spiders. In *Ecophysiology of Spiders* (ed. W. Nentwig). Heidelberg, Germany: Springer Verlag, pp. 133–141.

Pomiankowski, A. and Iwasa, Y. (1993). Evolution of multiple sexual preferences by Fisher runaway process of sexual selection. *Proceedings of the Royal Society of London, B*, **253**, 173–181.

Pourié, G., Ibarra, F., Franke, W. and Trabalon, M. (2005). Fatty acids mediate aggressive behavior in the spider *Tegenaria atrica*. *Chemoecology*, **15**, 161–166.

Prenter, J., Elwood, R. W. and Montgomery, W. J. (1994). Assessments and decisions in *Metellina segmentata* (Araneae: Metidae): evidence of a pheromone involved in mate guarding. *Behavioral Ecology and Sociobiology*, **35**, 39–43.

Prouvost, O., Trabalon, M., Papke, M. and Schulz, S. (1999). Contact sex signals on web and cuticle of *Tegenaria atrica* (Araneae, Agelenidae). *Archives of Insect Biochemistry and Physiology*, **40**, 194–202.

Pruitt, J. N. and Riechert, S. E. (2009). Male mating preference is associated with risk of pre-copulatory cannibalism in a socially polymorphic spider. *Behavioral Ecology and Sociobiology*, **63**, 1573–1580.

Ramírez, M. J., Lopardo, L. and Bonaldo, A. B. (2001). A review of the Chilean spider genus *Olbus*, with notes on the relationships of the Corinnidae (Arachnida, Araneae). *Insect Systematics and Evolution*, **31**, 441–462.

Reyes-Alcubilla, C., Ruiz, M. A. and Ortega-Escobar, J. (2009). Homing in the wolf spider *Lycosa tarantula* (Araneae, Lycosidae): the role of active locomotion and visual landmarks. *Naturwissenschaften*, **96**, 485–494.

Richman, D. B. (1982). Epigamic display in jumping spiders (Araneae, Salticidae) and its use in systematics. *Journal of Arachnology*, **10**, 47–67.

Richter, C. J. J., Stolting, C. J. and Vlijm, L. (1971). Silk production in adult females of the wolf spider *Pardosa amentata* (Lycosidae, Araneae). *Journal of Zoology*, **165**, 285–290.

Riechert, S. E. (1978). Games spiders play: behavioral variability in territorial disputes. *Behavioral Ecology and Sociobiology*, **3**, 135–162.

Riechert, S. E. (1979). Games spiders play. II. Resource assessment strategies. *Behavioral Ecology and Sociobiology*, **6**, 121–128.

Riechert, S. E. (1988). Game theory and animal conflict. In *Game Theory and Animal Behavior* (ed. L. A. Dugatkin and H. K. Reeve). New York: Oxford University Press, pp. 64–93.

Riechert, S. E. and Jones, T. C. (2008). Phenotypic variation in the social behaviour of the spider *Anelosimus studiosus* along a latitudinal gradient. *Animal Behaviour*, **75**, 1893–1902.

Riechert, S. E. and Singer, F. D. (1995). Investigation of potential mate choice in a monogamous spider. *Animal Behaviour*, **49**, 715–723.

Rivero, A., Alatalo, R. V., Kotiaho, J. S., Mappes, J. and Parri, S. (2000). Acoustic signalling in a wolf spider: can signal characteristics predict male quality? *Animal Behaviour*, **48**, 188–194.

Robbins, P. S., Nojima, S., Polavarapu, S., *et al.* (2009). Sex pheromone of the scarab beetle *Phyllophaga* (*Phytalus*) *georgiana* (Horn). *Journal of Chemical Ecology*, **35**, 336–341.

Roberts, J. A. and Uetz, G. W. (2004a). Chemical signaling in a wolf spider: a test of ethospecies discrimination. *Journal of Chemical Ecology*, **30**, 1271–1283.

Roberts, J. A. and Uetz, G. W. (2004b). Species-specificity of chemical signals: silk source affects discrimination in a wolf spider (Araneae: Lycosidae). *Journal of Insect Behavior*, **17**, 477–491.

Roberts, J. A., Taylor, P. W. and Uetz, G. W. (2007). Consequences of complex signaling: predator detection of multimodal cues. *Behavioral Ecology*, **18**, 236–240.

Robinson, M. B. and Robinson, B. (1980). Comparative studies of the courtship and mating behavior of tropical araneid spiders. *Pacific Insects Monograph*, **36**, 1–218.

Roland, C. (1984). Chemical signals bound to the silk in spider communication (Arachnida, Araneae). *Journal of Arachnology*, **11**, 309–314.

Roland, C. and Rovner, J. S. (1983). Chemical and vibratory communication in the aquatic pisaurid spider *Dolomedes triton* (Araneae: Pisauridae). *Journal of Arachnology*, **11**, 77–85.

Ross, K. and Smith, R. L. (1979). Aspects of courtship behavior of the black widow spider, *Latrodectus hesperus* (Araneae: Theridiidae) with evidence for the existence of a contact sex pheromone. *Journal of Arachnology*, **7**, 69–77.

Rovner, J. S. (1967). Acoustic communication in lycosid spider (*Lycosa rabida* Walckenaer). *Animal Behaviour*, **15**, 273–281.

Rovner, J. S. (1968). Territoriality in the sheet-web spider *Linyphia triangularis* (Clerck) (Araneae, Linyphiidae). *Zeitschschrift für Tierpsychologie*, **25**, 232–242.

Rovner, J. S. (1975). Sound production by nearctic wolf spiders: substratum-coupled stridulatory mechanism. *Science*, **190**, 1309–1310.

Rovner, J. S. (1980). Vibration in *Heteropoda venatoria* (Sparassidae): a 3rd method of sound production in spiders. *Journal of Arachnology*, **8**, 193–200.

Rovner, J. S. and Barth, F. G. (1981). Vibratory communication through living plants by a tropical wandering spider. *Science*, **214**, 464–466.

Rowe, C. (1999). Receiver psychology and the evolution of multicomponent signals. *Animal Behaviour*, **58**, 921–931.

Rundus, A. S., Santer, R. D. and Hebets, E. A. (2010). Multimodal courtship efficacy of *Schizocosa retrorsa* wolf spiders: implications of an additional signal modality. *Behavioural Ecology*, **21**, 701–707.

Rypstra, A. L., Schlosser, A. M., Sutton, P. L. and Persons, M. H. (2009). Multimodal signalling: the relative importance of chemical and visual cues from females to the behaviour of male wolf spiders (Lycosidae). *Animal Behaviour*, **77**, 937–947.

Rypstra, A. L., Wieg, C., Walker, S. E. and Persons, M. H. (2003). Mutual mate assessment in wolf spiders: differences in the cues used by males and females. *Ethology*, **109**, 315–325.

Santer, R. D. and Hebets, E. A. (2008). Agonistic signals received by an arthropod filiform hair allude to the prevalence of near-field sound communication. *Proceedings of the Royal Society of London, B*, **275**, 363–368.

Schäfer, M. A. and Uhl, G. (2002). Determinants of paternity success in the spider *Pholcus phalangioides* (Pholcidae: Araneae): the role of male and female mating behavior. *Behavioral Ecology and Sociobiology*, **51**, 368–377.

Schäfer, M. A., Misof, B. and Uhl, G. (2008). Effects of body size of both sexes and female mating history on male mating behavior and paternity success in a spider. *Animal Behaviour*, **76**, 75–86.

Schaible, U. and Gack, C. (1987). Zur Bedeutung der Kopfstrukturen bei einigen *Diplocephalus* – Arten (Erigoninae, Linyphiidae). *Abhandlungen des Naturwissenschaftlichen Vereins in Hamburg (NF)*, **9**, 171–180.

Scheffer, S. J., Uetz, G. W. and Stratton, G. E. (1996). Sexual selection, male morphology, and the efficacy of courtship signalling in two wolf spiders (Araneae: Lycosidae). *Behavioral Ecology and Sociobiology*, **38**, 17–23.

Schlegelmilch, B. (1974). Zur biologischen Bedeutung der Kopffortsätze bei Zwergspinnenmännchen (Micryphantidae). Diploma thesis. University of Freiburg, Germany.

Schmid, A. (1998). Different functions of different eye types in the spider *Cupiennius salei*. *Journal of Experimental Biology*, **201**, 221–225.

Schmitt, A., Friedel, T. and Barth, F. G. (1993). Importance of pause between spider courtship vibrations and general problems using synthetic stimuli in behavioural studies. *Journal of Comparative Physiology, A*, **172**, 707–714.

Schmitt, A., Schuster, M. and Barth, F. G. (1992). Male competition in a wandering spider (*Cupiennius getazi*, Ctenidae). *Ethology*, **90**, 293–306.

Schonewolf, K. W., Bell, R., Rypstra, A. L. and Persons, M. H. (2006). Field evidence of an airborne enemy avoidance kairomone in wolf spiders. *Journal of Chemical Ecology*, **32**, 1565–1576.

Schuch, W. and Barth, F. G. (1985). Temporal patterns in the vibratory courtship signals of the wandering spider *Cupiennius salei* Keys. *Behavioral Ecology and Sociobiology*, **16**, 263–271.

Schuch, W. and Barth, F. G. (1990). Vibratory communication in a spider: female responses to synthetic male vibrations. *Journal of Comparative Physiology, A*, **166**, 817–826.

Schulz, S. (1997). The chemistry of spider toxins and spider silk. *Angewandte Chemie International Edition in English*, **36**, 314–326.

Schulz, S. (2004). Semiochemistry of spiders. In *Advances in Insect Chemical Ecology* (ed. R. T. Cardé and J. G. Miller). Cambridge, UK: Cambridge University Press, pp. 110–150.

Schulz, S. and Toft, S. (1993). Identification of a sex pheromone from a spider. *Science*, **260**, 1635–1637.

Segoli, M., Harari, A. R. and Lubin, Y. (2006). Limited mating opportunities and male monogamy: a field study of white widow spiders, *Latrodectus pallidus* (Theridiidae). *Animal Behaviour*, **72**, 635–642.

Shamble, P. S., Wilgers, D. J., Swoboda, K. A. and Hebets, E. A. (2009). Courtship effort is a better predictor of mating success than ornamentation for male wolf spiders. *Behavioral Ecology*, **20**, 1242–1251.

Sheldon, B. C. (2000). Differential allocation: tests, mechanisms and implications. *Trends in Ecology and Evolution*, **15**, 397–402.

Shorey, H. (1976). *Animal Communication by Pheromones*. New York: Academic Press.

Singer, F. and Riechert, S. E. (1994). Tests for sex differences in fitness-linked traits in the spider *Agelenopsis aperta* (Araneae: Agelenidae). *Journal of Insect Behavior*, **7**, 517–532.

Singer, F. and Riechert, S. E. (1995). Mating system and mating success of the desert soldier *Agelenopsis aperta*. *Behavioral Ecology and Sociobiology*, **36**, 313–322.

Singer, F., Riechert, S. E., Xu, H., *et al.* (2000). Analysis of courtship success in the funnel web spider *Agelenopsis aperta*. *Behaviour*, **137**, 93–117.

Snow, L. S. E. and Andrade, M. C. B. (2004). Pattern of sperm transfer in redback spiders: implications for sperm competition and male sacrifice. *Behavioral Ecology*, **15**, 785–792.

Stoltz, J. A., Elias, D. O. and Andrade, M. C. B. (2008). Females reward courtship by competing males in a cannibalistic spider. *Behavioral Ecology and Sociobiology*, **62**, 689–697.

Stoltz, J. A., Elias, D. O. and Andrade, M. C. B. (2009). Male courtship effort determines female response to competing rivals in redback spiders. *Animal Behaviour*, **77**, 79–85.

Stoltz, J. A., McNeil, J. N. and Andrade, M. C. B. (2007). Males assess chemical signals to discriminate just-mated females from virgins in redback spiders. *Animal Behaviour*, **74**, 1669–1674.

Stowe, M. K., Tumlinson, J. H. and Heath, R. R. (1987). Chemical mimicry: bolas spiders emit components of moth prey species sex pheromones. *Science*, **236**, 964–967.

Stowe, M. K., Turlings, T. C. J., Loughrin, J. H., Lewis, W. J. and Tumlinson, J. H. (1995). The chemistry of eavesdropping, alarm, and deceit. *Proceedings of the National Academy of Sciences of the USA*, **92**, 23–28.

Stratton, G. E. (1983). Comparison of courtship behaviors and interspecific crosses in the *Schizocosa ocreata* species complex (Araneae, Lycosidae). *American Zoologist*, **23**, 967.

Stratton, G. E. (1991). A new species of wolf spider, *Schizocosa stridulans* (Araneae, Lycosidae). *Journal of Arachnology*, **19**, 29–39.

Stratton, G. E. (2005). Evolution of ornamentation and courtship behavior in *Schizocosa*: insights from a phylogeny based on morphology (Araneae, Lycosidae). *Journal of Arachnology*, **33**, 347–376.

Stratton, G. E. and Uetz, G. W. (1981). Acoustic communication and reproductive isolation in two species of wolf spiders (Araneae: Lycosidae). *Science Washington DC*, **214**, 575–577.

Stratton, G. E. and Uetz, G. W. (1983). Communication via substrate-coupled stridulation and reproductive isolation in wolf spiders (Araneae: Lycosidae). *Animal Behaviour*, **31**, 164–172.

Stratton, G. E. and Uetz, G. W. (1986). The inheritance of courtship behavior and its role as a reproductive isolating mechanism in two species of *Schizocosa* wolf spiders (Araneae, Lycosidae). *Evolution*, **40**, 129–141.

Stropa, A. A. (2007). Social encounters between male brown spiders, *Loxosceles gaucho* (Araneae, Sicariidae). *Journal of Arachnology*, **35**, 493–498.

Suter, R. B. and Hirscheimer, A. J. (1986). Multiple webborne pheromones in a spider *Frontinella pyramitela* (Araneae: Linyphiidae). *Animal Behaviour*, **34**, 748–753.

Suter, R. B. and Keiley, M. (1984). Agonistic interactions between male *Frontinella pyramitela* (Araneae, Linyphiidae). *Behavioral Ecology and Sociobiology*, **15**, 1–7.

Suter, R. B. and Renkes, G. (1982). Linyphiid spider courtship: releaser and attractant functions of a contact sex pheromone. *Animal Behaviour*, **30**, 714–718.

Suter, R. B. and Renkes, G. (1984). The courtship of *Frontinella pyramitela* (Araneae, Linyphiidae): patterns, vibrations and functions. *Journal of Arachnology*, **12**, 37–54.

Suter, R. B., Shane, C. M. and Hirscheimer, A. J. (1987). Communication by cuticular pheromones in a linyphiid spider. *Journal of Arachnology*, **15**, 157–162.

Suter, R. B., Shane, C. M. and Hirscheimer, A. J. (1989). Spider versus spider: *Frontinella pyramitela* detects *Argyrodes trigonum* via cuticular chemicals. *Journal of Arachnology*, **17**, 237–240.

Symonds, M. R. E. and Elgar, M. A. (2008). The evolution of pheromone diversity. *Trends in Ecology and Evolution*, **23**, 220–228.

Taylor, L. A. and McGraw, K. J. (2007). Animal coloration: sexy spider scales. *Current Biology*, **17**, R592–R593.

Taylor, P. W. and Jackson, R. R. (1999). Habitat-adapted communication in *Trite planiceps*, a New Zealand jumping spider (Araneae: Salticidae). *New Zealand Journal of Zoology*, **26**, 127–154.

Taylor, P. W., Hasson, O. and Clark, D. L. (2000). Body postures and patterns as amplifiers of physical condition. *Proceedings of the Royal Society of London, B*, **267**, 917–922.

Taylor, P. W., Hasson, O. and Clark, D. L. (2001). Initiation and resolution of jumping spider contests: roles for size, proximity, and early detection of rivals. *Behavioral Ecology and Sociobiology*, **50**, 403–413.

Taylor, P. W., Roberts, J. A. and Uetz, G. W. (2006). Mating in the absence of visual cues by *Schizocosa ocreata* (Hentz 1844) wolf spiders (Araneae, Lycosidae). *Journal of Arachnology*, **34**, 501–505.

Théry, M. and Casas, J. (2009). The multiple disguises of spiders: web colour and decorations, body colour and movement. *Royal Society Philosophical Transactions Biological Sciences*, **364**, 471–480.

Tichy, H., Gingl, E., Ehn, R., Papke, M. and Schulz, S. (2001). Female sex pheromone of a wandering spider (*Cupiennius salei*): identification and sensory reception. *Journal of Comparative Physiology, A*, **187**, 75–78.

Tiedemann, K. B., Ventura, D. F. and Ades, C. (1986). Spectral sensitivities of the eyes of the orb web spider *Argiope argentata* (Fabricius). *Journal of Arachnology*, **14**, 71–78.

Tietjen, W. J. (1977). Dragline-following by male lycosid spiders. *Psyche*, **84**, 165–178.

Tietjen, W. J. and Rovner, J. S. (1980). Trail-following behaviour in two species of wolf spiders: sensory and etho-ecological concomitants. *Animal Behaviour*, **28**, 735–741.

Tietjen, W. J. and Rovner, J. S. (1982). Chemical communication in lycosids and other spiders. In *Spider Communication: Mechanism and Ecological Significance* (ed. P. N. Witt and J. S. Rovner). Princeton, NJ: Princeton University Press, pp. 249–279.

Tietjen, W. J., Ayyagari, L. R. and Uetz, G. W. (1987). Symbiosis between social spiders and yeast: the role in prey attraction. *Psyche*, **94**, 151–158.

Townsend, Jr., V. R. and Felgenhauer, B. E. (1998). Cuticular scales of spiders. *Invertebrate Biology*, **117**, 318–330.

Townsend, V. R. and Felgenhauer, B. E. (1999). Ultrastructure of the cuticular scales of lynx spiders (Araneae, Oxyopidae) and jumping spiders (Araneae, Salticidae). *Journal of Morphology*, **240**, 77–92.

Trabalon, M. and Assi-Bessekon, D. (2008). Effects of web chemical signatures on intraspecific recognition in a subsocial spider, *Coelotes terrestris* (Araneae). *Animal Behaviour*, **76**, 1571–1578.

Trabalon, M., Bagnères, A. G. and Roland, C. (1997). Contact sex signals in two sympatric spider species, *Tegenaria domestica* and *Tegenaria pagana*. *Journal of Chemical Ecology*, **23**, 747–757.

Trabalon, M., Niogret, J. and Legrand-Frossi, C. (2005). Effect of 20-hydroxyecdysone on cannibalism, sexual behavior, and contact sex pheromone in the solitary female spider, *Tegenaria atrica*. *General and Comparative Endocrinology*, **144**, 60–66.

Tretzel, E. (1959). Zum Begegnungsverhalten von Spinnen. *Zoologischer Anzeiger*, **163**, 194–205.

Uetz, G. W. and Denterlein, G. (1979). Courtship behavior habitat and reproductive isolation in *Schizocosa rovneri* (Araneae, Lycosidae). *Journal of Arachnology*, **7**, 12–128.

Uetz, G. W. and Roberts, J. A. (2002). Multisensory cues and multimodal communication in spiders: insights form video/audio playback studies. *Brain, Behaviour and Evolution*, **59**, 222–230.

Uetz, G. W. and Smith, E. I. (1999). Asymmetry in a visual signaling character and sexual selection in a wolf spider. *Behavioral Ecology and Sociobiology*, **45**, 87–93.

Uetz, G. W. and Stratton, G. E. (1982). Acoustic communication and reproductive isolation in spiders. In *Spider Communication: Mechanism and Ecological Significance* (ed. P. N. Witt and J. S. Rovner). Princeton, NJ: Princeton University Press, pp. 123–129.

Uetz, G. W. and Stratton, G. E. (1983). Communication in spiders. *Endeavour*, **7**, 13–18.

Uetz, G. W., McClintock, W. J., Miller, D., Smith, E. I. and Cook, K. K. (1996). Limb regeneration and subsequent asymmetry in a male secondary sexual character influences sexual selection in wolf spiders. *Behavioral Ecology and Sociobiology*, **38**, 253–257.

Uetz, G. W., Roberts, J. A. and Taylor, P. W. (2009a). Multimodal communication and mate choice in wolf spiders: female response to multimodal versus unimodal signals. *Animal Behaviour*, **78**, 299–305.

Uetz, G. W., Roberts, J. A., Wrinn, K. M., Polak, M. and Cameron, G. N. (2009b). Impact of a catastrophic natural disturbance on fluctuating asymmetry (FA) in a wolf spider. *Ecoscience*, **16**, 379–386.

Uhl, G. (2000). Female genital morphology and sperm priority patterns in spiders. In *European Arachnology* (ed. S. Toft and N. Scharff). Aarhus, Denmark: Aarhus University Press, pp. 145–156.

Uhl, G. and Maelfait, J.-P. (2008). Male head secretion triggers copulation in the dwarf spider *Diplocephalus permixtus*. *Ethology*, **114**, 760–767.

Uhl, G. and Schmitt, M. (1996). Stridulation in *Palpimanus gibbulus* Dufour (Araneae: Palpimanidae). In *Proceedings of the XIIIth International Congress of Arachnology, Geneva, 1995*, Revue Suisse de Zoologie vol. hors série, pp. 649–660.

Uhl, G., Nessler, S. H. and Schneider, J. M. (2010). Securing paternity in spiders? A review on occurrence and effects of mating plugs and male genital mutilation. *Genetica*, **138**, 75–104.

Vakanas, G. and Krafft, B. (2004). Regulation of the number of spiders participating in collective prey transport in the social spider *Anelosimus eximius*. *Comptes Rendues Biologies*, **327**, 763–772.

VanderSal, N. D. and Hebets, E. A. (2007). Cross-modal effects on learning: a seismic stimulus improves color discrimination learning in a jumping spider. *Journal of Experimental Biology*, **210**, 3689–3695.

Vollrath, F. and Parker, G. A. (1992). Sexual dimorphism and distorted sex-ratios in spiders. *Nature*, **360**, 156–159.

Walla, P., Barth, F. G. and Eguchi, E. (1996). Spectral sensitivity of single photoreceptor cells in the eyes of the ctenid spider *Cupiennius salei* Keys. *Zoological Science*, **13**, 199–202.

Wanless, F. R. (1984). A revision of the spider genus *Cyrba* (Araneae; Salticidae) with the description of a new presumptive pheromone dispersing organ. *Bulletin of the British Museum of Natural History (Zoology)*, **47**, 445–481.

Watson, P. J. (1986). Transmission of a female sex pheromone thwarted by males in the spider *Linyphia litigiosa* (Linyphiidae). *Science*, **233**, 219–220.

Watson, P. J. (1993). Foraging advantage of polyandry for female Sierra Dome spiders (*Linyphia litigiosa*: Linyphiidae) and assessment of alternative direct benefit hypotheses. *American Naturalist*, **141**, 440–465.

Watson, P. J. (1998). Multi-male mating and female choice increase offspring growth in the spider *Neriene litigiosa* (Linyphiidae). *Animal Behaviour*, **55**, 387–403.

Wells, M. S. (1988). Effects of body size and resource value on fighting behaviour in a jumping spider. *Animal Behaviour*, **36**, 321–326.

Weygoldt, P. (1977). Communication in crustaceans and arachnids. In *How Animals Communicate* (ed. T. A. Seboek). Bloomington, IN: Indiana University Press, pp. 303–333.

Whitehouse, M. E. A. and Lubin, Y. (1999). Competitive foraging in the social spider *Stegodyphus dumicola*. *Animal Behaviour*, **58**, 677–688.

Whitehouse, M. E. A. and Lubin, Y. (2005). The functions of societies and the evolution of group living: spider societies as a test case. *Biological Reviews*, **80**, 347–361.

Wilson, E. O. (1975). *Sociobiology: The New Synthesis*. Cambridge, MA: Harvard University Press.

Wilson, E. O. and Bossert, W. H. (1963). Chemical communication among animals. *Recent Progress in Hormone Research*, **19**, 673–716.

Witt, P. N. and Rovner, J. S. (eds) (1982). In *Spider Communication: Mechanism and Ecological Significance*. Princeton, NJ: Princeton University Press.

Wood-Mason, J. (1876). On the gigantic stridulating spider. *Annals and Magazine of Natural History*, **16**, 96.

Wyatt, T. D. (2003). *Pheromones and Animal Behaviour: Communication by Smell and Taste*. Cambridge, UK: Cambridge University Press.

Xiao, Y., Zhang, J. and Li, S. (2009). A two-component female-produced pheromone of the spider *Pholcus beijingensis*. *Journal of Chemical Ecology*, **35**, 769–778.

Yamashita, S. (1985). Photoreceptor cells in the spider eye: spectral sensitivity and efferent control. In *Neurobiology of Arachnids* (ed. F. G. Barth). Berlin: Springer, pp. 103–117.

Yamashita, S. and Tateda, H. (1976). Spectral sensitivities of jumping spider eyes. *Journal of Comparative Physiology, A*, **105**, 29–41.

Yeargan, K. V. (1994). Biology of bolas spiders. *Annual Review of Entomology*, **39**, 81–99.

Yeargan, K. V. and Quate, L. W. (1996). Juvenile bolas spiders attract psychodid flies. *Oecologia*, **106**, 266–271.

6

Deceptive signals in spiders

MARIE E. HERBERSTEIN AND ANNE WIGNALL

Spiders are well known as prolific and efficient predators that overwhelm their prey with potent toxins or strong silks. The deployment of cunning tactics to lure and deceive their prey is less appreciated despite a considerable history of research into deceptive spider signals. In the early twentieth century, observations already suggested the presence of a moth-luring chemical in bolas spiders. More recent technological developments have enabled researchers to uncover and quantify deceptive visual, olfactorial and vibrational signals. The evolution of these signals is intriguing as a close association between spider and prey is often required. While deceptive colour signals seem to be generic, targeting a wide range of potential prey, deception via vibrational and olfactorial signals is often more specific. The specificity of the signal in turn requires a considerable degree of plasticity in order for the spider to target more than one prey type. Our review of deceptive signals makes use of several well-studied systems with fascinating plasticity and behavioural flexibility in the deployment of the signal.

6.1 The evolution of deceptive signals

Signals contain information that modulates the behaviour of the individuals that receive them (Bradbury and Vehrencamp, 1998). Some signals exploit pre-existing sensory biases in receivers. The neural responses to these signals may have evolved under different contexts but signal traits that exploit these biases are thought to be most effective (Endler and Basolo, 1998, Johnstone, 1997). When the sender of the signal as well as the receiver of the signal benefit from the interaction, the signal is said to be honest. However,

Spider Behaviour: Flexibility and Versatility, ed. Marie Elisabeth Herberstein. Published by Cambridge University Press. © Cambridge University Press 2011.

when signals are deceptive, the signaller benefits at the cost of the receiver that responds to the signal (Gaskett *et al.*, 2008, Johnson, 2000). The evolution and maintenance of honest communication is paradoxical as any form of communication can be corrupted by deceit: it is always in the interest of the signaller to manipulate the receiver (Dawkins and Guildford, 1991, Stuart-Fox, 2005).

Equally as vexing is the maintenance of dishonest communication, such as the use of deceptive signals by predators, as the cost of responding to these signals for the receiver can be death. Under this circumstance one expects the evolution of a strategy that might reduce the receiver's response to a deceptive signal. However, this is less likely to evolve if the frequency of encounter with deceptive signals is low and/or if the deceptive signal exploits a sensory bias in the receiver (Gaskett *et al.*, 2008). Deception at the cost of the receiver can be achieved in a number of ways, including aggressive mimicry or sensory exploitation. In aggressive mimicry the deceiver mimics a harmless model, such as some jumping spiders smelling like ants and thereby are not identified as a predator by their ant prey (Allan and Elgar, 2001). Other deceptive signals may not mimic a particular model but tap into a basal sensory bias (sensory exploitation) in their prey, such as reflecting light at particular wavelengths (see discussion below). In the absence of a known model, however, it is probably more conservative to talk about these phenomena more generally as deceptive signals. In this chapter, we describe several classic examples of deception via three different sensory modes: visual deception, olfactorial deception and vibrational deception.

6.2 Deception via colour

Most people do not associate spiders with bright, exuberant colour patterns, but there are examples of extraordinary colour displays including fluorescence, polymorphisms and colour change (Figure 6.1). The jumping spiders (Salticidae), for example, boast some of the most colourful examples, such as the peacock spider (*Maratus volans*). Furthermore, the ability to fluoresce is widespread among spiders, having evolved multiple times independently (Andrews *et al.*, 2007). The colour polymorphism of the Hawaiian happy face spider (*Theridion grallator*) is unsurpassed with up to 20 genetically determined colour patterns (Oxford and Gillespie, 1998, 2001). Finally, crab spiders (Thomisidae) show cunning plasticity by changing their colour over only a few days, often in response to the colour of the flower background on which they hunt (Oxford and Gillespie, 1998). In many of these examples, colour may have an anti-predatory function or facilitate communication between conspecifics (Lim *et al.*, 2007, Oxford and Gillespie, 1998). Some colour may also deceive and

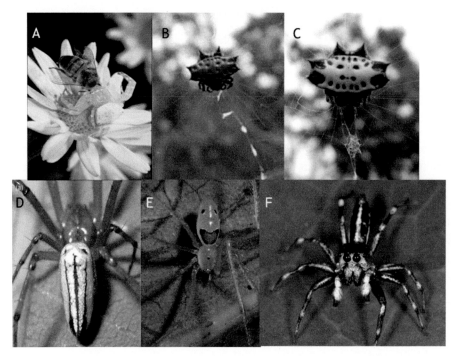

Figure 6.1 Examples of exuberantly coloured spiders. (A) Crab spider *Thomisus spectabilis* (photo credit: Ron Oldfield). (B and C) Different colour morphs of *Gasteracantha* (photo credit: F. Gawryszewski). (D) Orchid spider *Leucauge* (reprinted from Tso *et al.*, 2007, with kind permission from Elsevier). (E) Hawaiian happy face spider (photo credit: R. Gillespie). (F) *Cosmophasis* jumping spider from Singapore (photo credit: D. Li). See also colour plate.

attract prey, an important function especially for stationary predators such as web-building spiders and crab spiders. To fully understand deceptive signals, we have to consider colour vision in the prey of spiders, and possibly the spider itself, as well as how spiders produce these deceptive colours.

6.2.1   Colour vision in insects and spiders

Most insects have colour vision based on the presence of two or more different colour receptors, each sensitive to a specific range of light wavelengths. The ancestral state of winged insect colour vision appears to be an ultraviolet-blue-green trichromacy with colour receptors maximally sensitive in the UV (~350 nm), blue (~440 nm) and green (~530 nm) wavelengths (Briscoe and Chittka, 2001). Colour vision of most insects today is still based on this trichromacy. There are a few cases of insects where the blue receptor has been lost, such as some cockroaches and ants. In other insects, particularly in butterflies and moths, a fourth colour receptor sensitive in the red (>565 nm) is present

(Briscoe and Chittka, 2001). The identification of different receptor types and their sensitivity in insects is well advanced, but our understanding of how the insect brain processes the information conveyed by the receptors in the eye is limited to a few well-studied models such as the honey bee (Briscoe and Chittka, 2001, Chittka, 1996b). Yet, this information is crucial if we are to understand whether an object (such as a spider) is visible to an insect, or if it is indistinguishable from its background.

Colour vision in spiders is less well understood compared with the insects. Direct evidence from measuring receptor excitation at different wavelengths is limited to just a few species of spiders. For example, the orb-web spider *Araneus ventricosus* has two colour receptors, with maximal sensitivities in the green and the UV (Yamashita, 2002). Other orb-web spiders (*Argiope bruennichi* and *amoena*) are trichromatic (UV, blue and green; Yamashita, 2002). The wandering spider *Cupiennius* also has three different colour receptors (UV, blue, and green; Walla *et al.*, 1996) and the jumping spider *Menemerus fulvus* is tetrachromatic with a yellow receptor (~580 nm) in addition to a UV, blue and green receptor (in Yamashita, 2002). Other species of jumping spiders (e.g. *Phidippus* and *Plexippus*) seem to be dichromatic with only a green and a UV receptor (DeVoe, 1975).

Indirect behavioural evidence suggests widespread colour vision among spiders. For example, jumping spiders can discriminate between blue, green, yellow and red hues, although brightness may be additionally used to discriminate between differently coloured papers (Nakamura and Yamashita, 2000). Jumping spiders may also use UV vision to help locate insect prey, many of which have body parts that reflect in the UV (Li and Lim, 2005). Similarly, male jumping spiders of *Cosmophasis umbratica* display to females with UV-reflecting patches on the body (Li *et al.*, 2008, Lim *et al.*, 2007, 2008).

6.2.2   Colour production in spiders

Colour in animals is produced by pigments, surface structures, fluorophores or a combination of all three. Pigments consist of molecules (intra- or extracellular) that selectively absorb light at various wavelengths. The colour created by nanoscale surface structures results from light being scattered or refracted at specific wavelengths through layers. The most brilliant colours are often produced by a combination of both light scattered from surface structures as well as being absorbed by pigments underneath the surface (Grether *et al.*, 2004). Fluorophores are cells that absorb light at a particular (usually shorter) wavelength and emit the light at a different (usually higher) wavelength, a process that requires energy and results in a fluorescing spider (Andrews *et al.*, 2007).

To date only a few pigments have been identified as causing colour in spiders, which is more an indication of the lack of research focus in this area rather than a reflection of the true diversity in spider pigment (Oxford and Gillespie, 1998). Ommochromes are contained within intracellular granules in skin cells and are responsible for yellow, red, brown and black colours. Blue and green colours are associated with bilin pigments. Guanine is also sometimes considered a pigment, even though the guanine crystals deposited beneath the skin create a structural white colour (via diffracting light) rather than through selective absorption as in true pigments (Oxford and Gillespie, 1998). The guanine crystals are by-products of the digestive process in spiders and deposited in guanocyte cells. When the crystals are shaped into small plates they cause the silver metallic colour of some spiders such as *Argyrodes* (Oxford and Gillespie, 1998).

The metallic appearance of many jumping spiders (Salticidae) suggests a structural rather than a pigmentary colour. For example, in *Cosmophasis*, colour is produced by diffraction of light from its grated surface (ridges and grooves at nanoscales) as well as reflection of light from a multilayered exoskeleton with over 20 layers (Parker and Hegedus, 2003). Structural colours such as those in *Cosmophasis* can also extend into the UV (Land *et al.*, 2007) and represent important interspecific signals (Lim and Li, 2006, Lim *et al.*, 2007). Small hairs or setae on the surface of spiders may also create structural colours (Oxford and Gillespie, 1998).

The recently reported fluorescence in spiders has revealed intriguing patterns. Fluorescence seems surprisingly common in spiders, unlike other groups of animals, but is evolutionarily labile, having evolved multiple times independently. Moreover, spiders contain multiple types of fluorophores that are family specific, suggesting the evolution of novel fluorophores during the diversification of spiders. The function of spider fluorescence is unclear, but its evolution is likely to have been driven by predator–prey interactions (Andrews *et al.*, 2007) or sexual selection (Lim *et al.*, 2007).

6.2.3   *Deception with colour in spiders*

Diurnal web-building spiders, in particular orb-web spiders (Araneoidea), sit exposed in their webs, with seemingly little protection from visually hunting predators. Despite this, many orb-web spiders do not appear to be cryptic in coloration (to reduce detection and recognition by predators and prey). Instead they are often brightly coloured: white, yellow, red and in the UV, often quite conspicuous to human observers. Obvious functions for such bright colours include predator deterrence or prey attraction, with the latter idea drawing considerable experimental attention. Mate attraction via colour in orb-web spiders seems unlikely because of the lack of visual acuity of these spiders and the widespread use of pheromones for mate location (Gaskett, 2007). Methods that test for prey attraction include manipulating the visibility of the spider through shields, manipulating the actual colour by painting the spider or utilising natural variation in spider colour (Bush *et al.*, 2008, Craig and Ebert, 1994, Hauber, 2002, Tso *et al.*, 2002). The bright yellow and white stripes on the abdomen of *Argiope*, *Leucauge* and *Gasteracantha* (Araneidae; Figure 6.1) appear to increase prey capture: when these stripes were either coloured over or the entire spider obscured, webs intercepted fewer insects compared with a control (Bush *et al.*, 2008, Craig and Ebert, 1994, Hauber, 2002, Hoese *et al.*, 2006).

It is, however, important to show unambiguously that this effect is due to attraction rather than due to the effect of disruptive coloration. By painting over the stripes, the outline of the spider's body might become more obvious to approaching prey that subsequently avoid the web (Hoese *et al.*, 2006). However, using shields that obscure the entire spider suitably control for this possible confounding effect. Field studies on two *Argiope* species (*argentata* and *bruennichi*) both used such shields and found evidence that the bright colour of spiders attracts prey (Bush *et al.*, 2008, Craig and Ebert, 1994). However, a third field study using *A. bruennichi* found no such pattern: the presence of a brightly coloured spider did not increase prey capture compared with empty artificial webs (Václav and Prokop, 2006). Similarly, colouring over the brightly coloured abdomen of *Micrathena gracilis* did not affect prey capture compared with un-manipulated individuals, thus finding no support for either a prey attraction or crypsis function of bright coloration (Vanderhoff *et al.*, 2008). The different effects reported by these studies are difficult to interpret and may be due to variation in methods used or due to the identity and hence visual physiology of the potential prey in the various microhabitats.

Different colour morphs provide an excellent opportunity to test for the effect of colour on prey capture. The giant wood spider *Nephila pilipes* occurs in two colour morphs – a melanic form that is totally dark and a yellow morph with a dark abdomen decorated with white and yellow lines and spots (Tso *et al.*, 2002). Colour analysis and physiological modelling (using the honey bee model) showed that the melanic morph is entirely indistinguishable from its background, while the yellow morph is conspicuous (Tso *et al.*, 2004). If the yellow stripes and spots achieve disruptive coloration, both morphs should not be visible to prey and prey capture rates should be similar. However, the yellow morph captured almost twice as much prey as the melanic morph, suggesting that the conspicuous spider colour in *N. pilipes* lures prey to the web (Tso *et al.*, 2002).

While not immediately intuitive, deceptive colours may also be important for nocturnal foraging. Even under low light conditions, colour patterns such as the yellow stripes and spots of *N. pilipes* and *Leucauge celebesiana* or the bright spots of *Neoscona punctigera* can be detected by prey such as moths. Spiders with these colour patterns attracted more moth prey to the web compared with painted spiders (Chuang *et al.*, 2007a, 2007b, Tso *et al.*, 2007).

If a deceptive colour signal such as the yellow stripes in *Nephila or Argiope* is conspicuous to insect prey, it is also very likely that insect predators, with similar visual systems, are equally attracted to these signals. In which case, the colour signal becomes costly to the spider due to a greater likelihood of predatory attacks. Two studies have investigated if bright colours carry costs in terms of predator attraction. Hoese and colleagues (2006) observed the choice behaviour of praying mantid predators when offered naturally yellow or painted *Argiope*. They interpreted the preference of mantids for painted spiders as evidence that the conspicuous yellow stripe functions as disruptive coloration by obscuring the outline of the spider, thus providing an anti-predatory defence. A field study using *N. pilipes* dummies by contrast found that yellow dummies attracted more hymenoptera predators (as well as more prey) than black dummies, suggesting a trade-off between prey and predator attraction (Fan *et al.*, 2009). A limitation of predator studies, which explains their low frequency compared with prey studies, is that predatory attacks are generally infrequent and rarely witnessed and we often do not know the identity of spider predators.

While crab spiders (Thomisidae) do not build webs for prey capture, they hunt exposed on flowers or vegetation where they remain relatively motionless until an insect lands (Morse, 1981). Crab spiders are renowned for their colourful appearance (white, yellow, pink), and their ability to change colour over the course of a few days (Oxford and Gillespie, 1998, Théry and Casas, 2009). In most species of crab spiders, their colour and colour change is a case of background matching. The spiders change body colour according to the colour of their background. This renders them invisible to their insect prey and bird predators (Chittka, 2001, Théry and Casas, 2002, Théry *et al.*, 2005) with obvious advantages in terms of prey capture and predator avoidance. However, not all crab spiders are cryptic. Some Australian crab spider species differ substantially in colour from those studied in the Northern Hemisphere (Herberstein *et al.*, 2009). To the human observer they also seem to be matching their flower background, but in the UV range of light (invisible to humans) they form a strong contrast with the flower background (Heiling *et al.*, 2005a, 2005b; Figure 6.2). This UV contrast is attractive to insect prey such as bees (Heiling and Herberstein, 2004, Heiling *et al.*, 2003). As with colours in the visible range of light, these Australian species are able to vary the amount of UV light they reflect, possibly trading the advantage of attracting prey with the increased visibility to predators that are also sensitive to UV light (Heiling *et al.*, 2005b, Herberstein *et al.*, 2009). The evolutionary pattern of this trait is unknown: are only Australian species UV reflective or is this a broader phenomenon? It is also possible that UV reflection initially evolved as a protective

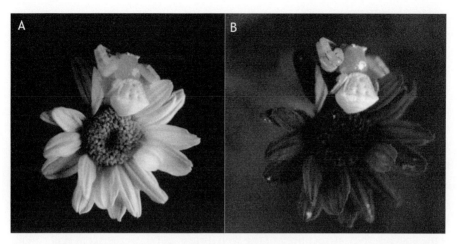

Figure 6.2 The crab spider *Thomisus spectabilis* when viewed under visible light (A) or only UV light (B). Under UV light, the spider forms a strong contrast against the non-UV-reflecting flower. (Reprinted from Heiling and Herberstein, 2004, with kind permission from the Royal Society, London.)

device against higher UV radiation in Australia (Herberstein *et al.*, 2009, Théry and Casas, 2009) although this trait clearly also functions as a deceptive colour signal.

The discovery of deceptive colour signals in spiders, while enormously exciting, raises the question of the exact mechanism that renders these signals attractive (and hence deceptive) for insect prey. Do these colour patterns represent a case of aggressive mimicry by mimicking existing rewarding signals, such as flowers, or are spiders exploiting a sensory bias without mimicking any specific model? Wavelength-specific attraction is an ancient behaviour in insects that preceded their ability to distinguish between colours (Briscoe and Chittka, 2001). Similarly, the visual system of insects, with receptor sensitivities to specific wavelengths (colours), is very old, evolving approximately 400 million years before flowering plants evolved. Thus, the colours of flowers exploit a sensory bias in pollinating insects (Chittka, 1996a). It is therefore more likely that deceptive colours in spiders also constitute a case of sensory exploitation rather than an example of flower mimicry. This is best illustrated when considering UV vision in insects. In honey bees, for example, the UV receptor is 16 times more sensitive than the blue or green receptor (von Helversen, 1972), and insects show an innate attraction to UV light (Briscoe and Chittka, 2001), which flowers exploit by using UV-bright markers on UV-dull petals (Chittka *et al.*, 1994). Similarly, it is most likely that UV-bright crab spiders exploit the visual system and sensory bias of their insect prey.

The colour of silk rather than the colour of the spider itself can also function as a deceptive signal that attracts prey to the web. Specifically, some spiders, such as

Nephila (Nephilidae), vary the colour of the silk they produce and incorporate into the web. Typically, the colours vary from white to a golden yellow. The yellow silks, rather than uncoloured, white silk, attract herbivorous and pollinating insects to the web. Moreover, pollinating hymenopterans have difficulty in learning the location of webs with yellow silk after they had been intercepted once compared with unpigmented webs (Craig *et al.*, 1996). However, the mechanism responsible for producing silks of different colours is not known (see Chapter 3 for a discussion). Another example of deceptive silks is the web decorations built by many orb-web spiders (Araneidae, Uloboridae). These conspicuous silk bands, spirals or discs reflect light in the UV and form strong contrasts against a typical green background (Bruce *et al.*, 2005). While numerous functions have been suggested for these intriguing structures, evidence suggests that, at least in some species, they attract prey to the web (Bruce, 2006, Herberstein *et al.*, 2000). Chapter 3 discusses silk decorations in greater detail.

6.2.4   *Colour variation in deceptive spiders*

Variation in deceptive signals, between and even within individuals, can almost be more interesting than the signal itself, as such variation points to significant costs of producing the signal in the first place. Several colour-deceptive spiders show intriguing intraspecific as well as intra-individual variation in the absence/presence of the signal as well as the quality of the signal. The basis of some of these polymorphisms may be genetic or due to environmental factors or reflect individual plasticity in switching on or off the signal.

The genetic basis for colour expression (deceptive or not) is best understood in the Hawaiian happy face spiders (*Theridion grallator*). Within populations, about 70% of individuals are yellow and the remaining 30% have additional red, black or white patches superimposed on a yellow background. Yellow is recessive to the other colour morphs, and the greater the amount of non-yellow pigments on the abdomen, the more dominant the morph (Oxford and Gillespie, 2001). Intriguingly, many of these colour morphs appear to have evolved independently on the different Hawaiian islands, where the colour morphs occupy similar niches (Oxford and Gillespie, 2001). How insect prey respond to the different colour morphs, however, is less well understood.

We know of two examples of colour polymorphisms that involve a deceptive signal: *Austracantha minax* (Hauber, 2002; Figure 6.1) and *Nephila pilipes* (Tso *et al.*, 2002). *Austracantha* occur in yellow, white, red and sometimes black morphs (Edmunds and Edmunds, 1986) and *N. pilipes* in a melanic and a yellow morph that is also UV reflective (Tso *et al.*, 2002). There has been some genetic characterisation of *N. pilipes*, which revealed no genetic differentiation between the two colour morphs, suggesting that environmental differences may be responsible for the colour morphs. It is tempting to speculate whether predation pressure on conspicuous signals in some environments is responsible for maintaining less conspicuous morphs.

The deceptive UV signal of Australian crab spiders is variable between individuals as well as within individuals. In the field, we find morphs of *Thomisus spectabilis* that appear white and yellow to the human observer. The main difference between them is that white morphs are UV reflective, while the yellow morphs are UV dull, reflecting little light below 400 nm (Heiling *et al.*, 2005b). The spiders clearly have information about their own colour state, as yellow *T. spectabilis* are found only on yellow flowers in the field and also prefer yellow flowers in choice experiments. White, UV-bright spiders are less selective and are found on white and yellow flowers (Heiling *et al.*, 2005b). Substrate choice is clearly important, as yellow UV-dull spiders that create strong contrasts against white flowers repulse prey while white UV-bright spiders are attractive to prey regardless of the flower colour. Prey seem to be indifferent to yellow spiders on yellow flowers (Heiling *et al.*, 2005b). The two colour morphs are not permanent states. Individuals can change their colour from UV dull (yellow) to UV bright (white) and vice versa over several days (F. Gawryszewski *et al.*, unpublished data).

Why are not all *T. spectabilis* spiders white? There is an obvious prey-capture advantage of UV-bright white spiders; white spiders have greater flexibility in flower choice and all individuals seem to be able to change colour to white. Furthermore, yellow UV-dull spiders are not cryptic on yellow flowers: they still form a visible colour contrast against the flower background (Heiling *et al.*, 2005b). Nevertheless, the strong contrast in the UV created by white *T. spectabilis* against white or yellow flowers may be more likely to attract the attention of predators that are sensitive to UV. Thus under higher predation pressure, yellow morphs may have lower costs, despite reduced prey-capture success. Moreover, white *T. spectabilis* are most attractive to European honey bees. Australian native bees, whilst still attracted to flowers with white crab spiders, seem to have evolved an anti-predatory response and are less likely to land on spider-occupied flowers (Heiling and Herberstein, 2004). The expression of yellow morphs may therefore reflect the presence of native bees. The physiological and perhaps structural basis for UV reflection in *T. spectabilis* and other UV-reflective Australian crab spiders is currently unexplored.

6.3   Deception via scent

Despite the excellent vision of insects, scents and pheromones from cuticular hydrocarbons play an important role in their inter- and intraspecific communication (Howard and Blomquist, 2005). The cuticular hydrocarbon bouquets of most insects are species and sex specific, facilitating the correct identification of conspecifics and potential mates. Among social insects, they play an additional role in nest-mate recognition, task decisions and in establishing dominance and reproductive hierarchies (Howard and Blomquist, 2005). Clearly, the facilitation of fundamental processes such as reproduction via scents in insects renders them vulnerable to exploitation via chemical deception. Among spiders, there are some classic examples of chemical deception that take advantage of insect pheromone communication.

6.3.1   Deception via chemicals in spiders

Spiders can take advantage of their prey via chemicals in two ways: they can use chemicals to remain undetected by their prey or to attract prey to their location. To remain undetected, spiders may mimic the chemical signature of a harmless model such as a conspecific of the targeted prey. To attract prey, spiders may mimic the scent of a mate that promises a benefit to the deceived prey. Both these examples are cases of aggressive mimicry as in most cases the model on which the mimicry is based has been identified. Not surprisingly, both these types of deception are broadly associated with the level of mobility of the spider. Those spiders that attract prey with chemicals are generally less mobile and sedentary than those that use chemicals to approach prey undetected.

Nelson and Jackson (Chapter 2) have described in some detail examples of aggressive mimicry in myrmecophagic jumping spiders (Salticidae). These spiders mimic the chemical signature of their ant prey to gain access to the ant nest and steal eggs and larvae. The chemical mimicry is apparently sufficient to blend in, as visually the spiders do not resemble the ants. Rather than reiterate the excellent descriptions in Chapter 2, we will here concentrate and expand on examples of chemical mimicry that attract prey to the spiders.

Several genera of orb-web spiders (Araneidae) attract prey with chemical lures including *Celaenia*, *Taczanowskia*, *Kaira*, and several genera of bolas spiders such as *Mastophora* (Yeargan, 1994). The best-studied of them, the bolas spiders, have reduced the web to only a sticky ball at the end of a short silk line and it seems almost implausible that they should be able to capture any prey at all with it. Early observations of the predatory behaviour of bolas spiders already suggested that they might attract their prey (Hutchinson, 1903). This suspicion was later confirmed: these spiders captured exclusively male moths of only two species that only approached the spider from downwind (Eberhard, 1977). The data suggested that the spiders mimic the pheromones of female moths. Three volatile compounds produced by the spider itself were later identified as identical to those of female moth sex pheromones. These compounds were not found on the silk but only on the spider, although a specific location for the scent production was not identified (Stowe *et al.*, 1987, Yeargan, 1994).

The interaction between the male moth prey and the bolas spider is dynamic. The spiders only produce the allomone when they have assumed a hunting position (hanging upside down suspended from a horizontal trapeze with out-stretched forelegs) with or without the bolas (Haynes *et al.*, 2001, Yeargan, 1994). Bolas construction tends to be initiated by the detection of a moth. It appears that the mechanical stimulation from the wing flap of the moth is the trigger for bolas construction (Haynes *et al.*, 2001). The ability to first sample prey avail-ability and modify predatory behaviour accordingly has clear advantages. First the energetic investment in the bolas itself can be optimised during periods of high prey activity. While the exact energetic costs of bolas construction are not known, the bolas itself is a complex silk structure consisting of curled fibres embedded within a viscous matrix (Eberhard, 1980). Second, it seems that the bolas has limited capture potential as spiders ingest the bolas after 20–30 minutes if they have not captured any prey, and the bolas shrinks in size over time (Eberhard, 1980, Yeargan, 1994). The wing flaps of nearby moths also elicit the swinging of the bolas, although there are some species where the spider continuously swings the bolas even in the absence of prey (Yeargan, 1994).

There are some intriguing ontogenetic changes in the hunting behaviour of bolas spiders. Juvenile spiders (of either sex) and adult males do not construct the bolas and do not capture male moths. They adopt the hunting position at the edge of a leaf with their front legs stretched out capturing small flies, which they snatch from the air (Yeargan, 1994, Yeargan and Quate, 1996, 1997). It is not until the female spiders are close to maturation that they start to construct the bolas. There are a number of other species in the *Mastophora* genus where the adults also do not construct the bolas but hunt by snatching prey from the air (Yeargan, 1994). Whether bolas construction has been lost in these species is unknown, but consid-ering the general trend in spiders, especially the Araneidae, to reduce the web and web-building behaviour it is likely that the bolas has been lost in these examples.

6.3.2   *Variation in deceptive chemical signals*

Chemical signals are thought to be relatively low in production costs as they are often by-products of metabolic processes, but this assumption needs to be supported by data. Chemical signals such as pheromones are under the control of one or a few genes, and it is not difficult to imagine the evolution of pheromone diversity due to small mutations (Symonds and Elgar, 2008). Intra-individual plasticity in the quality of chemical signals is less common and intriguingly complex. Nevertheless, we find two reasonably well studied examples of such plasticity in spiders.

As already described above (and in Chapter 2), myrmecophagic jumping spiders (Salticidae) rely on their cuticular hydrocarbon bouquet to remain undetected while raiding ant nests. Green tree ants (*Oecophylla smaragdina*) are generally highly aggressive and territorial but clearly mistake the jumping spider *Cosmophasis bitaeniata* for a nest mate. The mimicry is so convincing that the spider can remove larvae (their main prey) from the mandibles of minor workers (Allan and Elgar, 2001). The cuticular hydrocarbons are colony specific as green tree ants even react aggressively to the scent of conspecifics from another colony (Allan et al., 2002). So, how does *Cosmophasis* acquire these colony-specific scents – by direct contact with workers or are they able to synthesise the specific cuticular hydrocarbons independently of direct contact? *Cosmophasis* acquires colony-specific scents by ingesting the ant larvae, although it is unclear if the spider sequesters the ingested molecules or whether it distributes them via allogrooming. Moreover *Cosmophasis* has information about its own chemical profile and will avoid green tree ants from a different colony with a different chemical profile (Elgar and Allan, 2004, 2006). Thus intra- and interindividual plasticity in this deceptive signal is achieved by variation in the spider's diet.

Bolas spiders also appear to show intra-individual variation in the chemical signal they use to attract prey. These differences have not yet been characterised, but they are based on the different types of prey the spiders attract. Juvenile bolas spiders attract small flies, but adults attract moths, suggesting that different chemical signals are at work (Yeargan and Quate, 1996). How these chemicals are acquired is also unknown.

There is indirect evidence that adult female bolas spiders actively modify the chemical blends of their deceptive signals to attract different species of moths. *Mastophora cornigera* attracts up to 19 different species of moths, and it is unlikely that a single blend of volatiles is attractive to all of them (Stowe et al., 1987). However, to date, direct evidence based on the characterisation of these different blends has not been achieved, in part because it is very difficult to obtain large enough samples for gas chromatography. Adult *Mastophora hutchinsoni* attract two different moth species, each active at different times during the night, implying that the spider might alter its chemical bouquet throughout the night according to prey activity. However, an analysis of the cuticular hydrocarbons showed that the bolas spider produces a bouquet that contains components of both moth species simultaneously (Haynes et al., 2002).

6.4   Deception via vibrations

Spiders use vibratory communication for a diverse range of functions, including courtship and to mediate interactions with prey and predators. We

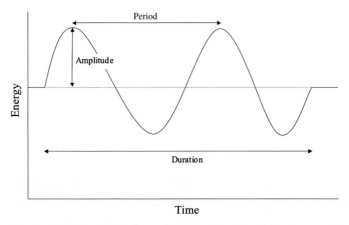

Figure 6.3 A hypothetical waveform of a vibration illustrating amplitude, period (used to calculate frequency) and duration.

know most about how spiders use vibrations to recognise prey, particularly prey ensnared in webs (Klärner and Barth, 1982, Landolfa and Barth, 1996, Masters, 1984) and about the male courtship vibrations of cursorial species (Baurecht and Barth, 1992, Elias *et al.*, 2003, Schmitt *et al.*, 1994). Several physical parameters of vibrations are usually quantified: amplitude (how 'loud' a vibration is), frequency (how high or low in 'pitch' a vibration is, measured in number of cycles/second) and duration (how long a vibration is; Figure 6.3). As vibrations travel along a substrate, they lose energy, resulting in an attenuation of amplitude (with some frequencies sometimes attenuated more than others).

6.4.1   Vibratory signals: purpose and perception in spiders

Spiders have adapted to living in a wide variety of habitats, and for effective communication vibratory signals must be capable of travelling through a range of substrate types while keeping the information contained intact. The propagation of information through substrates varies substantially due to the different properties of the media through which vibrations must travel (i.e. silk, plants, soil). It is not particularly surprising that the silk webs built by web-building spiders are excellent transmitters of vibratory stimuli, and are essentially extensions of the spider's sensory system (Landolfa and Barth, 1996). In spider webs, there are four types of web vibration that have different propagation properties. Longitudinal waves are vibrations that are parallel to the axis of the silk thread and are thought to be especially important for localising and recognising prey in orb webs (Klärner and Barth, 1982, Masters and Markl, 1981, Masters *et al.*, 1986). Transverse waves are vibrations perpendicular to both the silk thread and plane of the web, and are the most common type of vibration generated by prey in the web (Masters and Markl, 1981, Masters *et al.*, 1986). Lateral waves are vibrations perpendicular to the silk thread but in the same plane as the web (Masters and Markl, 1981, Masters *et al.*, 1986). Rotational, or torsional, waves are the most difficult type to measure and are vibrations involving twisting of the silk thread (Masters *et al.*, 1986).

Unlike web-building spiders that detect vibrations along silk threads, cursorial spiders need to detect vibratory stimuli along substrates such as rocks, soil, sand, water, bark and leaves. These substrates can vary substantially in their transmission properties (Elias *et al.*, 2004, Hebets *et al.*, 2008). This can present difficulties for spider species that inhabit multiple substrate types. The jumping spider *Habronattus dossenus* is found on rocks, sand and leaf litter. Leaf litter transmits vibrations most readily, with the other substrate types rapidly attenuating large parts of the courtship vibrations of the males. While males will readily court females on each of the three substrates, males were more successful when they courted on leaf litter (Elias *et al.*, 2004).

Courtship vibrations may function as species recognition, to stimulate the female to mate or be under sexual selection if they reflect male quality and influence female mate choice (see Chapters 5 and 7). The vibratory courtship of the wandering spiders, particularly *Cupiennius salei*, has been characterised in detail (Baurecht and Barth, 1992, 1993, Schimizu and Barth, 1996, Schmitt *et al.*, 1994). Jumping spiders and wolf spiders also show complex vibratory courtship behaviours. Female *Hygrolycosa rubrofasciata* wolf spiders prefer males that drum more, a behaviour that is a predictor of male viability (Kotiaho *et al.*, 1996). Generally, it is believed that more 'vigorous' male courtship vibrations are preferred by females. Courtship vibrations in web-building spiders have received surprisingly little research attention (but see Maklakov *et al.*, 2003, Suter and Renkes, 1984), especially considering that in some orb-web spiders, such as *Argiope*, the duration of courtship vibrations is an order of magnitude longer than the actual copulation (Herberstein *et al.*, 2002, Schneider and Lesmono, 2009).

6.4.2   Examples of vibratory deceptive spiders

Vibratory deception in spiders most commonly encompasses the use of aggressive mimicry. Araneophagic spiders that hunt web-building spiders often have difficulties in traversing the silk webs of other species (Whitehouse, 1988). This leaves the predatory spider at risk of being detected by the resident prey spider and even counter-attacked. By generating vibrations at the edge of the web that resemble insect prey caught in the web, the predatory spider can reduce this risk by luring the resident spider within attacking range.

Aggressive mimicry has been reported in the jumping spiders (Salticidae), tangle-web spiders (Theridiidae), pirate spiders (Mimetidae), gnaphosids (Gnaphosidae) and pholcids (Pholcidae). Given the diversity of families where aggressive mimicry has been described, this behaviour has obviously evolved multiple times. While araneophagy itself appears to be very common among spiders, with individuals taking advantage of opportunities during courtship and mating or aggressive encounters, aggressive mimicry is a less-documented phenomenon. Web-building spiders appear to be more vulnerable to exploitation by aggressive mimicry than cursorial spiders due to their poor vision and reliance on vibratory stimuli to provide information. Araneophagous jumping spiders consume a disproportionately large number of spiders and spider eggs in their diet although they also catch insects outside webs and, in the case of *Portia*, build webs themselves (Jackson, 1992b). However, few aggressive mimics rely on spiders as their main prey, instead relying more on insect prey (whether by building webs themselves or by kleptoparasitism).

Most non-salticid aggressive mimics prey on a small range of spider species, perhaps due to the poorer vision and less complex predatory strategies in non-salticids compared with the jumping spiders (Jackson, 1992b). There are some notable exceptions, however. *Mimetus notius* invades and preys on spiders from seven families (including Araneidae, Dictynidae, Tetragnathidae, Theridiidae; Kloock, 2001).

Without doubt the best-studied example of this form of deception by a spider is *Portia fimbriata*. This species is an aggressive mimic that preys on many species of spiders from a diverse range of families (see Chapter 2). Other species within the *Portia* genus that have been shown to use vibratory deception include *P. labiata*, another aggressive mimic (Jackson and Carter, 2001). Vibratory deception through aggressive mimicry appears to be remarkably common within the Spartaeinae jumping spiders, with species within the genera *Brettus*, *Cyrba* and *Gelotia* all also luring web-building spiders by generating vibrations to attract the resident within attacking distance (Jackson, 1990a, 1990b, 2002, Jackson and Hallas, 1986).

Outside the jumping spiders, vibratory deception is much rarer, or at least less documented, with *Pholcus phalangioides* (Jackson and Brassington, 1987), several species of pirate spiders (*Mimetus*; Jackson and Whitehouse, 1986) and spiders in the genera *Argyrodes* and *Zelanda* exhibiting deceptive behaviours (Jackson, 1992b, Jarman and Jackson, 1986). These species appear to have a smaller prey and signalling range than the jumping spiders, particularly when compared with *P. fimbriata*. These non-jumping spider species tend mostly to mimic the vibrations of ensnared insects. The exception is *Ero furcata* (Mimetidae) that has been reported to mimic male courtship vibrations (Czajka, 1963, cited in Jackson, 1992b). It is not surprising to find insect prey mimicry a more common deceptive strategy, as mimicry of male courtship would not be successful in luring juvenile or male spiders.

6.4.3   *Vibratory repertoire: different messages for different occasions*

The vibratory repertoires of spiders that use deception fall into two different strategies: trial and error or species-specific signals. Species-specific signals have only been reported in *P. fimbriata*, although it also commonly uses trial-and-error strategies (Jackson and Wilcox, 1990). Trial and error, the most common predatory strategy adopted by aggressive mimics, involves the spider generating random vibrations in the web until eliciting a response in the targeted spider, then repeating the signal that worked (Jackson and Wilcox, 1993; see Chapter 2). This method has been described in detail in jumping spiders (Jackson, 2002, Jackson and Carter, 2001, Jackson and Wilcox, 1993). There are several instances where different populations of a deceptive species exhibit differences in their vibratory repertoires. For example, the Queensland population of *P. fimbriata* spiders show much higher signalling diversity in their trial-and-error signal derivation and prey range than the Northern Territory population in Australia (Jackson, 1992c). While less is known about the signal-derivation strategies of other aggressive mimics, we can predict that trial and error is more likely to evolve in these generalist predators than species-specific tactics.

Species-specific deceptive signals have so far only been observed in *P. fimbriata* when hunting *Euryattus* (web-building spiders of the family Salticidae) female spiders. During these interactions, *Portia* will generate vibrations that resemble the male courtship signals in the webs, attracting the females within range of attack (Jackson *et al.*, 1997). This specific, deceptive signalling behaviour is not observed in populations of *Portia* that are not sympatric with *Euryattus* (Jackson, 1992a). It is probable that *Ero furcata* (see Section 6.4.2) may also use species-specific signalling, although this remains to be tested.

The flexibility of *Portia*'s deceptive signalling behaviour can be illustrated by the range of signals that *P. fimbriata* generates when hunting web-building spiders by mimicking prey. Tarsitano and colleagues (2000) measured the vibratory signals generated during hunts and observed three broad signal categories: signals that resemble prey snared in the web, signals that resemble an insect brushing against the periphery of the web and signals that simulate large web disturbances to mask the spider's approach. When hunting small spiders, *Portia* generates signals that closely resemble prey to lure the resident within range. When hunting large spiders, *Portia* generates signals resembling insects in the periphery of the web to prevent eliciting dangerous predatory behaviour. When moving through the resident spider's web, *Portia* generates large-scale disturbances as a form of self-generated smokescreen (Tarsitano *et al.*, 2000). The ability to generate such a wide range of vibratory signals that resemble different stimuli may be advantageous to *Portia* when hunting difficult or particularly dangerous prey.

While much is known of the predatory deception strategies of *Portia*, very little is known about the signal-choice strategies of other aggressive mimics. In particular, we may find similarities in signal structure between species that mimic insect prey, suggesting that the cues for eliciting predatory behaviour in the resident spider (that results in successful luring) may be common across species of web-building spiders.

6.5   Conclusions and outlook

Spiders deploy deceptive lures via three sensory modes: visual, olfactorial and tactile. Chemical deception in bolas spiders has had the longest and possibly the most intense research history. The most recent discovery in spider deception involves the use of spider colour as well as silk colour. The identification and quantification of these signals has been aided by the development of technologies such as gas chromatography, photospectrometry and laser vibrometry. As this equipment is increasingly becoming standard in many laboratories, it is anticipated that new deceptive signals will rapidly be discovered.

The deceptive colour signals appear to be tapping into a generic sensory bias in their insect prey, such as a general sensitivity to certain light wavelengths. While some vibratory deceptive signals appear quite specific, most have a more general trial-and-error signal-derivation strategy. The olfactorial signals identified so far are mostly more specific, targeting a more narrow range of prey. This is particularly the case in chemicals that mimic the female pheromone of prey insects or vibrations that mimic the courtship behaviour of male web-building spiders. This raises some interesting questions about the ability of deceptive spiders to vary their signal in order to target different prey. How quickly can the deceiver switch the signal to fit the available prey spectrum? This is clearly dependent on the nature of the signal: vibrational signals can be modified much faster than chemical signals. Does the deceiver require prior experience with the new prey to modify the signal? Finally, as deceptive strategies are being discovered in spiders, we can start addressing the evolutionary path of deceptive strategies. For example, have similar deceptive strategies evolved independently or only once followed by substantial speciation? What are the patterns of speciation in generic versus specific deceptive strategies? The diversity of deceptive signals in spiders makes them good models in which to address these questions.

Acknowledgements

We are grateful to I-Min Tso, Jutta Schneider and Daiqin Li for helpful and constructive comments on earlier drafts of the chapter. Many thanks to Felipe Gawryszewski, Rosie Gillespie and Ron Oldfield for the use of their photographs.

References

Allan, R. A. and Elgar, M. A. (2001). Exploitation of the green tree ant, *Oecophylla smaragdina*, by the salticid spider *Cosmophasis bitaeniata*. *Australian Journal of Zoology*, **49**, 129–137.

Allan, R. A., Capon, R. J., Brown, W. V. and Elgar, M. A. (2002). Mimicry of host cuticular hydrocarbons by salticid spider *Cosmophasis bitaeniata* that preys on larvae of the tree ants *Oecophylla smaragdina*. *Journal of Chemical Ecology*, **28**, 835–848.

Andrews, K., Reed, S. M. and Masta, S. E. (2007). Spiders fluoresce variably across many taxa. *Biology Letters*, **3**, 265–267.

Baurecht, D. and Barth, F. G. (1992). Vibratory communication in spiders. I. Representation of male courtship signals by female vibration receptor. *Journal of Comparative Physiology, A*, **171**, 231–243.

Baurecht, D. and Barth, F. G. (1993). Vibratory communication in spiders. II. Representation of parameters contained in synthetic male courtship signals by female vibration receptor. *Journal of Comparative Physiology, A*, **173**, 309–319.

Bradbury, J. W. and Vehrencamp, S. L. (1998). *Principles of Animal Communication*. Sunderland, MA: Sinauer.

Briscoe, A. D. and Chittka, L. (2001). The evolution of color vision in insects. *Annual Review of Entomology*, **46**, 471–510.

Bruce, M. (2006). Silk decorations: controversy and consensus. *Journal of Zoology*, **269**, 89–97.

Bruce, M. J., Heiling, A. M. and Herberstein, M. E. (2005). Spider signals: are web decorations visible to birds and bees? *Biology Letters*, **1**, 299–302.

Bush, A. A., Yu, D. W. and Herberstein, M. E. (2008). Function of bright coloration in the wasp spider *Argiope bruennichi* (Araneae: Araneidae). *Proceedings of the Royal Society of London, B*, **275**, 1337–1342.

Chittka, L. (1996a). Does bee colour vision predate the evolution of flower colour? *Naturwissenschaften*, **83**, 136–138.

Chittka, L. (1996b). Optimal sets of color receptors and color opponent systems for coding of natural objects in insect vision. *Journal of Theoretical Biology*, **181**, 179–196.

Chittka, L. (2001). Camouflage of predatory crab spiders on flowers and the colour perception of bees (Aranida: Thomisidae/Hymenoptera: Apidae). *Entomologia Generalis*, **25**, 181–187.

Chittka, L., Shmida, A., Troje, N. and Menzel, R. (1994). Ultraviolet as a component of flower reflections, and the colour perception of hymenoptera. *Vision Research*, **34**, 1489–1508.

Chuang, C.-Y., Yang, E.-C. and Tso, I. M. (2007a). Deceptive color signaling in the night: a nocturnal predator attracts prey with visual lures. *Behavioral Ecology*, **19**, 237–244.

Chuang, C.-Y., Yang, E.-C. and Tso, I. M. (2007b). Diurnal and nocturnal prey luring of a colorful predator. *Journal of Experimental Biology*, **210**, 3830–3838.

Craig, C. L. and Ebert, K. (1994). Colour and pattern in predator-prey interactions: the bright body colours and patterns of a tropical orbspinning spider attract flower-seeking prey. *Functional Ecology*, **8**, 616–620.

Craig, C. L., Weber, R. S. and Bernard, G. D. (1996). Evolution of predator-prey systems: spider foraging plasticity in response to the visual ecology of prey. *American Naturalist*, **147**, 205–229.

Dawkins, M. S. and Guildford, T. (1991). The corruption of honest signalling. *Animal Behaviour*, **41**, 865–873.

DeVoe, R. D. (1975). Ultraviolet and green receptors in principal eyes of jumping spiders. *Journal of General Physiology*, **66**, 193–207.

Eberhard, W. G. (1977). Aggressive chemical mimicry by a bolas spider. *Science*, **198**, 1173–1175.

Eberhard, W. G. (1980). Natural history and behavior of the bolas spider *Mastophora dizzydeani* sp. n. (Araneidae). *Psyche*, **87**, 143–169.

Edmunds, J. and Edmunds, M. (1986) The defensive mechanisms of orb weavers (Araneae: Araneidae) in Ghana, West Africa. In *Proceedings of the 9th International Congress of Arachnology, Panama, 1983* (ed. W. G. Eberhard, Y. D. Lubin and B. C. Robinson. Washington, DC: Smithsonian Institute Press.

Elgar, M. A. and Allan, R. A. (2004). Predatory spider mimics acquire colony-specific cuticular hydrocarbons from their ant model prey. *Naturwissenschaften*, **91**, 143–147.

Elgar, M. A. and Allan, R. A. (2006). Chemical mimicry of the ant *Oecophylla smaragdina* by the myrmecophilous spider *Cosmophasis bitaeniata*: is it colony-specific? *Journal of Ethology*, **24**, 239–246.

Elias, D. O., Mason, A. C. and Hoy, R. R. (2004). The effect of substrate on the efficacy of seismic courtship signal transmission in the jumping spider *Habronattus dossenus* (Araneae: Salticidae). *Journal of Experimental Biology*, **207**, 4105–4110.

Elias, D. O., Mason, A. C., Maddison, W. P. and Hoy, R. R. (2003). Seismic signals in a courting male jumping spider (Araneae: Salticidae). *Journal of Experimental Biology*, **206**, 4029–4039.

Endler, J. A. and Basolo, A. L. (1998). Sensory ecology, receiver biases and sexual selection. *Trends in Ecology and Evolution*, **13**, 415–420.

Fan, C.-M., Yang, E.-C. and Tso, I. M. (2009). Hunting effciency and predation risk shapes the color-associated foraging traits of a predator. *Behavioral Ecology*, **20**, 808–816.

Gaskett, A. (2007). Spider sex pheromones: emission, reception, structures, and functions. *Biological Reviews*, **82**, 26–48.

Gaskett, A. C., Winnick, C. G. and Herberstein, M. E. (2008). Orchid sexual deceit provokes ejaculation. *American Naturalist*, **171**, E206–212.

Grether, G. F., Kolluru, G. R. and Nersissian, K. (2004). Individual colour patches as multicomponent signals. *Biological Reviews*, **79**, 583–610.

Hauber, M. E. (2002). Conspicuous colouration attracts prey to a stationary predator. *Ecological Entomology*, **27**, 686–691.

Haynes, K. F., Gemeno, C., Yeargan, K. V., Millar, J. G. and Johnson, K. M. (2002). Aggressive chemical mimicry of moth pheromones by a bolas spider: how does this specialist predator attract more than one species of prey? *Chemoecology*, **12**, 99–105.

Haynes, K. F., Yeargan, K. V. and Gemeno, C. (2001). Detection of prey by a spider that aggressively mimics pheromone blends. *Journal of Insect Behavior*, **14**, 535–544.

Hebets, E. A., Elias, D. O., Mason, A. C., Miller, G. L. and Stratton, G. E. (2008). Substrate-dependent signalling success in the wolf spider, *Schizocosa retrorsa*. *Animal Behaviour*, **75**, 605–615.

Heiling, A. M. and Herberstein, M. E. (2004). Predator-prey coevolution: Australian native bees avoid their spider predators. *Proceedings of the Royal Society of London, B*, **271**, S196–S198.

Heiling, A. M., Cheng, K., Chittka, L., Goeth, A. and Herberstein, M. E. (2005a). The role of UV in crab spider signals: effects on perception by prey and predators. *Journal of Experimental Biology*, **208**, 3925–3931.

Heiling, A. M., Chittka, L., Cheng, K. and Herberstein, M. E. (2005b). Colouration in crab spiders: substrate choice and prey attraction. *Journal of Experimental Biology*, **208**, 1785–1792.

Heiling, A. M., Herberstein, M. E. and Chittka, L. (2003). Crab-spiders manipulate flower signals. *Nature*, **421**, 334.

Herberstein, M. E., Craig, C. L., Coddington, J. A. and Elgar, M. A. (2000). The functional significance of silk decorations of orb-web spiders: a critical review of the empirical evidence. *Biological Reviews*, **75**, 649–669.

Herberstein, M. E., Heiling, A. M. and Cheng, K. (2009). Evidence for UV-based sensory exploitation in Australian but not European crab spiders. *Evolutionary Ecology*, **23**, 621–634.

Herberstein, M. E., Schneider, J. M. and Elgar, M. A. (2002). Costs of courtship and mating in a sexually cannibalistic orb-web spider: female mating strategies and their consequences for males. *Behavioral Ecology and Sociobiology*, **51**, 440–446.

Hoese, F. J., Law, E. A. J., Rao, D. and Herberstein, M. E. (2006). Distinctive yellow bands on a sit-and-wait predator: prey attractant or camouflage? *Behaviour*, **143**, 763–781.

Howard, R. W. and Blomquist, G. J. (2005). Ecological, behavioral, and biochemical aspects of insect hydrocarbons. *Annual Review of Entomology*, **50**, 371–393.

Hutchinson, C. E. (1903). A bolas throwing spider. *Scientific American*, **89**, 172.

Jackson, R. R. (1990a). Predatory and silk utilisation behaviour of *Gelotia* sp. indet. (Araneae: Salticidae: Spartaeinae), a web-invading aggressive mimic from Sri Lanka. *New Zealand Journal of Zoology*, **17**, 475–482.

Jackson, R. R. (1990b). Predatory versatility and intraspecific interactions of *Cyrba algerina* and *Cyrba ocellata*, web-invading spartaeine jumping spiders (Araneae: Salticidae). *New Zealand Journal of Zoology*, **17**, 157–168.

Jackson, R. R. (1992a). Conditional strategies and interpopulation variation in the behaviour of jumping spiders. *New Zealand Journal of Zoology*, **19**, 99–111.

Jackson, R. R. (1992b). Eight-legged tricksters: spiders that specialize in catching other spiders. *BioScience*, **42**, 590–598.

Jackson, R. R. (1992c). Predator-prey interactions between web-invading jumping spiders and two species of tropical web-building pholcid spiders, *Psilochorus sphaeroides* and *Smeringopus pallidus*. *Journal of Zoology, London*, **227**, 531–536.

Jackson, R. R. (2002). Trial-and-error derivation of aggressive-mimicry signals by *Brettus* and *Cyrba*, spartaeine jumping spiders (Araneae: Salticidae) from Israel, Kenya, and Sri Lanka. *New Zealand Journal of Zoology*, **29**, 95–117.

Jackson, R. R. and Brassington, R. J. (1987). The biology of *Pholcus phalangioides* (Araneae, Pholcidae): predatory versatility, araneophagy and aggressive mimicry. *Journal of Zoology, London*, **211**, 227–238.

Jackson, R. R. and Carter, C. M. (2001). Geographic variation in reliance on trial-and-error signal derivation by *Portia labiata*, an araneophagic jumping spider from the Philippines. *Journal of Insect Behavior*, **14**, 799–827.

Jackson, R. R. and Hallas, S. E. A. (1986). Predatory versatility and intraspecific interactions of spartaeine jumping spiders (Araneae: Salticidae): *Brettus adonis, B. cingulatus, Cyrba algerina*, and *Phaeacius* sp. indet. *New Zealand Journal of Zoology*, **13**, 491–520.

Jackson, R. R. and Whitehouse, M. E. A. (1986). The biology of New Zealand and Queensland pirate spiders (Araneae, Mimetidae): aggressive mimicry, araneophagy and prey specialization. *Journal of Zoology, London*, **210**, 279–303.

Jackson, R. R. and Wilcox, R. S. (1990). Aggressive mimicry, prey-specific predatory behaviour and predator-recognition in the predator-prey interactions of *Portia fimbriata* and *Euryattus* sp., jumping spiders from Queensland. *Behavioral Ecology and Sociobiology*, **26**, 111–119.

Jackson, R. R. and Wilcox, R. S. (1993). Spider flexibly chooses aggressive mimicry signals for different prey by trial and error. *Behaviour*, **127**, 21–36.

Jackson, R. R., Li, D. and Robertson, M. B. (1997). Cues by which suspended-leaf nests of *Euryattus* (Araneae: Salticidae) females are recognised by conspecific males and by an aggressive-mimic salticid, *Portia fimbriata*. *Journal of Zoology, London*, **243**, 29–46.

Jarman, E. A. R. and Jackson, R. R. (1986). The biology of *Taieria erebus* (Araneae, Gnaphosidae), an araneophagic spider from New Zealand: silk utilisation and predatory versatility. *New Zealand Journal of Zoology*, **13**, 521–541.

Johnson, S. D. (2000). Batesian mimicry in the non-rewarding orchid *Disa pulchra*, and its consequences for pollinator behaviour. *Biological Journal of the Linnean Society*, **71**, 119–132.

Johnstone, R. A. (1997). The evolution of animal signals. In *Behavioural Ecology* (ed. J. R. Krebs and N. B. Davies). Oxford, UK: Blackwell Science.

Klärner, D. and Barth, F. G. (1982). Vibratory signals and prey capture in orb-weaving spiders (*Zygiella x-notata, Nephila clavipes*; Araneidae). *Journal of Comparative Physiology*, **148**, 445–455.

Kloock, C. T. (2001). Diet and insectivory in the 'araneophagic' spider, *Mimetus notius* (Araneae: Mimetidae). *American Midland Naturalist*, **146**, 424–428.

Kotiaho, J., Alatalo, R. V., Mappes, J. and Parri, S. (1996). Sexual selection in a wolf spider: male drumming activity, body size, and viability. *Evolution*, **50**, 1977–1981.

Land, M. F., Horwood, J., Lim, M. L. M. and Li, D. (2007). Optics of the ultra-violet reflecting scales of a jumping spider. *Proceedings of the Royal Society of London, B*, **274**, 1583–1589.

Landolfa, M. A. and Barth, F. G. (1996). Vibrations in the orb web of the spider *Nephila clavipes*: cues for discrimination and orientation. *Journal of Comparative Physiology, A*, **179**, 493–508.

Li, D. and Lim, M. L. M. (2005). Ultraviolet cues affect the foraging behaviour of jumping spiders. *Animal Behaviour*, **70**, 771–776.

Li, J. J., Zhang, Z. T., Liu, F. X., *et al.* (2008). UVB-based mate choice cues used by females of the jumping spider *Phintella vittata*. *Current Biology*, **18**, 699–703.

Lim, M. L. M. and Li, D. (2006). Extreme ultraviolet sexual dimorphism in jumping spiders (Araneae: Salticidae). *Biological Journal of the Linnean Society*, **89**, 397–406.

Lim, M. L. M., Land, M. F. and Li, D. (2007). Sex-specific UV and fluorescence signals in jumping spiders. *Science*, **315**, 481.

Lim, M. L. M., Li, J. and Li, D. (2008). Effect of UV-reflecting markings on female mate-choice decisions in *Cosmophasis umbratica*, a jumping spider from Singapore. *Behavioral Ecology*, **19**, 61–66.

Maklakov, A. A., Bilde, T. and Lubin, Y. (2003). Vibratory courtship in a web-building spider: signalling quality or stimulating the female? *Animal Behaviour*, **66**, 623–630.

Masters, W. M. (1984). Vibrations in the orbwebs of *Nuctenea sclopetaria* (Araneidae). II. Prey and wind signals and the spider's response threshold. *Behavioral Ecology and Sociobiology*, **15**, 217–223.

Masters, W. M. and Markl, H. (1981). Vibration signal transmission in spider orb webs. *Science*, **213**, 363–365.

Masters, W. M., Markl, H. S. and Moffat, A. J. M. (1986). Transmission of vibration in a spider's web. In *Spiders: Webs, Behavior, and Evolution* (ed. W. A. Shear). Stanford, CA: Stanford University Press.

Morse, D. H. (1981). Prey capture by the crab spider *Misumena vatia* (Clerck) (Thomisidae) on three common native flowers. *American Midland Naturalist*, **105**, 358–367.

Nakamura, T. and Yamashita, S. (2000). Learning and discrimination of colored papers in jumping spiders (Araneae, Salticidae). *Journal of Comparative Physiology, A*, **186**, 897–901.

Oxford, G. S. and Gillespie, R. G. (1998). Evolution and ecology of spider coloration. *Annual Review of Entomology*, **43**, 619–643.

Oxford, G. S. and Gillespie, R. G. (2001). Portraits of evolution: studies of coloration in Hawaiian spiders. *BioScience*, **51**, 521–528.

Parker, A. R. and Hegedus, Z. (2003). Diffractive optics in spiders. *Journal of Optics, A – Pure and Applied Optics*, **5**, S111–S116.

Schimizu, I. and Barth, F. G. (1996). The effect of temperature on the temporal structure of the vibratory courtship signals of a spider (*Cupiennius salei* Keys.). *Journal of Comparative Physiology, A*, **179**, 363–370.

Schmitt, A., Schuster, M. and Barth, F. G. (1994). Vibratory communication in a wandering spider, *Cupiennius getazi*: female and male preferences for features of the conspecific male's releaser. *Animal Behaviour*, **48**, 1155–1171.

Schneider, J. M. and Lesmono, K. (2009). Courtship raises male fertilization success through post-mating sexual selection in a spider. *Proceedings of the Royal Society of London, B*, **276**, 3105–3111.

Stowe, M. K., Tumlinson, J. H. and Heath, R. R. (1987). Chemical mimicry: bolas spiders emit components of moth prey species sex pheromones. *Science*, **236**, 964–967.

Stuart-Fox, D. (2005). Deception and the origin of honest signals. *Trends In Ecology and Evolution*, **20**, 521–523.

Suter, R. B. and Renkes, G. (1984). The courtship of *Frontinella pyramitela* (Araneae, Linyphiidae): patterns, vibrations and functions. *Journal of Arachnology*, **12**, 37–54.

Symonds, M. R. E. and Elgar, M. A. (2008). The evolution of pheromone diversity. *Trends in Ecology and Evolution*, **23**, 220–228.

Tarsitano, M., Jackson, R. R. and Kirchner, W. H. (2000). Signals and signal choices made by the araneophagic jumping spider *Portia fimbriata* while hunting the orb-weaving web spiders *Zygiella x-notata* and *Zosis geniculatus*. *Ethology*, **106**, 595–615.

Théry, M. and Casas, J. (2002). Predator and prey views of spider camouflage. *Nature*, **415**, 133.

Théry, M. and Casas, J. (2009). The multiple disguises of spiders: web colour and decorations, body colour and movement. *Philosophical Transactions of the Royal Society, B*, **364**, 471–480.

Théry, M., Debut, M., Gomez, D. and Casas, J. (2005). Specific color sensitivities of prey and predator explain camouflage in different visual systems. *Behavioral Ecology*, **16**, 25–29.

Tso, I. M., Huang, J.-P. and Liao, C.-P. (2007). Nocturnal hunting of a brightly coloured sit-and-wait predator. *Animal Behaviour*, **74**, 787–793.

Tso, I. M., Lin, C. W. and Yang, E. C. (2004). Colourful orb-weaving spiders, *Nephila pilipes*, through a bee's eyes. *Journal of Experimental Biology*, **207**, 2631–2637.

Tso, I. M., Tai, P. L., Ku, T. H., Kuo, C. H. and Yang, E. C. (2002). Colour-associated foraging success and population genetic structure in a sit-and-wait predator *Nephila maculata* (Araneae: Tetragnathidae). *Animal Behaviour*, **63**, 175–182.

Václav, R. and Prokop, P. (2006). Does the appearance of orbweaving spiders attract prey? *Annales Zoologici Fennici*, **43**, 65–71.

Vanderhoff, E., Byers, C. and Hanna, C. (2008). Do the color and pattern of *Micrathena gracilis* (Araneae: Araneidae) attract prey? Examination of the prey attraction hypothesis and crypsis. *Journal of Insect Behavior*, **21**, 469–475.

Von Helversen, O. (1972). Zur spektralen Unterschiedsempfindlichkeit der Honigbienen. *Journal of Comparative Physiology*, **80**, 439–472.

Walla, P., Barth, F. G. and Eguchi, E. (1996). Spectral sensitivity of single photoreceptor cells in the eyes of the ctenid spider *Cupiennius salei* Keys. *Zoological Science*, **13**, 199–202.

Whitehouse, M. E. A. (1988). Factors influencing specificity and choice of host in *Argyrodes antipodiana* (Theridiidae, Araneae). *Journal of Arachnology*, **16**, 349–355.

Yamashita, S. (2002). Efferent innervation of photoreceptors in spiders. *Microscopy Research and Technique*, **58**, 356–364.

Yeargan, K. V. (1994). Biology of bolas spiders. *Annual Review of Entomology*, **39**, 81–99.

Yeargan, K. V. and Quate, L. W. (1996). Juvenile bolas spiders attract psychodid flies. *Oecologia*, **106**, 266–271.

Yeargan, K. V. and Quate, L. W. (1997). Adult male bolas spiders retain juvenile hunting tactics. *Oecologia*, **112**, 572–576.

7

Mating behaviour and sexual selection

JUTTA SCHNEIDER AND MAYDIANNE ANDRADE

Spider mating behaviour is varied and often surprising. In the past few decades, there has been a shift from descriptive natural history approaches to a more manipulative, theory-based dissection of the behavioural and evolutionary ecology of mating. This approach has yielded evidence in support of important underlying themes of sexual selection. In this chapter, we summarise patterns of mating behaviour in spiders, and the conditions that underlie variation in this behaviour, with an emphasis on how sexual selection theory relates to observed patterns. We end by suggesting spiders may prove particularly tractable models for testing hypotheses regarding mechanisms of sexual selection, sex-specific mating tactics, and reciprocal links between these, and ecology, demography and life history.

7.1   Introduction

There are a number of traits common to the true spiders (Order Araneae) that lend unusual dimensions to their mating behaviour (e.g. Uhl and Elias, Chapter 5). Almost all spiders are predacious (for an exception see Meehan *et al.*, 2009), and have sensory systems exquisitely tuned to vibrational and pheromonal signals. Males transfer sperm via specialised intromittent organs (males' palps), not directly connected to the gonads, into females' sperm storage organs of variable number (spermathecae), often via independent insemination tubules (Foelix, 1996). In addition, although the mating season holds risks similar to those for all sexual species (e.g. mate rejection, competitive injury, predation), male spiders (and rarely, females; Aisenberg *et al.*, 2009, Cross *et al.*, 2007b, Jackson and Pollard, 1990, Schutz and Taborsky, 2005) also face the additional risk of mortality through their predacious potential mate. While

Spider Behaviour: Flexibility and Versatility, ed. Marie Elisabeth Herberstein. Published by Cambridge University Press. © Cambridge University Press 2011.

risks of injury during mating exist in other taxa such as dung flies (Hammer, 1941) and toads (Davies and Halliday, 1979), there is only a handful of other taxa in which males are killed by the female during courtship, copulation or after copulation (e.g. praying mantids, ceratopogonid midges, reviewed in Elgar, 1992). The risk and occurrence of cannibalism in spiders has three important consequences. First, foraging and mating considerations are likely to have intertwined effects on variation in female reproductive decisions, allowing interesting linkages to be made between ecology and mating behaviour (e.g. Elgar, 1998, Johnson, 2005a, Newman and Elgar, 1991). Secondly, the risk of cannibalism may impose strong selection on behavioural, morphological and life history traits that influence male reproduction. Thus, spiders may be particularly useful subjects for testing evolutionary ecology hypotheses regarding how these phenotypic traits respond to sexual selection. Thirdly, the evolutionary interests of females may have a particularly strong influence on mating outcomes, allowing more direct tests of theory underlying female reproductive decisions than is possible in other systems. For these reasons, despite unique aspects of their reproductive biology, spiders may nevertheless provide excellent models for investigating a range of general questions and debates regarding the evolution and maintenance of sexual strategies (Huber, 2005). Some of these issues have been reviewed recently (e.g. sperm competition and cryptic choice, Eberhard, 2004; genital evolution, Eberhard and Huber, 2010, Huber, 2003, Ramos *et al.*, 2005; sexual cannibalism, Wilder *et al.*, 2009; sexual size dimorphism, Foellmer and Moya-Larano, 2007, Mas *et al.*, 2009).

Here we step through the diverse and complex mating behaviours of spiders in sequence by starting with initial mate attraction and ending with postcopulatory processes that affect paternity. We focus primarily on solitary species, as the bulk of research on mating behaviour has been in these taxa (see Chapter 8 for more information on social spiders). We provide a summary of the theory and key empirical studies that are important at each stage of sexual interactions between males and females. As we summarise our current knowledge about the reproductive strategies of spiders, we also suggest areas where more study is important, and highlight those areas where new work on Araneae may illuminate broadly applicable areas of theory.

7.2   Mate attraction and approach

7.2.1   *Sex pheromones and attracting potential mates*

The first step in successful reproduction is finding a potential mate, and this may not be trivial for spiders since most are solitary (Foelix, 1996; for exceptions see Avilés, 1997). In one crab spider species (Thomisidae: *Misumena vatia*) mate-searching males are induced by mechanical cues to follow silk lines left on the substrate, a method that can lead them to relatively immobile conspecific females (Anderson and Morse, 2001). This method is error prone, however, as males follow very old lines as well as those of heterospecifics. Nevertheless, because females are sparsely distributed, rarely move, and do not build webs, chemical cues may be available only transiently. This is an exception to the usual pattern, however, as in most species receptive females produce chemicals to which males are attracted (pheromones). Some web-bound and/or cuticular pheromones are emitted as airborne volatiles while others are detected only on contact (Gaskett, 2007, Schulz, 2004). In at least two wolf spiders (*Allocosa brasiliensis* and *A. alticeps*: Lycosidae), females approach males that defend burrows in which females oviposit (Aisenberg *et al.*, 2009, 2010). Even in this sex-role-reversed species attraction and discrimination among potential mates is mediated by volatile pheromones, in this case emitted by males (Aisenberg *et al.* 2008, 2009, 2010).

The mode of pheromone transmission (airborne or contact) varies across taxa. Pheromones requiring direct contact with silk or cuticle have been found in all species studied to date, but airborne pheromones have been mainly documented in web-building species (Gaskett, 2007). This pattern may reflect the fact that an airborne gradient would not yield reliable information about mate location in species where females move frequently, so there would be little selection on males (receivers) to use airborne chemicals for mate searching in cursorial spiders. Regardless of transmission mode, the chemicals themselves encode a wide range of information that can be used by males (reviewed in Gaskett, 2007, Schulz and Toft, 1993), including location and identity of conspecifics (but see Kasumovic and Andrade, 2004, Ross and Smith, 1979), female mating status, mass (which is usually related to fecundity), age and even morphotype (Aisenberg and Costa, 2008, Pruitt and Riechert, 2009). Since females are voracious hunters, a male that mistakenly approaches a heterospecific or a non-receptive conspecific female increases the risk of being killed, so correct identification of potential mates is critically important for male spiders. Using pheromones that are airborne or on silk allows this to occur at a safe distance (Gaskett, 2007, Schulz, 2004). Strong selection to detect and respond to chemicals produced by females has resulted in very sensitive tuning of male responses. For example, *Anelosimus studiosus* (Theridiidae) are behaviourally polymorphic with social and asocial forms. Asocial females have a higher probability of attacking and killing males whereas social females are more likely to tolerate males and mate (Pruitt and Riechert, 2009, Pruitt *et al.*, 2008). Males of both morphotypes preferentially approach and court social females, and this discrimination is based on pheromones released from the female's web or from her body (Pruitt and Riechert, 2009).

Once males are in close proximity to females, their webs or burrows, phero-mones elicit courtship activity (Anava and Lubin, 1993, Maklakov et al., 2003, Papke et al., 2001) and/or induce males to remain on or near the web (Andrade and Kasumovic, 2005, Prenter et al., 1994a). This often requires direct contact with the chemicals on the female's cuticle or silk (Gaskett, 2007, Pruitt and Riechert, 2009, Schulz, 2004, Stoltz et al., 2007, Wu et al., 2007). In diurnal, mobile species such as jumping spiders (Salticidae), visual contact with females may also be necessary or may augment effects of pheromonal courtship triggers (Elias et al., 2003, Maddison and Hedin, 2003).

While it is clearly advantageous for males to detect and respond appropri-ately to chemical information produced by females, females do not always benefit from male responses. From the female's perspective, there may be significant costs associated with the presence of courting males (e.g. kleptopara-sitism, decreased foraging success, increased exposure to predation, damage to the web (Anava and Lubin, 1993, Forster, 1995, Herberstein et al., 2002, Pruden and Uetz, 2004, Rovner, 1968, Watson, 1986). Moreover, pheromone-mediated discrimination among females by males may limit female opportunities for polyandry (see Sections 7.2.4 'Male mate choice' and 7.4 'Consequences of polyandry'). Although attracting males often increases female fitness despite these costs (particularly for virgin females), it is not always clear whether pheromones are true signals (products of sender–receiver coevolution, opti-mised for information transfer), or whether they are cues (produced as a side-effect of females' physiological processes) exploited by males (see Bradbury and Vehrencamp, 2000, for discussion of the relationship between these). If phero-mones are cues that lead to male responses not favourable to females, an evolutionary arms race could result with females evolving to conceal cues that males evolve to detect. A recent study on wolf spiders (Lycosidae: *Schizocosa malitiosa*) suggests this question may be interesting. Baruffaldi and Costa (2010) show that male *S. malitiosa* have sexual responses to chemicals on females' silk even when those females are not sexually receptive. Most intriguing, males show low response to the silk of recently moulted adult females even though these females are receptive and present a low risk of sexual cannibalism. This apparent mismatch between receiver response and information content of the pheromone suggests males are detecting cues inadvertently produced by females rather than chemical signals. Although the distinction between cues and signals has received considerable theoretical attention (e.g. Bradbury and Vehrencamp, 2000), no studies on spiders have examined this question directly.

If pheromones are true signals, strategic production by females is expected. Given the costs of attracting males, and possible physiological costs associated with sex pheromone synthesis (Chinta et al., 2010, Jerhot et al., 2010, Johansson

and Jones, 2007, Schulz, 2004), females should only produce attractive pheromones when the direct (material) or indirect (genetic) benefits of mating or
remating (Andersson, 1994) outweigh these costs. For virgin females, costs
should be balanced by the risk of remaining unfertilised, and for previously
mated females, potential benefits of additional matings should be important
mediators of pheromone production (see Sections 7.2.3 'Female mate choice'
and 7.4 'Consequences of polyandry'). Consistent with this prediction, pheromone production by females is typically related to mating status (Gaskett, 2007,
Schulz, 2004). Studies suggest virgin females initially produce pheromones and
cease production after mating, and females of some species recommence production after depositing a number of egg sacs, perhaps when sperm supplies are
depleted (Anava and Lubin, 1993, Maklakov *et al.*, 2003, Perampaladas *et al.*,
2008, Roberts and Uetz, 2005, Stoltz *et al.*, 2007). However, the possibility that
pheromone production might be more flexibly related to variation in the benefits of polyandry has not been studied to date.

In addition to 'all or none' production tactics, there is intriguing evidence
that experience may lead to graded variation in females' pheromone production
tactics. In at least one species, *Neriene litigiosa* (Linyphiidae), virgin females that
are isolated from males (reared in the laboratory) apparently produce more
concentrated (or more attractive) airborne pheromones than those reared in
the presence of males (Watson, 1986). Such sensitivity to the proximity or
density of potential mates may be critically important in the field, where
females' webs or burrows may be located in areas where males are unlikely to
detect them, but the accumulation of males on females' webs results in costly
web destruction (Watson, 1986).

Summary

Mate attraction and the initiation of sexual behaviour are mediated by
pheromones in most spiders. For males, a wide range of information about
potential mates can be derived from sex pheromones, and using chemicals to
identify receptive conspecifics reduces the risk of sexual cannibalism. Through
pheromone production, females control this first step of mating interactions.
Since the attraction of courting males is costly to females, females may engage
in strategic advertisement, only producing sex pheromones when sperm is
needed (e.g. virgin females, females that are sperm depleted). Graded variation
in pheromone production is also possible, but this has not been well studied. It
is currently unclear whether sex pheromones of most species are properly
considered true signals, or whether they are cues produced inadvertently by
females and exploited by males. The distinction has important evolutionary
implications, but has received little attention to date.

7.2.2   *Courtship*

Here we consider pre-copulatory interactions that affect whether or not mating occurs. Courtship clearly affects mating success in many species; it also affects post-copulatory processes (e.g. sperm-use patterns), but we consider the latter independently below (Section 7.4 'Consequences of polyandry').

As males approach conspecific females, there is likely to be strong selection for effective courtship signalling to suppress the hunting behaviour of predatory females, which requires males to identify themselves as conspecifics while attracting the female's attention. Males must also induce receptivity and/or trigger favourable choice by females. Failure at either of these steps could be fatal. Thus adaptations in males to avoid female aggression may manifest in striking ways during approach and courtship. In web-building spiders (Orbiculariae), courtship usually begins when males move across the female's web, and frequently involves male modifications of the web that could impede the female's movements and decrease the risk of cannibalism (Robinson and Robinson, 1980), or reduce the attraction of rivals by damaging pheromone-bearing silk (i.e. 'web reduction'; e.g. Theridiidae: Anava and Lubin, 1993, Forster, 1995; and Linyphiidae: Rovner, 1968, Watson, 1986). In addition, males of some web-building and cursorial species drape their own silk directly across the female's abdomen (i.e. 'bridal veils'; e.g. Theridiidae: Forster, 1995; Nephilidae: Robinson and Robinson, 1980; Lycosidae: Aisenberg *et al.*, 2008, Kaston, 1970; Pisauridae: Merrett, 1988; Thomisidae: Bristowe, 1958; Ctenidae: Schmitt, 1992). Although the function of these 'veils' is unclear, they may expose females to tactile and/or chemical cues that induce quiescence (see 'Catalepsy' in Section 7.3.2). Despite some claims to the contrary, these veils do not appear to function by physically restraining the female.

Courtship generally involves sequences of movements that create visual and vibratory signals, and may also facilitate chemical communication (see Chapter 5). Courtship signalling in spiders is often interpreted as a way to prevent sexual cannibalism before mating. Such a premature death is detrimental for the male's reproductive success but may also be so for females if they remain unmated as a result (Arnqvist and Henriksson, 1997, Johnson and Sih, 2005, 2007). Pre-copulatory sexual cannibalism has been discussed for years and several explanations have been proposed and tested (reviewed in: Elgar, 1992, Elgar and Schneider, 2004, Prenter *et al.*, 2006). One of these ideas connected with courtship is that pre-copulatory cannibalism occurs when females confuse males with prey. The correct display should prevent or reduce these recognition errors. One critical prediction of this hypothesis is that variation in male signals should be linked to the likelihood of sexual cannibalism. A similar prediction derives from an alternative hypothesis – that females assess males during court-ship and use pre-copulatory cannibalism to reject inferior males (reviewed in Prenter *et al.*, 2006). While some studies show that variation in the phenotype or behaviour of courting males affects the frequency of pre-copulatory sexual cannibalism (reviewed in Prenter *et al.*, 2006), there is little definitive evidence for the importance of courtship in preventing cannibalism.

Although spiders in many taxa identify conspecifics at a distance by phero-mones (Gaskett, 2007), close-range vibratory or visual signals of courtship also have elements that allow species recognition by females (e.g. Ctenidae, *Cupiennius* species; Barth and Schmitt, 1991, Schmitt *et al.*, 1994, Schüch and Barth, 1990). It is worth noting that female preference for species-specific signal features could also be beneficial if the ability to produce these features reliably is heritable (e.g. 'sexy sons' benefits of female choice; Hedrick, 1988) but this possibility has not been examined in spiders. Nevertheless, courtship signals clearly function pri-marily in sexual selection in many species. For example, phylogenetic and empir-ical analyses suggest that the species-specific courtship signals of salticids (jumping spiders) are most consistent with rapid evolutionary divergence driven by sexual selection (e.g. Elias *et al.*, 2007, Maddison and Hedin, 2003, Maddison and Stratton, 1988, Masta and Maddison, 2002; see Chapter 5). In the salticid genus *Habronattus*, relatively recent divergence among species is accompanied by striking divergence in male sexual displays (morphology and behaviour) and genitalia. Moreover, a study on recent divergence among isolated populations of *Habronattus pugilis* shows divergent female preference for male display traits that differ between populations, and genetic evidence of directional selection on those same male traits (Elias *et al.*, 2007, Masta and Maddison, 2002). The same process may explain the diverse signals of some wolf spiders (Lycosidae, *Schizocosa*; e.g. Stratton, 2005). In general it is not yet clear why courtship signals may be important primarily for species recognition in some taxa but an impor-tant element of female choice in others (see Section 7.2.3 'Female mate choice').

Even among species where courtship signalling is under sexual selection, there is variability in the importance of the details of the signal itself. Whereas signal characteristics are reliable indicators of male phenotype and predict mating success in some species, in others it has been argued that it is simply the presence of the signal that affects male attractiveness. For example, while seismic signal frequency is condition dependent, related to male viability, and strongly affects female mating propensity in some wolf spiders (Lycosidae; Ahtiainen *et al.*, 2004, Kotiaho *et al.*, 1996, 1999b), in other species, simply the presence of a signal is a critical mediator of female receptivity to mating (Elias *et al.*, 2005, Jackson, 1981, Maklakov *et al.*, 2003). Male *Stegodyphus lineatus* (Eresidae) produce relatively simple vibratory signals in the female's cob web.

Not all males vibrate, but vibration is more common in pairings with virgin females rather than mated females, and vibrating males copulate with virgins more rapidly and more frequently than those that do not. Vibratory frequency had no effect on female aggression or male mating success (also see Quirici and Costa, 2005, Rivero *et al.*, 2000, for comparable results in wolf spiders and tarantulas). Similarly, in some *Schizocosa* species (Lycosidae), mating success is increased by the presence (rather than absence) of leg tufts, which increase the ease with which females visually detect males (Hebets and Uetz, 2000, Scheffer *et al.*, 1996). Some of the diversity in the function of courtship signals may thus be driven by variation in signalling microhabitats and substrates, as this affects the detectability of males, the efficacy and attenuation of signal components (this is particularly true of signals transmitted through variable webs; Singer *et al.*, 2000), and thus the potential information content for females (e.g. Elias *et al.*, 2004, Hebets *et al.*, 2008a). Whether the details of signal traits are generally unimportant in spiders is unclear, since most work has been done on lycosids and salticids. Moreover, in general, there have been relatively few sophisticated analyses of the information content of signals in spiders.

In addition to the diversity of signal modalities, there is a stunning range of behavioural elements and sequences in the courtship of spiders, even among closely related species (Elias *et al.*, 2007, Robinson and Robinson, 1980) and geographically separated populations of single species (Elias *et al.*, 2007, Maddison and Stratton, 1988, Masta and Maddison, 2002). Visual signals have been said to resemble 'dancing', 'posturing', 'sidling' or 'waving', and seismic signals may range from simple taps to complex sequences of 'groans', 'thumps' and vibratory trills that sound like motorcycle engines when transduced into auditory stimuli. Broad comparative analyses may be useful to determine whether, for example, interspecific variation in these elements and their sequence reflects differences in selection on courtship elements correlated with heritable high fitness versus phylogenetic canalisation of arbitrary attractive traits or trait sequences that diverge in allopatry.

Impressive variation also exists in courtship behaviours and sequences within populations. In one particularly well studied example of intraspecific variation, alternative male courtship behaviours appear tailored to maximise detectability of two male morphs of the jumping spider *Maevia inclemens* (Salticidae; Clark and Biesiadecki, 2002, Clark and Morjan, 2001, Clark and Uetz, 1993; see Chapter 5). Each morphotype signals at a different distance from the female, and is more easily detected than the other morphotype at that distance. There is no difference in the fitness of the two types of males, suggesting disruptive selection for conspicuousness at each courtship distance may have produced the two morphotypes (Clark and Biesiadecki, 2002, Clark and Uetz, 1992). This type of morph-specific alternative strategy appears to be relatively rare (but see description of size-dependent sneaking behaviour in Section 7.2.5 'Male–male competition'), but context-dependent variation in individual signalling behaviours may be common, at least in salticids (Jackson, 1997). For example, in a number of Salticidae (e.g. *Phidippus johnsoni*, *Mopsus mormon*, *Natta horizontalis*, *Plexippus paykulli*) the form of courtship depends on where it occurs. When males encounter females outside their nests, visual signalling and posturing are important elements of courtship, but inside the nest, where visual signals are impossible because of physical limitations on movement and female vision, courtship is mainly vibratory (Jackson, 1978, 1983, 1986, Jackson, 1997, Jackson and Macnab, 1989a, 1989b).

Another feature of courtship that shows wide variation is courtship duration. The average duration of courtship prior to the initial mating attempt or successful copulation differs by an order of magnitude between taxa. For example, mating occurs after only a few seconds or minutes in hypochilids (Catley, 1993), mygalomorphs (e.g. Costa and Pérez-Miles, 1998, Jackson and Pollard, 1990), and lycosids (Jiao *et al.*, 2009) but after several hours in some theridiids (e.g. Forster, 1995, Harari *et al.*, 2009), linyphiids (Watson and Lighton, 1994) and agelenids (Singer *et al.*, 2000). One can speculate that average differences in courtship duration between taxa may reflect the evolutionary balance between costs of prolonged courtship for males (e.g. risk of interruption by rivals, increased energy use) and the benefits of increased investment prior to attempting mating (e.g. increases in paternity mediated by pre- or post-copulatory female preferences (Schneider and Lesmono, 2009, Stoltz and Andrade, 2010, Stoltz *et al.*, 2008), moderated by the extent to which females shape the outcome of intersexual interactions (see Section 7.4.3 'Sexual conflict'). These factors can also shape intraspecific variation in duration if they affect context-dependent male decisions about investment in courtship. In the simplest case, courtship duration may be variable because some males are rebuffed repeatedly in their attempt to convince females to mate while others are accepted quickly. In this case, courtship duration will be negatively correlated with male attractiveness or indicators of male quality and with female receptivity (e.g. Huber and Eberhard, 1997).

Even more intriguing from the perspective of understanding male behavioural plasticity is the intraspecific variation in courtship duration that is unrelated to immediate female responses (i.e. the time invested prior to the first mating attempt). As might be predicted, males vary courtship effort as a function of their own condition or size (Kotiaho, 2000, but see Johnson, 2005b), the likely reproductive value of the female (Hoefler, 2008), and the risk of usurpation by another male (Stoltz *et al.*, 2008, 2009, Whitehouse, 1991). Changing

abiotic factors such as temperature may also affect variation in courtship duration (Jiao *et al.*, 2009). In *Pardosa astrigera*, courtship (and copulation) duration
decrease with increasing temperature, but the rate of pedipalp insertion
increases (Jiao *et al.*, 2009). These effects may arise through global, temperature-
dependent changes in the rate of physiological processes, but such changes in
courtship or copulation duration could affect post-copulatory sexual selection.
Moreover, it is possible that male decisions about how to best expend effort may
change with external conditions, as temperature-dependent changes in female
receptivity are known in other taxa (e.g. crickets; Kindle *et al.*, 2006). In general,
female mate-choice decision rules and criteria are likely to be important mediators of male courtship duration regardless of temperature. For example, if
females have an absolute standard for choice (a 'threshold' criterion; Kotiaho
et al., 2004, Real, 1990, Stoltz and Andrade, 2010), males that attempt mating
before satisfying this criterion risk failure or worse (e.g. cannibalism; Stoltz and
Andrade, 2010, Stoltz *et al.*, 2009). This may lead to the evolution of limited
variation in male courtship duration. In contrast, if females follow a 'best of *n*'
rule, trade-offs in the likelihood of being the 'best male' versus the risk of
usurpation by a newly arrived rival may lead to briefer or more variable courtship durations. An interesting twist on this effect is seen in the wolf spider
Rabidosa punctulata, in which males court females prior to mating, mount
females directly with no courtship, or use a combination of these tactics.
Wilgers *et al.* (2009) showed that males in poor body condition were more likely
to use the courtship tactic whereas males in good body condition were more
likely to forgo courtship and attempt a direct mount. While this may initially
seem counterintuitive, it could represent divergent optimal male tactics with
cannibalistic females. In this species, direct mounts lead to higher mating
success, but also entail a higher risk of sexual cannibalism, particularly for
males in poor condition. Thus a high-condition male may derive highest fitness
from the direct mount, whereas males in poor condition may do better to take
the less risky, but lower pay-off option (Wilgers *et al.*, 2009).

Summary

Effective courtship is critically important for male success as males
approach potential mates that are also potential cannibals. Courtship signals
occur in multiple modalities but there is currently little evidence that fine
details of attractive signals are heritable, or transmit reliable information
about male phenotype, although the presence of signals often increases mating
success. However, studies of signal elements in arachnids lag far behind the
sophisticated work in insects and birds, so no general patterns can be asserted.
In addition to variable signal elements, extensive plasticity in courtship

behaviours, sequence and duration exists within and across species, and in some cases this has been linked to conditions that affect signal detection, or costs and benefits of investing effort in courtship. There is a critical need for more studies of courtship variation in a wider range of spider taxa.

7.2.3   Female mate choice

Differential response of females to courting males suggests that female choice may impose sexual selection on males and that choosing males of particular behavioural or morphological phenotypes may carry some benefit for females (Andersson, 1994). In spiders, there is no paternal care and nuptial gifts are rare, so there is little chance that female choice provides material benefits to offspring or to the females themselves (but see nuptial gift-giving spiders in Section 7.3.1). This does not rule out the possibility that the timing of female mating may hinge on the avoidance of male-imposed costs (e.g. Herberstein *et al.*, 2002). However, if female spiders are demonstrated to favour males of a particular phenotype, one of the main candidate explanations is that genetic benefits (either heritable high viability or heritable attractiveness) may accrue to offspring of choosy females (Andersson, 1994). The likelihood that genetic benefits of choice are sufficiently large to allow female preferences to evolve and be maintained despite costs of choosiness has been the subject of considerable debate (see review in Puurtinen *et al.*, 2009; Andersson, 1994, Kotiaho and Puurtinen, 2007). However, it is possible that even minimal benefits are sufficient to maintain choice if costs of choice are similarly low (Alatalo *et al.*, 1998). For us, a definitive demonstration of female choice for genetic benefits requires evidence that female preference for male traits confers heritable fitness benefits (e.g. viability, fecundity or attractiveness) to offspring. As in other taxa, evidence from various spider species supports different parts of this hypothesis (Prenter *et al.*, 2006). Studies showing female preference as a function of male phenotype and condition dependence of male signals are the most common of these, possibly because these are commonly tested relationships. To our knowledge, however, only the body of work on *Hygrolycosa* provides convincing evidence for female choice driven by indirect benefits in spiders. Females of *Hygrolycosa rubrofasciata* are attracted to male seismic signals and prefer high drumming rates (Kotiaho *et al.*, 1996, Parri *et al.*, 1997, 2002) that are positively correlated with male longevity (Mappes *et al.*, 1996) and immunocompetence (Ahtiainen *et al.*, 2004). The benefit of selecting males of above average quality is slightly better offspring viability (Alatalo *et al.*, 1998). Drumming activity is condition dependent and costly for males (Kotiaho, 2000) and is thus an honest signal of heritable viability, supporting a good genes model of sexual selection. In contrast to the common examination of predictions underlying good genes models, few studies have asked whether attractive males have more attractive offspring (a critical prediction of 'sexy sons' models). This may be a productive line of research, particularly in taxa with flamboyant and apparently arbitrary variation in male decorations (e.g. salticids) or conspicuous copulatory courtship (e.g. pholcids).

While increased attention to courtship signalling may reveal additional variation in female preference in response to male phenotype, recent studies highlight the critical importance of other female-specific factors, such as nutrition, past experience and age for explaining variation in female choice. *Schizocosa* females consistently show a preference for tufted males over males with reduced leg tufts over three weeks post maturity (Uetz and Norton, 2007) but the preference changes with age and female mating status (Persons and Uetz, 2005). In a striking study of *Schizocosa* females, Hebets (2003) showed that females exposed to males of a given signal intensity as juveniles were more likely to prefer such males as adults (also see Hebets and Vink, 2007). Although it is not clear why selection would favour alteration of female choice behaviour based on this type of experience, this study does suggest that juvenile experience can be an important mediator of mating dynamics.

Other types of variations in female life history affect choosiness in ways that could increase female fitness. For example, there is evidence that females use their body condition to gauge their relative attractiveness as a mate and shift their degree of choosiness accordingly (e.g. Buston and Emlen, 2003). This reduces the risk of delayed mating in species where males prefer females in better body condition (see Section 7.2.4 'Male mate choice'). In a classic example of this type of assortative mating mediated by female choice, high-diet female *Schizocosa* preferentially mated with high-diet males while low-diet females expressed no choice (Hebets *et al.*, 2008b). Similarly, high-diet female *Pardosa* (Lycosidae) are more likely to engage in sexually cannibalistic attacks on potential mates than are low-diet females (Wilder and Rypstra, 2008a). This type of effect can also lead to assortative mating if a subset of males (e.g. larger males) are more likely to survive female attacks (e.g. Wilder and Rypstra, 2008d, Wilder *et al.*, 2009). These examples are consistent with the idea that high-diet females can afford to be more choosy than low-diet females. For example, although the aggressive behaviour of high-diet *Pardosa* females raises a 'bar' that males must surpass to mate and so makes mating less likely, their increased choosiness may not have a net fitness cost because they will be preferred by males (see Section 7.2.4 'Male mate choice'). The female's perception of likelihood of mating may also affect the expression of choosiness. For example, in the lycosid *Hogna helluo* females are more likely to accept a mating if a previous encounter with a male ended without copulation (Wilder and Rypstra, 2008b). Such an experience may suggest the female is of relatively low quality or in a habitat with choosy males, either of which may decrease the probability of successful insemination. In fishing spiders (*Dolomedes*, Pisauridae) females that cohabit with males as juveniles are more likely to cannibalise (rather than mate with) suitors they encounter as adults. This is consistent with the hypothesis that females can use cohabitation to assess the relative utility of a male as a 'mate or a meal' (Johnson, 2005a). The interpretation that female choice depends on female and male relative quality is also consistent with the finding that pre-mating sexual cannibalism appears to occur more with old males (Morse and Hu, 2004) and against relatively small males (Elgar and Jones, 2008). In the wolf spider *Hogna helluo*, hungry females were more likely to attack a male but only if the size difference was relatively large (Wilder and Rypstra, 2008c). Hence at least in a few cases, pre-copulatory sexual cannibalism likely imposes selection on male body size, age, and on male sensitivity to the potential danger imposed by the female he is about to approach (Prenter *et al.*, 2006).

Summary

Female choice may impose selection for honest signals of good genes or for heritable attractiveness, but the former has been convincingly demonstrated in only one spider species and the latter has rarely been studied. General principles underlying female decision rules is a hot area of recent work, and one general insight seems to be the likely importance of past experience, which is rarely factored into conventional tests for mate choice.

7.2.4   *Male mate choice*

Male mate choice in a sex-role-reversed system is expected if males are the sex with the higher reproductive investment and/or if the operational sex ratio (OSR) is sufficiently female biased (Bonduriansky, 2001). There are only two spider species where male reproductive investment approaches or exceeds that of females (e.g. Aisenberg and Costa, 2008). However, male mate choice within otherwise conventional sex roles in spiders is most likely where (a) males are severely sperm limited or (b) males have only a single mating opportunity (monogyny) while females mate multiply and (c) females vary in quality. Preferences of males for virgins, and for larger and fecund females, have been found in a number of species (see review by Huber, 2005; Andrade and Kasumovic, 2005). Males may be particularly likely to prefer virgin females when there is strong first-male sperm precedence and defending penultimate-instar females until they moult takes longer than finding virgins (Elgar, 1998). However, a virgin-female mating bias may also reflect female-mediated reduction in the production of attractive pheromones after mating (Gaskett, 2007). In most of the studies showing a preference for female fecundity, it is not clear why males are under selection to allocate their mating efforts strategically because they do not seem to be limited in mating frequency.

Male choice should be more likely in species where one or more of the following factors limit male mating frequencies. Firstly, adult males of web-building spiders no longer build webs and are less able than cursorial species to maintain the body condition necessary for mate search and competition for long periods. Since mating itself also holds the risk of cannibalism, there may be strong selection to ensure matings with high-quality females. However, if choosy males must forgo females to search for other potential mates, these same factors may mediate against male choice. Secondly, some species may have a limited supply of sperm. This is likely true for males of species that are adapted to mate with one or two females only (monogynous or bigynous) (see Section 7.3.2 'Male mating rates'). Fourteen species with low male mating rates have been tested for the presence of male mate choice, but there is little evidence for mate choice based on female phenotypic traits (Andrade and Kasumovic, 2005). One exception is males of the bigynous *Argiope keyserlingi* (Araneidae) in which males prefer females with slim opisthosomas over fat females even though slim females are likely to be less fecund. The preference presumably arises because in a natural setting the latter are likely mated already while the former are more likely to have recently moulted and be virgin (Gaskett *et al.*, 2004, Herberstein *et al.*, 2005b). A third reason for male mate choice may be pre-copulatory sexual cannibalism. As a counter-adaptation, males are expected to modulate their behaviour or even reject a female according to the risk of sexual cannibalism. Indeed, small and satiated lycosid females (*Lycosa tarantula*) have more male visitors than large and hungry ones (Moya-Larano *et al.*, 2003).

Male mate choice may yield patterns of size-assortative mating. In jumping spiders (Salticidae), binary choice experiments showed that males of all sizes preferred large and early maturing females (Hoefler, 2007). Subsequent tests only using silk of penultimate females suggest that time until maturation is more important than female size probably because of a first male advantage, or an advantage in mating quickly rather than waiting. The sex ratio early in the season is heavily male biased and large males win contests over access to females. These dynamics produce a size-assortative mating pattern (Hoefler, 2007). Size-assortative mating mediated by male mate choice has also been reported in the common orb-web spider *Zygiella x-notata* (Araneidae) where male mating preferences shift with the degree of competition (Bel-Venner *et al.*, 2008). When competition is intense larger males guard more fecund females. Smaller males then avoid these females and thus avoid the cost of losing competitions. When competition is relaxed, males of all sizes mate indiscriminately rather than being choosy. Accordingly, size-assortative mating was only found at a field site with high competition, where males selected females based on their own size and RHP (resource holding potential; see Section 7.2.5 'Male–male competition'). This observational data set could also arise if intermale competition mediated mate-guarding patterns (e.g. larger males were better able to defend all females). Bel-Venner and colleagues (2008) argue this is not the case as data include only pairs found early in the morning, and additional observations suggest these pairs form without intermale competition. Moreover, a recent model suggests this type of mate choice may arise under a range of ecological and social conditions (Venner *et al.*, 2010). Nevertheless, experimental confirmation of this study would be beneficial.

Summary

Although male mate choice is expected to be most likely in species with low male mating rates, the benefits of mating with a virgin and the competition over this privilege may override any benefits gained through mating with the most fecund female. For this reason, although males prefer fecund females in many species, variation in social conditions that affect the likelihood of successfully copulating (e.g. degree of competition) can have significant effects on male choosiness.

7.2.5   *Male–male competition*

When female spiders advertise their receptivity they commonly attract more than one male (Miller, 2007). These males may then engage in combat. As in most species, the outcome of a fight is usually decided by phenotypic differences between combatants (differences in resource holding potential, RHP). In spiders victory may be predicted by RHP asymmetries based on body size (Austad, 1983, Christenson and Goist, 1979, Elias *et al.*, 2008b, Hack *et al.*, 1997, Hoefler, 2002, Jackson and Cooper, 1991, Schaefer and Uhl, 2003, Schmitt *et al.*, 1992, Stoltz *et al.*, 2008, Watson, 1990) or handicaps such as missing legs (e.g. Salticidae: Taylor and Jackson, 2003; Agelenidae: Riechert, 1988; Thomisidae: Dodson and Beck, 1993, but see Dodson and Schwaab, 2001; Pholcidae: Johnson and Jakob, 1999) and early detection of rivals (Taylor *et al.*, 2001). Asymmetries can be assessed through vibratory or visual signalling (Elias *et al.*, 2008b). Escalation of fights is costly in terms of energy expenditure (DeCarvalho *et al.*, 2004) as well as risk of injury or death, and is expected only if the two opponents are very similar in size and vigour (Enquist and Leimar, 1983, 1990) or if the value of the contested resource is sufficiently high (Enquist and Leimar, 1987, Hack *et al.*, 1997, Jackson *et al.*, 2006, Schmitt *et al.*, 1992, Wells, 1988). In most cases however, interactions are brief and settled by a quick flurry of signals that facilitate assessment, followed by the retreat of the inferior individual (Elias *et al.*, 2008a, Taylor *et al.*, 2001).

In his classic study, one of the first to test the basic theory underlying this area of game theory, Austad (1983) manipulated both relative male RHP (size) and female value and showed that both affect fight outcomes in the bowl and doily spider (*Frontinella communis*: Linyphiidae). In these spiders, body size differences above 1 mm clearly determined the winner of fights over females. These fights were generally very brief as the larger male won quickly. In contrast, contestants that differed by less than 1 mm in body length fought for variable, usually longer, durations. The outcome of these 'evenly matched' fights was mainly predicted by the value of the female for each male, consistent with game theory models (Leimar *et al.*, 1991). In this species, the value of females is initially high for a resident male, but declines as copulation proceeds and fertilisation success reaches an asymptote. For an intruder with no opportunity to assess the female, however, the best estimate of female value is the population average, and this does not change over time. As predicted, copulating males usually won fights initiated during the early part of sperm transfer. In contrast, intruders frequently won as copulation duration approached the fertilisation asymptote. Moreover, when RHP was closely matched, asymmetries in the value of the female led to smaller residents winning up to 60% of fights. Even more striking was the finding that smaller residents won up to 20% of fights when the intruder was significantly larger, showing that female value can trump RHP in determining contest outcomes.

Game theoretical models (Enquist and Leimar, 1983, 1987, 1990) predict that a contestant's expected value of future reproduction should also influence his investment in combat, but this parameter is notoriously difficult to manipulate. Fromhage and Schneider (2005a) capitalised on useful aspects of the natural history of *Nephila fenestrata* (Nephilidae) to provide a rare test of this prediction by comparing the contest behaviour of mated and virgin males (Fromhage and Schneider, 2005b). Male *N. fenestrata* damage their embolus and are functionally sterile after mating with females (Fromhage and Schneider, 2006). The broken embolus functions as a mating plug but can be removed by rivals unless the female is guarded (Fromhage and Schneider, 2005b). Thus, the expectation of future reproduction for mated (sterile) males is nil, and males should be motivated to risk injury to guard a mated female, whereas this may not be the case for virgin (fertile) males. In staged encounters, as predicted, virgin males rarely fought, whereas sterile males were more likely to escalate and win fights, even against slightly larger opponents. In general, escalation of fights until combatants are severely injured or killed occurs frequently in some species under conditions that generally match predictions from theory (e.g. Austad, 1983, Cross *et al.*, 2007a, Leimar *et al.*, 1991, Whitehouse, 1991). However, in other spiders, escalation is rare despite predictions (Cross *et al.*, 2007a, Stoltz *et al.*,

2008). Negative responses of females to combat (Stoltz *et al.*, 2008, 2009) or male adoption of alternative tactics (Whitehouse, 1991) may explain this variation.

As in other taxa, observed contest dynamics raise the question of how males assess their own RHP in relation to an opponent (Enquist and Leimar, 1983) or whether self-assessment is sufficient to explain observed contest dynamics (Taylor and Elwood, 2003). Studies on assessment in spiders support a variety of models (Bridge *et al.*, 2000, Elias *et al.*, 2008b, Hack *et al.*, 1997, Hoefler, 2002, Kotiaho *et al.*, 1999a, Leimar *et al.*, 1991, Taylor *et al.*, 2001), and recent work suggests contests may be best understood by considering stage-dependent assessment strategies by which the mode of assessment changes as the fight progresses (Elias *et al.*, 2008b).

There has been very little work on how experience might affect combat tactics in spiders, although these phenomena are important in other taxa (Hsu and Wolf, 2001, Hsu *et al.*, 2006). Such studies may have been limited in the past by a perception that the relatively simple nervous system of spiders is unlikely to allow sophisticated memory effects. However, several experiments now demonstrate that experience (Dodson and Schwaab, 2001, Hoefler, 2002, Kasumovic *et al.*, 2009, Whitehouse, 1997), residency (Hoefler, 2002, Jackson and Cooper, 1991, Stoltz and Andrade, 2010) and the presence of an eavesdropping female (Jackson *et al.*, 2006) can interact with RHP to affect contest progress or outcomes. Depending on the spatiotemporal distribution of competitors, these factors could amplify or dampen the effects of individual phenotypes on contest outcomes (but see Kasumovic *et al.*, 2009). More critically, experience effects may allow males to modulate their aggressive behaviour as a function of their own RHP relative to a running average of local competitors (Hsu and Wolf, 2001, Hsu *et al.*, 2006). Thus consideration of tactics that depend on memory may expose dynamics important to the resolution of combat in the field.

In spiders, past performance has been linked to winner effects (previous winners do better than expected; Theridiidae, *Argyrodes antipodianus*: Whitehouse, 1997; Thomisidae, *Misumenoides formosipes*: Dodson and Schwaab, 2001; Hoefler, 2002; Salticidae, *Phidippus clarus*: Kasumovic *et al.*, 2009), and loser effects (previous losers do worse than expected; Salticidae, *Phidippus clarus*: Kasumovic *et al.*, 2009). In influential early work on experience effects, Whitehouse (1997) trained similarly sized *Argyrodes* males as winners or losers by pairing them repeatedly with larger or smaller competitors. Under normal conditions, each size-matched male had a 50% chance of winning a fight, but when trained males were paired, the trained winner beat the trained loser 94% of the time. Similarly, Dodson and Schwaab (2001) showed that male crab spiders with a single winning experience beat previous losers in 83% of contests, and Hoefler's (2002) work on the same species showed that these winner effects can overcome a demonstrated residency advantage. Recent work on a jumping spider (*Phidippus clarus*: Salticidae) has allowed a dissection of the relative influence and pattern of winner and loser effects with intriguing results. When Kasumovic and colleagues (2010) paired experienced males with size-matched inexperienced males, independent winner and loser effects were measurable (Elias *et al.*, 2008a). Experience had substantial effects on contest behaviour (>20% change in the probability of winning or losing). Interestingly, loser effects were sustained over a longer period (at least 2 hours) than winner effects (less than 2 hours), which may suggest males have a risk-averse tactic for adjusting behaviour with past experience (Kasumovic *et al.*, 2010). This supports a recent proposal that experience effects may allow males to adjust estimates of their own RHP relative to shifting population averages while minimising costs associated with assessment and losing fights (Hsu and Wolf, 2001, Hsu *et al.*, 2006).

While assessment and experience effects may explain variable male behaviour in a number of species, in others alternative competitive behaviours are linked to absolute differences in male size or condition. Typically, while larger males court and guard females, smaller males attempt to sneak copulations. In *Nephila* species, for example, variation in instar number results in a wide range of male sizes with some individuals being 10 times heavier than their competitors (e.g. Elgar and Fahey 1996). Large male *N. clavipes* (Christenson and Goist, 1979), *N. edulis* (Elgar and Jones, 2008, Elgar *et al.*, 2003, Schneider *et al.*, 2000), and *N. plumipes* (Elgar and Fahey 1996) hold the central position at the web hub, usually opposite or above the female. Small males are chased by large males, but they can sneak copulations if they manage to approach and mount the female undetected. Small male *N. edulis* copulate for several minutes while copulations of large males are much shorter (Elgar and Jones, 2008, Schneider *et al.*, 2000), and small males have higher paternity when males are mated in sequence (Schneider *et al.*, 2000). However, relative paternity is apparently equal for both size classes if large and small males compete simultaneously (Elgar and Jones, 2008) which may mean that a large-male advantage in direct competition can balance the copulation duration advantage of small males (also see Kasumovic and Andrade, 2009).

Similar alternative competitive behaviours exist in species with continuous size distributions (Stoltz *et al.*, 2008, Whitehouse, 1991), but these tactics may vary significantly as a function of the context in which males find themselves (e.g. with a larger, smaller, or size-matched competitor). Relatively smaller males generally adopt some form of 'sneaking' behaviour while larger males court or guard females (Elgar and Jones, 2008, Elgar and Fahey, 1996, Stoltz *et al.*, 2008, Whitehouse, 1991, 1997). For example, in *Latrodectus hasselti*, male behaviour changes markedly with the relative size of the competitor, so that males in the same absolute size class court for almost 210 minutes in the presence of a smaller competitor or scramble to mate within 50–80 minutes when a competitor is larger or of similar size (Stoltz and Andrade, 2010, Stoltz *et al.*, 2008, 2009).

Summary

Although fights frequently involve competitive signals and end without significant injury to either combatant, the rules mediating contest resolution are not entirely clear. Spider contests match basic game theory predictions. Recent exploration of how various types of experience and memory effects shape contest outcomes suggest these may provide important additional ways for individuals to tune their competitive strategies to fit local competitive conditions and minimise costs of injury and energy expenditure.

7.3   Mating

The previous section concerned processes that occur prior to mating and that largely determine whether and with whom a spider is going to mate. Since Parker's (1970) and Eberhard's (1996) seminal papers on post-copulatory processes, many studies have addressed adaptations to sperm competition and cryptic female choice in spiders.

Post-copulatory sexual selection requires, at a minimum, the potential for multiple mating by the female. The relative mating frequencies of females and males largely determine selection on both sexes and they determine whether the sexes are in conflict. Therefore, we will start by discussing female and then male mating frequencies before we explore the details of post-copulatory processes.

7.3.1   Female mating rates

Strict monogamy in the sense that both sexes mate with a single partner is rare in spiders. A lack of monogamy is not surprising because monogamy is mostly associated with bi-parental care (Kokko and Jennions, 2008, Trivers, 1972). Spiders do not tend to commit to intensive brood care (with a few exceptions; Chapter 8) and only one case of paternal care has been reported in an arachnid (Mora, 1990). Even in species with extreme forms of maternal care such as many subsocial spiders, males do not contribute to care and hence generally benefit from attempts to mate multiple times (for exceptions from this rule see below).

Female mating rates vary within and between taxa (Elgar, 1998). Species that show variation in re-mating rates are of interest in identifying factors affecting re-mating (Norton and Uetz, 2005, Pérez-Miles *et al.*, 2007, Schaefer and Uhl,

2005, Singer and Riechert, 1995), which include manipulation by males and strategic decisions by females (Elgar, 1998). Male-induced monogamy may occur if the first male to mate employs defences against sperm competition that either influence female receptivity or attractiveness (Aisenberg and Costa, 2005, Hosken *et al.*, 2009). While post-mating declines in female receptivity and attractiveness have been observed in several spider species (e.g. Austad, 1982, Elgar and Bathgate, 1996), the mechanisms involved and which sex is in control are mostly unknown. When Aisenberg and Costa (2005) prevented sperm uptake to the pedipalps in experimental males, they found that these males did not induce the reduction in receptivity seen in females mated to normal males. They suggested that substances in the seminal fluid are responsible, although mechanisms related to the presence of the sperm in the spermatheca have not been excluded.

Males may also influence female mating rates by applying mating plugs. Mating plugs are particularly common among entelegyne species, likely because the application of a plug into or onto the insemination duct does not interfere with egg laying as it would in haplogyne spiders (Uhl *et al.*, 2010). Some mating plugs completely prevent remating (Suhm *et al.*, 1996) while in others the plug can be removed by subsequent males (see discussion below on sperm competition). Female contributions to plug formation may also play a role, suggesting plugs sometimes benefit both sexes (Aisenberg and Eberhard, 2009, Knoflach, 1998, Uhl *et al.*, 2010).

Variation in remating rates of females and low mating rates may also arise from female tactics that reflect the benefits of polyandry relative to costs of remating and sexual conflict. Such costs include increased predation risk and decline in foraging success due to damage to the web and kleptoparasitism (reviewed in Schneider and Lubin, 1998). In *Stegodyphus lineatus* (Eresidae) males cohabit with females for several days: during this time they steal prey from the female and the female no longer maintains her web. A field experiment showed that females lose weight during cohabitation while males gain weight (Erez *et al.*, 2005). Extreme costs of remating due to infanticide (see below) have been reported from the same species (Schneider and Lubin, 1996, 1997b). Potential indirect benefits of polyandry would have to be large to compensate for these costs, but good genes effects were not found to be very pronounced (Maklakov and Lubin, 2004, Maklakov *et al.*, 2005). Nevertheless, despite these massive costs and the regular occurrence of resistance by mated females, conflict with males sometimes ends in female re-mating in up to 50% of the cases (Maklakov *et al.*, 2003).

Benefits of polyandry versus monandry have been looked at in only a few spider species. A theoretical benefit that balances the costs is the avoidance of inbreeding through multiple mating (Cornell and Tregenza, 2007) and there is some support for this in spiders. Sedentary web spiders are particularly vulnerable to inbreeding but active inbreeding avoidance prior to mating has not been documented in spiders. However, several studies propose general mechanisms that reduce the risk of inbreeding such as asynchronous maturation of the sexes (Bukowski and Avilés, 2002) or natal dispersal (Bonte *et al.*, 2007, Li and Kuan, 2006). *Stegodyphus lineatus* is distributed in clusters that often consist of family groups (Johannesen and Lubin, 2001). Males show a tendency to mate initially within a cluster, suggesting that the risk of inbreeding is high. Inbreeding results in a 10% reduction in the quality of first generation offspring under semi-natural conditions, suggesting that inbreeding depression is present, although moderate (Bilde *et al.*, 2005). Mating with more than one male can reduce the risk and cost of inbreeding. This has been convincingly shown in a breeding study on *Oedothorax apicatus* (Linyphiidae) where negative effects of inbreeding are also moderate in the F1 generation, but increase drastically in the F3 (Bilde *et al.*, 2007a). Polyandrous mating with a combination of related and unrelated males completely rescued these negative effects. There exists the interesting possibility that females can assess the risk of inbreeding and remate if appropriate but, at least for *S. lineatus*, this does not appear to be the case. Rather, whether a female remates or not is determined by the body size of subsequent males relative to the female. If the male is larger than the female he can overcome her resistance and the female will mate (Maklakov *et al.*, 2004, Schneider and Lubin, 1997b). Potential indirect benefits through sexy sons that inherit the ability to overcome female resistance have not been tested in *S. lineatus* or in any other spider.

Good genes benefits of multiple mating are reported in two studies, one on bowl and doily spiders (*Neriene litigiosa*, Linyphiidae: Uhl *et al.*, 2005, Watson, 1998) and the second one on cellar spiders (*Pholcus phalangioides*, Pholcidae: Uhl *et al.*, 2005). Offspring sired by multiple fathers had better growth rates and larger body sizes in *N. litigiosa* (Watson, 1998). In the cellar spider, daughters of multiply mated females were in better body condition (Uhl *et al.*, 2005) while female choice had no detectable effect on offspring. Many more studies are needed to be able to draw conclusions about the relevance of additive or non-additive indirect benefits for the evolution of polyandry in spiders. A first useful approach may be the comparison of the risk of inbreeding in monandrous versus polyandrous species.

Other, direct benefits of polyandry include the prevention of sperm depletion as well as the provision of resources, such as nuptial gifts. The latter is probably the most general reason for multiple mating in insects (Arnqvist and Nilsson, 2000). Sperm depletion is likely in spider species with a long reproductive period and a large number of eggs. Indeed *Latrodectus hasselti* females readvertise their receptivity again later in their reproductive life, possibly to replenish or renew sperm supplies before overwintering (Perampaladas *et al.*, 2008), although spermathecal contents were not determined and a single copulation can be sufficient to fertilise all eggs of a female in this species (Andrade and Banta, 2002). Unfortunately, there are extremely few systematic studies available on the problem of sperm depletion in spiders.

The male soma may qualify as a direct benefit of multiple mating if males are consumed after mating. However, in most species where cannibalism after mating is a regular occurrence, males are much smaller than the females and no benefits of consumption on female reproductive success were detected (Andrade, 1996, Elgar *et al.*, 2000, Schneider *et al.*, 2005b). However, so far only fecundity effects (numbers of eggs, not sizes of eggs) have been considered. No study has looked at effects on female survival, or the viability of the offspring as a function of whether or not the father was eaten.

Few spider species present nuptial gifts. Until the recent discovery of nuptial gifts in Trechaleidae, South American cursorial spiders (Costa-Schmidt *et al.*, 2008), only the hunting spiders (Pisauridae) were known for such behaviour. The only well-studied species is *Pisaura mirabilis*. The male approaches the similar-sized female cautiously carrying a prey item in his chelicerae. The size of the gift and the amount of silk in which the gift is wrapped correlate with the duration of copulation (Lang, 1996) which predicts paternity success under sperm competition (Stalhandske, 2001). Females are polyandrous and the degree of polyandry determines relative paternity of all males except the last one to mate, which always achieves about the same fraction of paternity (Drengsgaard and Toft, 1999). Females produce a large egg sac that they carry around in their chelicerae for a period of several weeks. The nuptial gift is often wrapped in white silk and has a similar form as an egg sac. The gift influences mating success, suggesting that the gift works as a sensory trap exploiting the maternal care instinct of the female (Stalhandske, 2002). Bilde *et al.* (2007b) challenged this idea and performed elegant gift-switching experiments so that males presented females with wrapped and unwrapped gifts as well as true egg sacs. Male mating success did not vary with the type of gift presented and females accepted and fed on egg sacs as well. In addition, they found female hunger was most critical for gift acceptance, a result that was supported by a study on another population (Prokop, 2006). Experimental variations of gift shape showed that males benefited from round and wrapped gifts not because of improved acceptance as a mate but because a round wrapped gift facilitated his ability to gain and retain physical access to female genitalia (Andersen *et al.*, 2008). While it is intuitive that the gift somehow benefits the female, there is no evidence that presence or size of the gift influences female reproductive output or offspring size.

Summary

Moderate female multiple mating is common in female spiders but direct benefits are probably rare. Unlike in the insects (Arnqvist and Nilsson, 2000), there is very little evidence that direct benefits provide the most general explanation for polyandry in spiders. Indirect benefits are likely connected to inbreeding avoidance (Maklakov and Lubin, 2006). Selection on polyandry due to indirect benefits requires post-mating selection processes (but see Cornell and Tregenza, 2007). Evidence for cryptic female choice is rare but a few first accounts are encouraging (see below).

7.3.2   Male mating rates

Males are generally described as promiscuous and indeed in many spiders, male fitness is a linear function of his number of mates, consistent with Bateman's rule (Bateman, 1948). Only a few studies looked at natural male mating rates and found that they are limited by search mortality and are rather low (between 1 and 2 on average) (Andrade, 2003, Fromhage *et al.*, 2007, Maklakov *et al.*, 2005, Morse, 2007, Schneider, 1997, Schneider and Lubin, 1996, Singer and Riechert, 1995). The generality of this conclusion is unclear, however, as three of these species were studied partly because their mating systems suggest infrequent male re-mating (*Stegodyphus lineatus*, *Nephila fenestrata* and *Latrodectus hasselti*).

Male mating rates are extremely low, even to the point of monogyny, in a number of species in several families (Miller, 2007). In monogynous species males mate with a single female only and have adaptations for this life history. Such a peculiar mating system can evolve under a restricted set of conditions even in the absence of paternal care (Fromhage *et al.*, 2005). Two major requirements are that monogyny yields some paternity benefit and that in the population more males than females get to mate so that the average male mating success is below one. In a large comparative analysis (Miller, 2007) found that the accumulation of multiple males with individual females co-occurs with male sacrifice across web-building spiders, lending support to the theory.

There are a few monogynous species that are particularly well studied, for example the Australian redback spider *Latrodectus hasselti* (Theridiidae), which will be described in more detail below. The family Theridiidae contains several curious species in which males mate with one female only; the most peculiar are perhaps the one-palped *Tidarren* and *Echinotheridion* species. Male *Tidarren* curtail their own reproductive potential by removing one of their two copulatory organs at sexual maturity (see Chapter 1 for an explanation of male genital morphology). Subsequently, males have only one organ remaining for copulation. In some species, males become 'catatonic' and die during their only copulation (Knoflach and Benjamin, 2003); in others, cannibalism occurs (Knoflach and Van Harten, 2000) so it is unclear whether the female actively kills the male or if she just consumes the dead body.

Other monogynous species occur within the family Nephilidae (see below) and Araneidae such as the genus *Argiope*. The latter genus is interesting because some species show a mixture of a monogynous and a bigynous mating system (Fromhage *et al.*, 2008, Herberstein *et al.*, 2005a). Apart from *Tidarren* and *Echinotheridion* all known examples for monogynous mating systems include males with two pedipalps that are both functional.

After the successful use of their second pedipalp, males of some monogynous species within the families described above will not or cannot reuse a pedipalp – hence they are functionally sterile. While some cases are known where sterile males survive (see below), they die in others. Death of the male can have several causes: males may just perish while still attached to the copulatory opening of the female (Foellmer and Fairbairn, 2003, Sasaki and Iwahashi, 1995) or sacrifice themselves by inviting sexual cannibalism by placing their body on the female chelicerae (Forster, 1992, Segoli *et al.*, 2008a). In *Argiope bruennichi*, female aggression appears to be responsible for male death as females stereotypically attack males within a second of the onset of copulation. While 30% of males survive the attack during the use of their first pedipalp, the male is always killed after his second copulation (Schneider *et al.*, 2006). After the use of the second pedipalp, males simply do not attempt escape and are wrapped and consumed.

In those species in which males use each pedipalp only once but can only insert a single pedipalp during copulation, it is in the male's interest to survive the first mating to use his second pedipalp. Nevertheless females of some species, including *L. hasselti* and *A. bruennichi* threaten the survival of their mating partner during his first mating. Hence, while death after the second insertion may benefit the male, death after the first insertion is costly. Counter-adaptations of males that prevent premature sexual cannibalism are expected and have been demonstrated in a small number of cases; they include abdominal constriction, opportunistic mating and perhaps the induction of catalepsy.

Abdominal constriction

One of the most extensively documented cases of male self-sacrifice occurs in the genus *Latrodectus*. During mating, diminutive *L. hasselti* and *L. geometricus* males (Figure 7.1) twist through 180° such that the dorsal surface of the male's abdomen presses directly against the female's fangs while

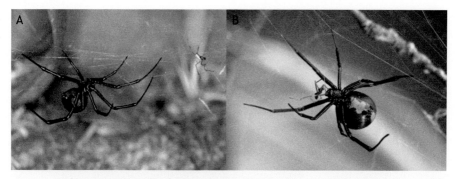

Figure 7.1 (A) Female redback spider (left) with much smaller, courting male (right) (photo credit: A. C. Mason). (B) Female redback spider with cannibalised male (photo credit: K. Jones). See also colour plate.

copulation proceeds (i.e. copulatory somersault; Andrade, 1996, Forster, 1992, Segoli *et al.*, 2008a). Females cannibalise males while they are in this posture in both species (65% of the time in *L. hasselti*, 29% of the time in *L. geometricus*). In both species, at least some males are partially cannibalised during mating while in the somersault posture, but nevertheless frequently dismount, court again, then return for a second mating with their second pedipalp. The somersault occurs again and most males are killed during this second insertion.

A remarkable trait that counters effects of female attacks is the abdominal constriction of *L. hasselti*. During courtship, male redbacks develop a mid-dorsal constriction across their abdomen (Forster, 1992, 1995) likely from the contraction of the muscles attached to the apodemes (Andrade *et al.*, 2005). The constriction was hypothesised to allow males to survive partial cannibalism by shifting abdominal contents away from the site of damage (Forster, 1992). Experimental wounding of males confirmed that constricted males survive injury longer than non-constricted males, but only when wounding is in the location typically damaged by the female (Andrade *et al.*, 2005). Moreover, a congener which is not typically cannibalised (*L. hesperus*) showed no constriction and succumbed quickly to experimental wounding regardless of the location of the wound (Andrade *et al.*, 2005). Although the somersault behaviour invites sexual cannibalism, death during the first copulation is not in the interest of the male. Abdominal constriction evolved to facilitate male survival after the first insertion so that both pedipalps can be discharged.

Opportunistic mating

The term opportunistic mating includes copulations while the female is occupied because she is hunting, feeding or moulting (termed 'soft mating'). In orb-web spiders (Araneidae, Nephilidae), opportunistic mating is regularly

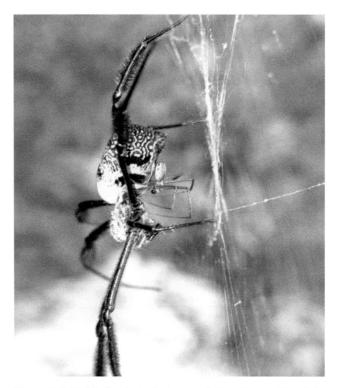

Figure 7.2 *Nephila fenestrata* during copulation. The small male inserts one of his pedipalps into one genital opening of the female. (Photo credit: J. M. Schneider.) See also colour plate.

observed (Robinson and Robinson, 1980) and in several species (e.g. *Nephila plumipes*, *N. inaurata*, *Metellina segmentata*) mating exclusively occurs while the female is hunting (Elgar and Fahey, 1996, Schneider *et al.*, 2005a) or feeding (Prenter *et al.*, 1994b). In *N. plumipes*, for example, males copulate with the female during the process of prey capture. As soon as the prey is motionless and the female starts wrapping it, copulation ends (Elgar and Fahey, 1996, Schneider and Elgar, 2002). In *N. fenestrata* (Figure 7.2), however, males mate with and without the female having prey. Males that mated without prey had more injuries and were more often cannibalised than males that mated opportunistically (Fromhage and Schneider, 2005a). Sexual cannibalism prevented males from mate guarding so that a second mate could gain an average of 50% paternity as opposed to roughly 25% if the first male survived (Fromhage and Schneider, 2005a).

During moulting the female is very vulnerable and totally defenceless until the exoskeleton has hardened. Soft matings may be more common than currently known because they are difficult to observe. In *Argiope aurantia*, the majority of copulations occur while the female is moulting (Foellmer and Fairbairn, 2005). The costs and benefits of soft copulations for males and females have not been investigated in any spider yet, but the obvious benefit for males is that females cannot cannibalise the male and he can mate uninterrupted. Female costs may include harm inflicted by males as the female exoskeleton has not yet hardened (Foellmer and Fairbairn, 2005) as well as the loss of control over who mates and for how long. However, there is no solid evidence for female costs due to soft matings (Schneider and Lubin, 1998). This exciting question will hopefully be addressed soon.

Catalepsy

In *Agelenopsis aperta* females fall into a cataleptic posture (lack of response to external stimuli, legs curled) during courtship as soon as the pair makes physical contact. In all pairings where males court females in the laboratory, the females enter a cataleptic state (Singer *et al.*, 2000). Catalepsy is apparently triggered by airborne chemicals released by the male (Becker *et al.*, 2005), and these chemicals can affect both sexes (Singer *et al.*, 2000). During courtship, rapid drumming of the male's pedipalps may waft these chemicals towards females. The male mates with the female while she is immobile then rapidly retreats. Males may copulate immediately after inducing catalepsy for the first time or more commonly the male will resume courtship and repeatedly induce catalepsy. Males differed in their success at inducing catalepsy and active, vigorous males were more successful. It is not entirely clear whether inducing catalepsy protects the male from female aggression, whether it is a means to control copulation or whether it is a trait under female choice.

Summary

In species where it has been measured, male mating rates are often low due to a number of reasons including sexual cannibalism. However, this conclusion is from studies on only five species. Low mating prospects of some species resulted in curious adaptations that evolved to secure male mating success, a few of which we described. There are further male behaviours and features that may have evolved under the threat of sexual cannibalism, such as mate binding (but see Section 7.2.2 'Courtship') or the large chelicerae of Tetragnathidae, but experimental evidence is lacking.

7.4   Consequences of polyandry

Polyandry extends the scope for sexual selection and sexual conflict beyond the act of mating. Female multiple mating selects for mechanisms that allow males to either avoid or win post-copulatory competition (sperm competition) and it selects for traits that are favoured by choosy females.

Below we will first describe adaptations in males that are consequences of sperm competition. However, females are unlikely passive vessels for storage of ejaculates and fertilisation success is probably a result of the interaction of post-copulatory sexual selection imposed by males and females (cryptic female choice). Female contributions have been rarely explored to date and we will list a few case studies in this context that may encourage further studies. Another major influence on post-copulatory processes may be sexual conflict – which arises because the evolutionary interests of females and males rarely coincide. We describe several examples where spider behaviour is shaped by sexual conflict. However, we will not enter the debate about which type of coevolution is more relevant in spiders, as there are currently insufficient data to draw broad conclusions.

7.4.1   *Post-copulatory adaptations in males*

Female spiders lay their eggs in batches and copulation and oviposition are generally separated by a period of time during which sperm remains stored inside specialised storage organs, the spermathecae. Under polyandry, females may store sperm from two or more males. In order to evaluate fertilisation patterns, we need to measure relative paternity. There are several possible methods for paternity analyses and in most vertebrates genetic methods using DNA fingerprinting or microsatellites have been applied. Most spiders produce very large clutches and genetic methods can be expensive, requiring using subsamples or destroying entire clutches, so the use of the sterile-male technique has been the method of choice (see Box 7.1).

In many species, a general order effect exists such that the first or the last male to mate fathers the majority of the offspring – first or last male sperm precedence. Sperm precedence patterns vary from last-male sperm precedence in some haplogynes (e.g. Schaefer and Uhl, 2002) and sperm mixing or first-male precedence in many entelegynes (Elgar, 1998). While many studies found order effects, variation in the distribution of paternity success is generally very high. Austad (1984) realised these general patterns and explained them as the result of the relative position of ejaculates inside the spermathecae (Elgar, 1998). Austad classified sperm storage organs in first-in-first-out (conduit) and in first-in-last-out (cul-de-sac) categories and related this pattern to the relative positioning of insemination and fertilisation exits from the sperm store. While Austad's study has stimulated a lot of research, his explanation has been largely discarded (Uhl, 2000).

Box 7.1   The sterile male technique

First proposed for pest control by (Knipling, 1955), the **sterile male technique for assessing paternity** was developed and formalised by Parker (1970) and Boorman and Parker (1976) and has been used extensively in spiders (Table 7.1) and other invertebrates. Although there are limitations on the type of data that can be collected (e.g. it cannot be used for field-collected egg sacs), the sterile male technique remains widely used because it is a relatively simple and low-cost method that can produce high-quality data when used properly. Most commonly used to quantify paternity when females are mated to pairs of males, it also allows assessment of paternity of a focal male when a female mates with a series of competitors (Elgar *et al.*, 2003, Schneider and Elgar, 2005).

Technique

In the **paired-male design**, experimental females are mated to one **'irradiated' male** (R, exposed to low doses of radiation) and one **'normal' male** (N, not irradiated) and the proportion of eggs that hatch in egg sacs produced after the second mating is quantified. Radiation doses must be sufficiently low that the phenotypes of males and competitiveness of their sperm are unaffected, but sufficiently high that eggs fertilised by irradiated sperm are inviable due to mutations induced in the germ-line (Parker, 1970). Determining the appropriate radiation dose for a given species (Table 7.1) may require trial and error and examination of sperm phenotype (e.g. Austad, 1984). Mating order of experimental males is randomised (i.e. **RN** or **NR** mating order). Paternity of irradiated males can be estimated as the proportion of males that do not hatch, once controls are used to adjust this for the success of the irradiation treatment (irradiation control, females mated to two **R** males) and average rates of infertility (the fertility control, females mated to two **N** males; see calculations below, Boorman and Parker, 1976). In the **multi-male design**, experimental treatments should include focal males that are **R** or **N** and all other competitors should be of the opposite treatment (e.g. paternity of third of four males, treatments are **RRNR** and **NNRN**). Controls must include as many different males as the chosen experimental treatment to avoid fertility effects associate with number of copulations (e.g. **RRRR** and **NNNN**).

Testing a critical assumption

The assumption that sperm phenotype is unaffected by irradiation must be tested. This is done by assessing whether the estimated paternity of the second male (P2) depends on mating order of experimental males (e.g. **NR** or **RN**). If P2 is different between experimental treatments, then a critical assumption underlying the technique has failed and paternity results are suspect. Recent work shows that irradiation can affect fertilisation success as a function of whether or not competing ejaculates are in the same sperm storage organ (Jones and Elgar, 2008). Thus, if there is variation in whether or not competing males inseminate the same spermatheca, this must be factored into this analysis. Ideally, insemination patterns should be controlled when possible (e.g. Jones and Elgar, 2008, Snow and Andrade, 2005).

Estimating paternity

After Boorman and Parker (1976), if x is the proportion of eggs that hatch after **RN** or **NR** matings, we can estimate the proportion of eggs fertilised by the **R** male as:

$$P_R = (1 - x/p) + (z/p \times (1 - x/p)/1 - z/p)), \qquad (1)$$

where p is the proportion of eggs that hatch after the fertility control (**NN**) and z is the proportion of eggs that hatch after the irradiation control (**RR**). If irradiation is completely successful and $z = 0$ then this reduces to:

$$P_R = 1 - x/p. \qquad (2)$$

The potential of losing paternity to a rival selects for male behavioural and morphological strategies that either protect or defend the ejaculate against future rivals (defensive strategies) or that remove or dilute ejaculates already present from a predecessor (offensive strategies). Female genital morphology is crucial in setting the rules for male strategies; for example, haplogynes store sperm in a single receptaculum to which the male genitalia have direct access from the outside. Such accessibility makes it possible for males to use their genitalia to remove sperm from previous males (physically or by other means, see Peretti and Eberhard, 2010) and offensive strategies and last-male sperm precedence are expected. In the haplogyne cellar spider, Schaefer and Uhl (2002)

Table 7.1 *Overview of studies on spiders that were published after Elgar's (1998) review of sperm competition in arachnids in which paternity was estimated*

Species	Paternity assessment	Irradiation dose (S) or number of loci (G, P)	References
Argiope bruennichi	S	1. 40 Gy (X-ray source @ 0.8 to 1.2 Gy/min)	Schneider and Lesmono, 2009
		2. 40 Gy (γ source)	Schneider et al., 2006
Argiope lobata	S	40 Gy (γ source @ 0.8 Gy/min)	Nessler et al., 2007
Argiope keyserlingi	S	100 Gy (γ source)	Elgar et al., 2000
Latrodectus hasselti	S	90 Gy (γ source, @ 8.2 Gy/min)	Snow and Andrade, 2005, Snow et al., 2006
Nephila edulis	S (2 and 3 males)	100 Gy (γ source)	Schneider et al., 2000, Schneider and Elgar, 2005, Jones and Elgar, 2008, Elgar and Jones, 2008
Nephila plumipes	S (3 males)	100 Gy (γ source)	Elgar et al., 2003, Schneider et al., 2001
Nephila fenestrata	S	60 Gy (γ source)	Fromhage and Schneider, 2005
Pholcus phalangioides	G P	7 microsatellite loci 5 allozyme loci	Schaefer and Uhl, 2002, Schaefer et al., 2008
Pisaura mirabilis	S	50 Gy (X-rays)	Drengsgaard and Toft, 1999
Tetragnatha extensa	S	30 Gy	West and Toft, 1999

S, sterile male; G, genetic analysis; P, protein analysis.

found a pronounced last-male advantage which could be explained by males removing sperm from previous suitors through the movements of their pedipalps during copulation. However, an alternative explanation is that pedipalp movements induce females to selectively dump rival sperm, as shown in another pholcid (Peretti and Eberhard, 2010). In another haplogyne species, *Silhouettella loricatula* (Oonopidae), males were also observed to rhythmically move their pedipalps during copulation. Morphological studies revealed that ejaculates are packaged into sacs consisting of secretions of unknown origin. If the female mated with a second male, the sperm sac containing the ejaculate from the previous male was expelled. Even though selective sperm dumping by the female is a tempting interpretation, experiments are required to determine whether the male, the female or both are responsible (Burger, 2007).

Behavioural strategies expected in a species with a last-male advantage are the guarding of females until they produce the egg sac. However, at least in the cellar spider (*Pholcus phalangioides*) and another pholcid, *Physocyclus globosus*, this expectation was not met (Huber and Eberhard, 1997, Uhl and Vollrath, 1998). Individually marked males were equally likely to be found in the proximity of females that had already laid eggs as they were with females prior to oviposition. However, since many other factors can affect the pay-offs for guarding (e.g. risk of a take-over, cost of guarding), this is not necessarily inconsistent with last-male precedence. For example, if guarding is costly or unlikely to be effective, males may do better to mate with as many females as possible and minimise investment in each one.

Under first-male sperm precedence, virgin females are most valuable for males and mate guarding is most likely before females mature. Guarding males maximise the chances of being the first to mate with the female and securing the highest paternity. Indeed, pre-copulatory mate guarding was observed in a number of entelegyne species (e.g. Bel-Venner and Venner, 2006, Hoefler, 2007, Prenter *et al.*, 1994a). In *Neriene litigiosa* males guard virgin females and take down the web of these females to prevent further pheromone emission (Watson, 1986). In *Phidippus clarus*, males guard penultimate instar females early in the season and attempt to mate once these females mature. Later in the season, when most females are mated, males roam in search of additional mating opportunities and no longer guard females (Hoefler, 2007).

Other defensive mechanisms may include physiological manipulation of female receptivity and post-copulatory mate guarding. For example, in *A. keyserlingi*, males copulate once with a female and then guard her for a while, perhaps until her attractivity or accessibility for rivals is reduced. Guarding males can prevent rivals from mating (Herberstein *et al.*, 2005a).

Sperm precedence of the first male is often associated with the application of a mating plug. Plugs can consist of a secretion or of a fragment from the male pedipalp (reviewed in Uhl *et al.*, 2010). Using parts of their genitalia to plug the insemination duct of a female has evolved in several taxa independently. In the genus *Latrodectus* males lose the terminal sclerite of the curved embolus and a plug is effective if the sclerite is placed in the entrance to the spermatheca (Berendonck and Greven, 2005, Snow *et al.*, 2006, Segoli *et al.*, 2008b; Figure 7.3). In the genus *Argiope* genital damage occurs in a number of species and prevalence as well as effectiveness at plugging varies (Nessler *et al.*, 2007, 2009a, Sasaki and Iwahashi, 1995, Uhl *et al.*, 2007). Interestingly, mating plugs consisting of parts of male genitalia appear common in species with low male mating rates and sexual cannibalism (Foellmer, 2008, Fromhage and Schneider, 2006, Kuntner *et al.*, 2009b, Miller, 2007, Nessler *et al.*, 2007, Schneider *et al.*, 2001,

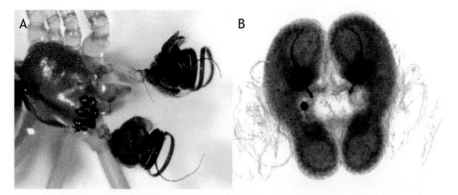

Figure 7.3 (A) Cephalothorax and pedipalps of male redback spider with both
emboli partly uncoiled. The top pedipalp has been used in copulation and the apical
sclerite has broken off inside the female. The lower pedipalp has not yet been used
and is intact. (B) Spermathecae and associated tubules of female redback spider
(macerated with KOH to visualise the spermathecal contents). Two plugs are visible
(dark curved lines), one in each spermatheca. Each is the apical sclerite of a male's
pedipalp. (Photo credit: M. B. C. Andrade.) See also colour plate.

Snow *et al.*, 2006) a pattern which has been confirmed in a comparative study
(Miller, 2007).

Recent studies on *N. plumipes* and *A. bruennichi* tested the plugging function of
genital damage by predetermining that a first male inseminated and plugged
only one of the paired genital openings. A second male was then experimentally
induced (e.g. by selective amputation of one pedipalp) to mate into the used or
the unused genital opening (Nessler *et al.*, 2007, Schneider *et al.*, 2008). In
A. bruennichi, males that mate into a used spermatheca gain no paternity in
most cases (Schneider and Lesmono, 2009). Only when the previous male
belonged to the 3% that do not plug successfully are copulation duration and
relative paternity the same as when mating into a virgin duct (Nessler *et al.*,
2007, Schneider and Lesmono, 2009).

Nephila plumipes males regularly break the tip of the sperm transferring
embolus during mating (Schneider *et al.*, 2001). However, this does not prevent
a future male from mating and from transferring sperm (Schneider *et al.*, 2008).
The function of this damage may be to prevent females from prematurely
dislodging the male from her epigyne, although other interpretations, such as
genital stimulation, are also conceivable (Schneider *et al.*, 2001). Hence, genital
damage per se does not always imply a mating plug function. Interestingly, in
the congener *N. fenestrata*, a species at the base of the genus *Nephila* (Kuntner
et al., 2008), the broken-off fragment functions as a mating plug and prevents
rivals from using the same insemination duct in subsequent copulations

(Fromhage and Schneider, 2006). Below we outline insights from a recent comparative study of genital damage (in Nephilidae) as we hope it may stimulate similar analyses in other interesting groups.

Evolution of genital damage in Nephilidae

The family Nephilidae shows intriguing variation in the presence and absence of genital damage and the effectiveness of broken genitalia as mating plugs. The family consists of four genera in which sexual size dimorphism, genital mutilation and plugging all evolved at the same node, distal from the basal genus *Clitaetra* (Kuntner *et al.*, 2008). In the genera *Herennia* and *Nephilengys*, males evolved complex pedipalps. In both genera, part of the embolic conductor or the entire pedipalp (eunuch phenomenon) breaks off and remains inside the female's genital opening, effectively preventing future copulations. The fourth (and most derived) genus, *Nephila*, partly reversed the pattern. In females, the lumen of the genital openings increased, perhaps to prevent embolic plugs from blocking the entrance completely. At the same time, male emboli lost their complexity and became thinner. In some *Nephila* this results in the possibility that emboli of rival males can bypass existing plugs. In *N. pilipes* for example, up to five plugs are found simultaneously in single genital openings (Kuntner *et al.*, 2009a). The observed genital complexity is correlated between the sexes and Kuntner *et al.* (2009a) conclude the evidence best supports an antagonistic arms race (but see Eberhard and Huber, 2010).

Polyandry and the resulting sperm competition selects for male measures to protect their sperm and secure maximal paternity with a single female. Male monopolisation may oppose female interests if females benefit from polyandry and plugs cause them to lose the potential to cryptically favour certain males over others. Females then benefit from evolving counter-adaptations against male monopolisation. Interestingly, *N. fenestrata* is sister to all other *Nephila* and has plugs that close the genital opening completely, although plugs can be removed by rivals (Fromhage and Schneider, 2006, Kuntner *et al.*, 2008, 2009a). All other distal *Nephila* (e.g. *N. plumipes*) do not show effective plugs, and some species no longer break their emboli. Broken emboli can cause sterility in Nephilidae, thus constraining males to monogyny (Fromhage and Schneider, 2006). The reversion of genital damage suggests males of some species may regain the potential to inseminate multiple females if there are no other constrains that prevent this.

Sperm transfer

Male spiders can vary in how they use their pedipalps at mating (one or both may be used) and sperm release may vary as well (whether sperm is released at all and if so, how much). Thus a copulating male may fill one or both of a female's spermathecae. *Gasteracantha cancriformis* males fill both of the female's spermathecae but only if she is virgin (Bukowski *et al.*, 2001). Males that copulate into a used spermatheca often do not release sperm and leave the female. Hence the second male either avoids sperm competition or the previous male protected his ejaculate well. *Micrathena gracilis* males release sperm early during copulation and the time after sperm transfer appears to influence how much sperm is stored (Bukowski and Christenson, 1997). Copulation duration in such species is not directly related to sperm transfer and lasts longer than it takes to empty the pedipalps (see also Snow and Andrade, 2004 for a similar pattern in *L. hasselti*). It is important to acknowledge that the duration of copulation may not equal sperm transfer, which may not equal sperm storage which may not equal sperm use for fertilisation (Linn *et al.*, 2007). Hence, it is problematic to consider individual processes such as copulation duration or number of sperm transferred in isolation because cryptic processes that occur between sperm transfer and fertilisation may affect relative paternity. Ideally, all investigations of male success in competition should include data on relative paternity. The processes that occur inside the female are intriguingly complex and we still know very little about whether and how males are able to influence their success in sperm competition. However, in several species with very short copulations, copulation duration directly affects the number of sperm found in the spermatheca (Schneider and Elgar, 2001, Schneider *et al.*, 2006) and predicts male paternity. These species are particularly suitable to study the influence of sperm competition on male mating strategies and fitness.

Summary

Defence and offence mechanisms selected by sperm competition depend on female genital morphology. The differences between female morphology may explain the prevalence of last-male sperm precedence in haplogynes where physical barriers cannot be applied and first-male precedence in entelegynes where plugs are common. While behavioural mechanisms such as pre- or post-copulatory mate guarding and web reduction depend on the sperm precedence pattern, others determine the priority: for example, if mating plugs are applied, first-male sperm precedence is the result but not the precondition. The latter is evidenced by high paternity that second males can win if the plugs are not successful. Comparative data sets are revealing but still very rare. The case of the family Nephilidae illustrates how the interaction of sexual conflict and sperm competition yields dynamic patterns of gain and loss of adaptations over evolutionary time. We know very little about plasticity of males in the allocation of their ejaculates. Species that have regained their ability to mate with more than one female and no longer damage their genitalia may be particularly promising for the study of strategic sperm allocation patterns.

7.4.2   Post-copulatory adaptations in females

Cryptic female choice in the broad sense includes all processes during and after copulation that bias paternity of males in favour of candidates preferred by females (Birkhead, 1998, Eberhard, 1996, 1998, 2000, Pitnick and Brown, 2000). Although the inclusion of 'female' in the term implies an active role of the female, the definition does not exclude male adaptations (Eberhard, 1998). Many if not most of the male traits described in the previous section are the result of interacting selection pressures from both sexes. Defined in this way, the term cryptic female choice is synonymous with the overall term of post-copulatory sexual selection. Unfortunately, there are still very few studies available in this context. In particular, the consequences for females through a paternity bias towards males with specific adaptations would be revealing as cryptic female choice and other coevolutionary models make different predictions in that respect. So far, there is no experimental work on benefits for females that mate with males that stimulate, manipulate or monopolise them best ('sexy sons' models), although there are behaviours in some species that may suggest these processes (Huber and Eberhard, 1997, Peretti and Eberhard, 2010, Peretti *et al.*, 2006).

Despite the coevolutionary interactions of male and female influences, there is still some utility in disentangling the relative role of the male and female in these processes. A limited number of experimental studies revealed an unambiguous female contribution to post-copulatory sexual selection in spiders. Females can achieve a paternity bias in favour of a preferred male, for example through selective termination of copulation if copulation duration is related to paternity success. For example, in *A. keyserlingi* females are in control of copulation duration because they terminate copulation by attacking the male (Elgar *et al.*, 2000). In *A. bruennichi* males skip courtship in the presence of a competitor and scramble instead for first access to the female. Whether a male courts or not has no influence on his mating success or on the duration of copulation but males that did not court fathered fewer eggs than courting males (Schneider and Lesmono, 2009). The mechanism that produced this cryptic bias is unknown. Another example is found in *L. hasselti* where females are more likely to kill males after their first copulation if these males courted for a relatively shorter time (Stoltz *et al.*, 2008, 2009). Females apply a threshold rule to courtship length (Stoltz and Andrade, 2010). Interestingly, this threshold can be exploited by intruder males that parasitise the courtship already performed by the resident male.

There is some evidence that spiders might discriminate between ejaculates. Welke and Schneider (2009) investigated the potential for cryptic female choice to reduce negative effects of inbreeding in *A. lobata*. Through selective amputation of pedipalps two males were induced to inseminate different spermathecae. Thereby direct interactions of ejaculates while in storage were excluded. Females were mated to siblings and unrelated males in varying orders and into left or right spermathecae. While females stored similar sperm quantities from their first mate regardless of whether he was a brother or not, more sperm was stored from a second unrelated male if the first one was a sibling. The patterns of sperm storage were reflected in the relative paternity values, with siblings obtaining fewer offspring than non-siblings (Welke and Schneider, 2009).

Recent evidence shows that at least some haplogyne females separate male ejaculates by coating the spermatozoa with secretions (Burger *et al.*, 2003). This may enable the female to selectively eject sperm of unfavoured males (Burger *et al.*, 2006). Morphological analyses suggest haplogyne species have a particularly high potential for sperm selection (Burger, 2007, Burger *et al.*, 2003, 2006), but double mating studies have not been conducted to test this prediction. Future studies that combine morphology and behavioural studies promise exciting insights into the causes and mechanisms of male and female control of sperm storage and fertilisation.

Summary

Spiders are ideal for studies of post-copulatory sexual selection (Eberhard, 2004). While male adaptations to sperm competition are well covered in a number of species, the female role in cryptic female choice is hardly explored. In particular, haplogyne spiders appear promising candidates for future research on cryptic choice because of their potential to eject sperm. Entelegyne spiders are promising because of their two independent sperm storage organs that can be filled by different males. Sperm counts and paternity studies are easily applicable because the ejaculates are stored separately inside the female.

7.4.3   *Sexual conflict*

Sexual conflict occurs if the evolutionary optima of females and males diverge and if a reproductive strategy of one sex imposes costs on the other sex (Arnqvist and Rowe, 2005, Chapman, 2006). As male spiders do not invest in brood care, conflicts occur over mating, including frequency of mating and mating duration. Resolutions of the conflict will depend on many factors including which sex is in control. Spiders are cannibalistic predators and it is often dangerous to act against the interest of another spider. Conflicts in spiders that lead to aggression may end with injury or even death of one opponent. Who wins a conflict will in most cases be decided by relative body sizes, and conflicts between males and females are no exception. Control over mating in spiders is often a question of physical strength of the opponents.

Sexual cannibalism is usually directed towards the male that is attacked and killed by the female. Sexual cannibalism is often called the pinnacle of sexual conflict obviously because a male's reproductive future is brutally limited by female aggressiveness (Elgar and Schneider, 2004). The degree of conflict depends on the timing of sexual cannibalism. Male attempts to escape female's attacks are often successful and there is evidence that large males are more likely to escape than smaller conspecifics (Wilder and Rypstra, 2008c, Wilder *et al.*, 2009). However, small males may be better in avoiding sexual cannibalism if they are less likely to be detected by the female (Elgar and Fahey, 1996). Within species, females may use sexual cannibalism to discriminate against males and may favour small body size (Schneider *et al.*, 2000). In general, however, relative dominance determined through the differences in male and female body size correlates with the occurrence of sexual cannibalism within and between taxa (Wilder and Rypstra, 2008d).

Conflict over copulation duration

How much time to spend in copula may have different optima for males and females. Prolonged copulation may increase relative paternity of a given male or facilitate male control of female remating. Females may benefit if copulation is terminated after sufficient sperm is transferred, perhaps to retain control or to prevent further costs of mating. Females have means of terminating copulation often through an aggressive attack on the mating male or by leaving the mating position or location. In response, males evolved measures to overcome female control. Such mechanisms include the already described copulatory somersault that prolongs copulation duration as well as other male mating strategies that involve self-sacrifice. In addition, elaborate genitalia that facilitate genital coupling and copulatory courtship strategies may prolong copulation, which can oppose female interest. While selection favours male strategies that prolong copulation beyond female interests, sexual cannibalism and its effects on terminating copulation will at the same time select for rapid sperm transfer (Foellmer and Fairbairn, 2004). Indeed copulations last just a few seconds in *A. aurantia* or *A. bruennichi* but still enough sperm to fertilise hundreds of eggs are transferred (Foellmer and Fairbairn, 2004, Schneider *et al.*, 2005b). Extremely rapid sperm transfer may be the result of an arms race over controlling the duration of copulation and with it the transfer of sperm and perhaps accessory fluids. Interestingly, male *A. bruennichi* are able to influence the risk of

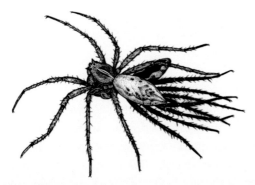

Figure 7.4 Male and female *Pisaura mirabilis*. The female is holding a nuptial gift in her chelicerae, while the male is also hanging onto it while being in a state of thanatosis (death feigning). (Drawn by Monika Hänel from a photo by T. Bilde.)

cannibalism during their first copulation through modifying the duration of copulation (Nessler *et al.*, 2009b). In the presence of female pheromones males tended to opt for a long first copulation that invariably ended with sexual cannibalism. In the absence of female pheromones more males survived their first copulation because they jumped off before the female could capture them and won a higher chance of using both of their pedipalps (Nessler *et al.*, 2009b). However, the latter tactic still includes a probability of dying after a very short copulation. While the adaptive values of the behavioural options are not clear, the study uncovered male flexibility in avoiding or accepting death and invites further experimental studies that target male and female costs and benefits through variation in the duration of copulation.

The curious death-feigning behaviour (thanatosis) of *Pisaura mirabilis* males may have evolved for the same reason of prolonging the duration of copulation (Figure 7.4). Some spiders show a remarkable ability to 'feign death', a behaviour that is evident in several insects where it typically functions as an anti-predator adaptation (Miyatake *et al.*, 2004, Nishino and Sakai, 1996). In the nursery web spider *P. mirabilis* it is sometimes seen in the context of mating. Copulation starts once the female bites into the nuptial gift that the male offers. The gift is then held by both mating partners. Females may, however, attempt to run away with the gift fixed tightly between her chelicerae. The male then risks losing the gift and the mate and may even be attacked by the female. In such a situation some males play dead (Bilde *et al.*, 2006). They somehow decrease their internal hydrolic pressure so they are suddenly completely limp, but without losing their tight grip on the gift. Once the female stops moving the male 'reanimates' and cautiously attempts mating. While it is tempting to speculate that thanatosis may be used by males to prevent sexual cannibalism, data currently only support the explanation that it reduces the risk for the male of losing the gift and his chances to achieve a copulation (Hansen *et al.*, 2008).

Infanticide

A particularly clear example of sexual conflict occurs in the semelparous eresid spider, *Stegodyphus lineatus*. Females produce a single egg sac that they guard for several weeks until they open the cocoon and release the spiderlings. Females feed their brood and invariable die due to matriphagy. Accordingly, females invest maximally into a single brood (Schneider and Lubin, 1997a). The mating season overlaps with the egg-laying season so that late males encounter females that already have egg sacs (Schneider and Lubin, 1997b). These males can only expect reproductive success with such a female if they force her to produce a replacement clutch. Females that lose their egg sac will replace it after a long period (over 10 days). Females with egg sacs are very aggressive towards visiting males but not all succeed in inducing a male to leave (Schneider and Lubin, 1997b). Some males will gain entry to the silken nest and cut the egg sac off the inner wall and drop it to the ground where the female is unable to recover it (Schneider and Lubin, 1996). The male then copulates with the female and leaves her. Females pay large costs mainly because they lose time and accumulate an increased risk of not surviving until brood care is completed. There is an additional fecundity cost as the second egg sac contains fewer eggs. Males gain much by committing infanticide as they can expect to encounter an average of two females in their lifetime. Hence discarding the option to reproduce with one of them reduces their expected reproductive success by half. Success of the infanticidal male is determined by his size relative to the female who defends her eggs: if male prosoma width is larger than that of the female, the probability of his winning a fight is high and he will lose the fight if his prosoma is smaller than that of the female (Schneider and Lubin, 1997b). A suggested counter-adaptation that reduces the risk of infanticide is that early maturing females delay their oviposition until males become less common (Schneider, 1999) even though they are larger than late maturing females (Schneider, 1997).

Summary

Sexual conflict is widespread in spiders and can be fairly dramatic. The interests of the sexes likely diverge over the frequency and duration of copulation and may get resolved through drastic means such as sexual cannibalism or infanticide. Relative body sizes of females and males appear to play an important role in intersexual conflict resolution.

7.5   Conclusions and outlook

Early work on spider mating behaviour described courtship sequences and reproductive morphologies, and highlighted average traits of a wide range of species. The advent of behavioural ecology led to an explosion of studies examining factors affecting sources of variation in reproductive behaviour. The combination of these bodies of work has yielded insights into a widely variable group with often flamboyant and lurid mating innovations shaped by life history, morphology and cannibalistic females. There is a growing appreciation of the extent to which spider mating behaviour is tuned in ecological time by intrinsic and extrinsic variables that affect fitness. Our understanding of fine-tuned flexibility in reproductive behaviours whose fitness effects depend on context is developing rapidly. However, our picture of spider mating behaviour is currently based largely on insights from a handful of species from (roughly) seven families (Araneidae, Ctenidae, Linyphiidae, Lycosidae, Pholcidae, Salticidae, Theridiidae) – a very poor sample in a group with over a hundred recognised families with a wide range of life histories, mating systems and ecological roles.

As the volume of work on the behavioural ecology of mating expands, new and promising areas of research are appearing, and increased effort could yield major breakthroughs in understanding in the next few years. Here we suggest three areas where spider models could be at the forefront of research in mating behaviour.

Control of polyandry and genetic benefits of choice

This is currently a major area of debate and study. Tests of existing models for pre- and post-copulatory choice and polyandry are facilitated by the wide range of manipulative treatments possible due to the unusual genitalia of spiders (Eberhard, 2004). In many species females control mating access (due to female-biased size dimorphism) so the outcome of intersexual interactions may reflect female preferences more directly than in other taxa. In some taxa, laboratory rearing would allow studies of inheritance of male traits (indicators of good genes or attractiveness) using half-sib designs or pedigree analyses and animal models. Finally, the field conditions under which polyandry or choosiness are important can be established using patterns of sex pheromone production as a proxy for female availability or receptivity. This grounding of laboratory manipulations in the natural context is not possible in many systems.

Effects of adaptive secretions in seminal fluids on paternity and female fitness

The majority of work in this area is on model systems (particularly *Drosophila*, e.g. Chapman *et al.*, 1995, Snook and Hosken, 2004), so the generality of conclusions about functions of secretions in seminal fluids in sexual conflict is unclear. Two studies of lycosids suggest seminal secretions affect female physiology (Aisenberg and Costa, 2005, Estramil and Costa, 2007). This may be widespread as sperm transfer occurs rapidly but copulation is prolonged in several groups and female receptivity changes after mating. Interaction between ejaculates may affect paternity, and the option of physically separating or combining ejaculates in the female's genitalia allows for powerful study design.

Effects of experience and learning on female choice and
male competition

Spiders can glean social or ecological information about changing local conditions throughout their life history. These changing conditions may have large effects on fitness pay-offs for different behavioural tactics (Kasumovic et al., 2008). For example, cursorial species and mate-searching males can interact directly with conspecifics; juveniles and females can detect the presence and perhaps density of conspecifics of both sexes using chemical cues (Gaskett, 2007, Kasumovic and Andrade, 2006); and juvenile and adult females often cohabit with one or more males. Existing work suggests such information may change competitive behaviour and choice. Generally, flexibility in spider behaviour has been largely ignored and this may be particularly true in the context of mating. Hence, future studies should pay more attention to variants in female and male behaviour and investigate the causes and consequences of this variation.

Acknowledgements

We thank Bill Eberhard, Matthias Foellmer, Lutz Fromhage, Klaas Welke, Nicole Ruppel, Helma Roggenbuck, Steffi Zimmer, Michael Kasumovic, Jeff Stoltz, Emily MacLeod, Maria Modanu and Janice Ting for reading the chapter and for comments. Monika Hänel did the drawing of *Pisaura* and Trine Bilde provided the photograph.

References

Ahtiainen, J. J., Alatalo, R. V., Kortet, R. and Rantala, M. J. (2004). Sexual advertisement and immune function in an arachnid species (Lycosidae). *Behavioral Ecology*, **15**, 602–606.

Aisenberg, A. and Costa, F. G. (2005). Females mated without sperm transfer maintain high sexual receptivity in the wolf spider *Schizocosa malitiosa*. *Ethology*, **111**, 545–558.

Aisenberg, A. and Costa, F. G. (2008). Reproductive isolation and sex-role reversal in two sympatric sand-dwelling wolf spiders of the genus *Allocosa*. *Canadian Journal of Zoology*, **86**, 648.

Aisenberg, A. and Eberhard, W. G. (2009). Female cooperation in plug formation in a spider: effects of male copulatory courtship. *Behavioral Ecology*, **20**, 1236–1241.

Aisenberg, A., Baruffaldi, L. and González, M. (2010). Behavioural evidence of male volatile pheromones in the sex-role reversed wolf spiders *Allocosa brasiliensis* and *Allocosa alticeps*. *Naturwissenschaften*, **97**, 63–70.

Aisenberg, A., Estramil, N., Gonzalez, M., Toscano-Gadea, C. A. and Costa, F. G. (2008). Silk release by copulating *Schizocosa malitiosa* males (Araneae, Lycosidae): a bridal veil? *Journal of Arachnology*, **36**, 204–206.

Aisenberg, A., González, M., Laborda, Á., Postiglioni, R. and Simó, M. (2009). Reversed cannibalism, foraging, and surface activities of *Allocosa alticeps* and *Allocosa brasiliensis*: two wolf spiders from coastal sand dunes. *Journal of Arachnology*, **37**, 135–138.

Alatalo, R. V., Kotiaho, J., Mappes, J. and Parri, S. (1998). Mate choice for offspring performance: major benefits or minor costs? *Proceedings of the Royal Society of London, B*, **265**, 2297–2301.

Anava, A. and Lubin, Y. (1993). Presence of gender cues in the web of a widow spider, *Latrodectus revivensis*, and a description of courtship behaviour. *Bulletin of the British Arachnological Society*, **9**, 119–122.

Andersen, T., Bollerup, K., Toft, S. and Bilde, T. (2008). Why do males of the spider *Pisaura mirabilis* wrap their nuptial gifts in silk: female preference or male control? *Ethology*, **114**, 775–781.

Anderson, J. T. and Morse, D. H. (2001). Pick-up lines: cues used by male crab spiders to find reproductive females. *Behavioral Ecology*, **12**, 360–366.

Andersson, M. (1994). *Sexual Selection*. Princeton, NJ: Princeton University Press.

Andrade, M. C. B. (1996). Sexual selection for male sacrifice in the Australian redback spider. *Science*, **271**, 70–72.

Andrade, M. C. B. (2003). Risky mate search and male self-sacrifice in redback spiders. *Behavioral Ecology*, **14**, 531–538.

Andrade, M. C. B. and Banta, E. M. (2002). Value of male remating and functional sterility in redback spiders. *Animal Behaviour*, **63**, 857–870.

Andrade, M. C. B. and Kasumovic, M. M. (2005). Terminal investment strategies and male mate choice: extreme tests of Bateman. *Integrative and Comparative Biology*, **45**, 838–847.

Andrade, M. C. B., Gu, L. and Stoltz, J. A. (2005). Novel male trait prolongs survival in suicidal mating. *Biology Letters*, **1**, 276–279.

Arnqvist, G. and Henriksson, S. (1997). Sexual cannibalism in the fishing spider and a model for the evolution of sexual cannibalism based on genetic constraints. *Evolutionary Ecology*, **11**, 255–273.

Arnqvist, G. and Nilsson, T. (2000). The evolution of polyandry: multiple mating and female fitness in insects. *Animal Behaviour*, **60**, 145–164.

Arnqvist, G. and Rowe, L. (2005). *Sexual Conflict*, Princeton, NJ: Princeton University Press.

Austad, S. N. (1982). 1st male sperm priority in the bowl and doily spider, *Frontinella pyramitela* (Walckenaer). *Evolution*, **36**, 777–785.

Austad, S. N. (1983). A game theoretical interpretation of male combat in the bowl and doily spider (*Frontinella pyramitela*). *Animal Behaviour*, **31**, 59–73.

Austad, S. N. (1984). *Evolution of Sperm Priority Patterns in Spiders*, London: Academic Press.

Avilés, L. (1997). Causes and consequences of cooperation and permanent-sociality in spiders. In *Evolution of Social Behaviour in Insects and Arachnids* (ed. J. Choe and B. Crespi). Cambridge, UK: Cambridge University Press.

Barth, F. G. and Schmitt, A. (1991). Species recognition and species isolation in wandering spiders (*Cupiennius* spp.; Ctenidae). *Behavioral Ecology and Sociobiology*, **29**, 333–339.

Baruffaldi, L. and Costa, F. (2010). Changes in male sexual responses from silk cues of females at different reproductive states in the wolf spider *Schizocosa malitiosa*. *Journal of Ethology*, **28**, 75–85.

Bateman, A. J. (1948). Intra-sexual selection in *Drosophila*. *Heredity*, **2**, 349–368.

Becker, E., Riechert, S. and Singer, F. (2005). Male induction of female quiescence/catalepsis during courtship in the spider, *Agelenopsis aperta*. *Behaviour*, **142**, 57–70.

Bel-Venner, M. C. and Venner, S. (2006). Mate-guarding strategies and male competitive ability in an orb-weaving spider: results from a field study. *Animal Behaviour*, **71**, 1315–1322.

Bel-Venner, M. C., Dray, S., Allaine, D., Menu, F. and Venner, S. (2008). Unexpected male choosiness for mates in a spider. *Proceedings of the Royal Society of London, B*, **275**, 77–82.

Berendonck, B. and Greven, H. (2005). Genital structures in the entelegyne widow spider *Latrodectus revivensis* (Arachnida; Araneae; Theridiidae) indicate a low ability for cryptic female choice by sperm manipulation. *Journal of Morphology*, **263**, 118–132.

Bilde, T., Lubin, Y., Smith, D., Schneider, J. M. and Maklakov, A. A. (2005). The transition to social inbred mating systems in spiders: role of inbreeding tolerance in a subsocial predecessor. *Evolution*, **59**, 160–174.

Bilde, T., Maklakov, A. A. and Schilling, N. (2007a). Inbreeding avoidance in spiders: evidence for rescue effect in fecundity of female spiders with outbreeding opportunity. *Journal of Evolutionary Biology*, **20**, 1237–1242.

Bilde, T., Tuni, C., Elsayed, R., Pekar, S. and Toft, S. (2006). Death feigning in the face of sexual cannibalism. *Biology Letters*, **2**, 23–25.

Bilde, T., Tuni, C., Elsayed, R., Pekar, S. and Toft, S. (2007b). Nuptial gifts of male spiders: sensory exploitation of the female's maternal care instinct or foraging motivation? *Animal Behaviour*, **73**, 267–273.

Birkhead, T. R. (1998). Cryptic female choice: criteria for establishing female sperm choice. *Evolution*, **52**, 1212–1218.

Bondurianskzy, R. (2001). The evolution of male mate choice in insects: a synthesis of ideas and evidence. *Biological Reviews*, **76**, 305–339.

Bonte, D., Van Belle, S. and Maelfait, J. P. (2007). Maternal care and reproductive state-dependent mobility determine natal dispersal in a wolf spider. *Animal Behaviour*, **74**, 63–69.

Boorman, E. and Parker, G. A. (1976). Sperm (ejaculate) competition in *Drosophila melanogaster*, and reproductive value of females to males in relation to female age and mating status. *Ecological Entomology*, **1**, 145–155.

Bradbury, J. W. and Vehrencamp, S. L. (2000). Economic models of animal communication. *Animal Behaviour*, **59**, 259–268.

Bridge, A. P., Elwood, R. W. and Dick, J. T. A. (2000). Imperfect assessment and limited information preclude optimal strategies in male-male fights in the orb-weaving spider *Metellina mengei*. *Proceedings of the Royal Society of London, B*, **267**, 273–279.

Bristowe, W. S. (1958). *The World of Spiders*. London: Collins.

Bukowski, T. C. and Avilés, L. (2002). Asynchronous maturation of the sexes may limit close inbreeding in a subsocial spider. *Canadian Journal of Zoology*, **80**, 193–198.

Bukowski, T. C. and Christenson, T. E. (1997). Determinants of sperm release and storage in a spiny orbweaving spider. *Animal Behaviour*, **53**, 381–395.

Bukowski, T. C., Linn, C. D. and Christenson, T. E. (2001). Copulation and sperm release in *Gasteracantha cancriformis* (Araneae: Araneidae): differential male behaviour based on female mating history. *Animal Behaviour*, **62**, 887–895.

Burger, M. (2007). Sperm dumping in a haplogyne spider. *Journal of Zoology*, **273**, 74–81.

Burger, M., Michalik, P., Graber, W., *et al.* (2006). Complex genital system of a haplogyne spider (Arachnida, Araneae, Tetrablemmidae) indicates internal fertilization and full female control over transferred sperm. *Journal of Morphology*, **267**, 166–186.

Burger, M., Nentwig, W. and Kropf, C. (2003). Complex genital structures indicate cryptic female choice in a haplogyne spider (Arachnida, Araneae, Oonopidae, Gamasomorphinae). *Journal of Morphology*, **255**, 80–93.

Buston, P. and Emlen, S. (2003). Cognitive processes underlying human mate choice: the relationship between self-perception and mate preference in Western society. *Proceedings of the National Academy of Sciences of the USA*, **100**, 8805–8810.

Catley, K. (1993). Courtship, mating and post-oviposition behaviour of *Hypochilus pococki* Platnick (Araneae, Hypochilidae). *Memoirs of the Queensland Museum*, **33**, 469–474.

Chapman, T. (2006). Evolutionary conflicts of interest between males and females. *Current Biology*, **16**, R744–R754.

Chapman, T., Liddle, L. F., Kalb, J. M., Wolfner, M. F. and Partridge, L. (1995). Cost of mating in *Drosophila melanogaster* females is mediated by male accessory-gland products. *Nature*, **373**, 241–244.

Chinta, S. P., Goller, S., Lux, J., et al. (2010). The sex pheromone of the wasp spider *Argiope bruennichi*. *Angewandte Chemie International Edition*, **49**, 2033–2036.

Christenson, T. E. and Goist, K. C. (1979). Costs and benefits of male-male competition in the orb-weaving spider *Nephila clavipes*. *Behavioral Ecology and Sociobiology*, **5**, 87–92.

Clark, D. L. and Biesiadecki, B. (2002). Mating success and alternative reproductive strategies of the dimorphic jumping spider, *Maevia inclemens* (Araneae, Salticidae). *Journal of Arachnology*, **30**, 511–518.

Clark, D. L. and Morjan, C. L. (2001). Attracting female attention: the evolution of dimorphic courtship displays in the jumping spider *Maevia inclemens* (Araneae: Salticidae). *Proceedings of the Royal Society of London, B*, **268**, 2461–2465.

Clark, D. L. and Uetz, G. W. (1992). Morph-independent mate selection in a dimorphic jumping spider: demonstration of movement bias in female choice using video-controlled courtship behavior. *Animal Behaviour*, **43**, 247–254.

Clark, D. L. and Uetz, G. W. (1993). Signal efficacy and the evolution of male dimorphism in the jumping spider, *Maevia inclemens*. *Proceedings of the National Academy of Sciences of the USA*, **90**, 11 954–11 957.

Cornell, S. J. and Tregenza, T. (2007). A new theory for the evolution of polyandry as a means of inbreeding avoidance. *Proceedings of the Royal Society of London, B*, **274**, 2873–2879.

Costa, F. G. and Pérez-Miles, F. (1998). Behavior, life cycle and webs of *Mecicobothrium thorelli* (Araneae, Mygalomorphae, Mecicobothriidae). *Journal of Arachnology*, **26**, 317–329.

Costa-Schmidt, L. E., Carico, J. E. and De Araujo, A. M. (2008). Nuptial gifts and sexual behavior in two species of spider (Araneae, Trechaleidae, Paratrechalea). *Naturwissenschaften*, **95**, 731–739.

Cross, F., Jackson, R. R., Pollard, S. D. and Walker, M. (2007a). Cross-modality effects during male–male interactions of jumping spiders. *Behavioural Processes*, **75**, 290–296.

Cross, F. R., Jackson, R. R. and Pollard, S. D. (2007b). Male and female mate-choice decisions by *Evarcha culicivora*, an East African jumping spider. *Ethology*, **113**, 901–908.

Davies, N. B. and Halliday, T. M. (1979). Competitive mate searching in male common toads, *Bufo bufo*. *Animal Behaviour*, **27**, 1253–1267.

DeCarvalho, T. N., Watson, P. J. and Field, S. A. (2004). Costs increase as ritualized fighting progresses within and between phases in the sierra dome spider, *Neriene litigiosa*. *Animal Behaviour*, **68**, 473–482.

Dodson, G. N. and Beck, M. W. (1993). Pre-copulatory guarding of penultimate females by male crab spiders, *Misumenoides formosipes*. *Animal Behaviour*, **46**, 951–959.

Dodson, G. N. and Schwaab, A. T. (2001). Body size, leg autotomy, and prior experience as factors in the fighting success of male crab spiders, *Misumenoides formosipes*. *Journal of Insect Behavior*, **14**, 841–855.

Drengsgaard, I. L. and Toft, S. (1999). Sperm competition in a nuptial feeding spider, *Pisaura mirabilis*. *Behaviour*, **136**, 877–897.

Eberhard, W. G. (1996). *Female Control: Sexual Selection by Cryptic Female Choice*. Princeton, NJ: Princeton University Press.

Eberhard, W. G. (1998). Female roles in sperm competition. In *Sperm Competition and Sexual Selection* (ed. T. R. Birkhead and A. P. Moller). London: Academic Press.

Eberhard, W. G. (2000). Criteria for demonstrating postcopulatory female choice. *Evolution*, **54**, 1047–1050.

Eberhard, W. G. (2004). Why study spider sex: special traits of spiders facilitate studies of sperm competition and cryptic female choice. *Journal of Arachnology*, **32**, 545–556.

Eberhard, W. G. and Huber, B. A. (2010) Spider genitalia: precise maneuvers with a numb structure in a complex lock. In *Evolution of Primary Sexual Characters in Animals* (ed. J. Leonard and A. Córdoba-Aguilar). Oxford, UK:Oxford University Press.

Elgar, M. A. (1992). Sexual cannibalism in spiders and other invertebrates. In *Cannibalism: Ecology and Evolution among Diverse Taxa* (ed. M. A. Elgar and B. J. Crespi). New York: Oxford University Press.

Elgar, M. A. (1998). Sperm competition and sexual selection in spiders and other arachnids. In *Sperm Competition and Sexual Selection* (ed. T. R. Birkhead and A. P. Moller). London: Academic Press.

Elgar, M. A. and Bathgate, R. (1996). Female receptivity and male mate-guarding in the jewel spider *Gasteracantha minax* Thorell (Araneidae). *Journal of Insect Behavior*, **9**, 729–738.

Elgar, M. A. and Fahey, B. F. (1996). Sexual cannibalism, competition, and size dimorphism in the orb-weaving spider *Nephila plumipes* Latreille (Araneae: Araneoidea). *Behavioral Ecology*, **7**, 195–198.

Elgar, M. A. and Jones, T. M. (2008). Size-dependent mating strategies and the risk of cannibalism. *Biological Journal of the Linnean Society*, **94**, 355–363.

Elgar, M. A. and Schneider, J. M. (2004). Evolutionary significance of sexual cannibalism. *Advances in the Study of Behavior*, **34**, 135–163.

Elgar, M. A., de Crespigny, F. E. C. and Ramamurthy, S. (2003). Male copulation behaviour and the risk of sperm competition. *Animal Behaviour*, **66**, 211–216.

Elgar, M. A., Schneider, J. M. and Herberstein, M. E. (2000). Female control of paternity in the sexually cannibalistic spider *Argiope keyserlingi*. *Proceedings of the Royal Society of London, B*, **267**, 2439–2443.

Elias, D. O., Hebets, E. A., Hoy, R. R., Maddison, W. P. and Mason, A. C. (2007). Regional seismic song differences in Sky Island populations of the jumping spider *Habronattus pugillis* Griswold (Araneae, Salticidae). *Journal of Arachnology*, **34**, 545–556.

Elias, D. O., Hebets, E. A., Hoy, R. R. and Mason, A. C. (2005). Seismic signals are crucial for male mating success in a visual specialist jumping spider (Araneae: Salticidae). *Animal Behaviour*, **69**, 931–938.

Elias, D. O., Kasumovic, M. M., Andrade, M. C. B., Mason, A. C. and Punzalan, D. (2008a). Assessment during aggressive contests between male jumping spiders. *Animal Behaviour*, **76**, 901–910.

Elias, D. O., Kasumovic, M. M., Punzalan, D., Andrade, M. C. B. and Mason, A. C. (2008b). Assessment during aggressive contests between male jumping spiders. *Animal Behaviour*, **76**, 901–910.

Elias, D. O., Mason, A. C. and Hoy, R. R. (2004). The effect of substrate on the efficacy of seismic courtship signal transmission in the jumping spider *Habronattus dossenus* (Araneae: Salticidae). *Journal of Experimental Biology*, **207**, 4105–4110.

Elias, D. O., Mason, A. C., Maddison, W. P. and Hoy, R. R. (2003). Seismic signals in a courting male jumping spider (Araneae: Salticidae). *Journal of Experimental Biology*, **206**, 4029–4039.

Enquist, M. and Leimar, O. (1983). Evolution of fighting behaviour: decision rules and the assessment of relative strength. *Journal of Theoretical Biology*, **102**, 387–410.

Enquist, M. and Leimar, O. (1987). Evolution of fighting behaviour: the effect of variation in resource value. *Journal of Theoretical Biology*, **127**, 187–205.

Enquist, M. and Leimar, O. (1990). The evolution of fatal fighting. *Animal Behaviour*, **39**, 1–9.

Erez, T., Schneider, J. M. and Lubin, Y. (2005). Is male cohabitation costly for females of the spider *Stegodyphus lineatus* (Eresidae)? *Ethology*, **111**, 693–704.

Estramil, N. and Costa, F. G. (2007). Female sexual receptivity after partial copulations in the wolf spider (*Schizocosa malitiosa*). *Journal of Zoology*, **271**, 148–153.

Foelix, R. F. (1996). *Biology of Spiders*. Oxford, UK: Oxford University Press.

Foellmer, M. and Moya-Larano, J. (2007). Sexual size dimorphism in spiders: patterns and processes. In *Sex, Size and Gender Roles: Evolutionary Studies of Sexual Size Dimorphism* (ed. D. J. Fairbairn, W. Blanckenhorn and T. Székely). Oxford, UK: Oxford University Press.

Foellmer, M. W. (2008). Broken genitals function as mating plugs and affect sex ratios in the orb-web spider *Argiope aurantia*. *Evolutionary Ecology Research*, **10**, 449–462.

Foellmer, M. W. and Fairbairn, D. J. (2003). Spontaneous male death during copulation in an orb-weaving spider. *Proceedings of the Royal Society of London, B*, **270**, S183–S185.

Foellmer, M. W. and Fairbairn, D. J. (2004). Males under attack: sexual cannibalism and its consequences for male morphology and behaviour in an orb-weaving spider. *Evolutionary Ecology Research*, **6**, 163–181.

Foellmer, M. W. and Fairbairn, D. J. (2005). Competing dwarf males: sexual selection in an orb-weaving spider. *Journal of Evolutionary Biology*, **18**, 629–641.

Forster, L. M. (1992). The steroryped behaviour of sexual cannibalism in *Lactrodectus hasselti* Thorell (Araneae, Theridiidae), the Australian redback spider. *Australian Journal of Zoology*, **40**, 1–11.

Forster, L. M. (1995). The behavioral ecology of *Latrodectus hasselti* (Thorell), the Australian redback spider (Araneae: Theridiidae): A review. *Records of the Western Australian Museum, Supplement*, **52**, 13–24.

Fromhage, L., Jacobs, K. and Schneider, J. M. (2007). Monogynous mating behaviour and its ecological basis in the golden orb spider *Nephila fenestrata*. *Ethology*, **113**, 813–820.

Fromhage, L., Mcnamara, J. M. and Houston, A. I. (2008). A model for the evolutionary maintenance of monogyny in spiders. *Journal of Theoretical Biology*, **250**, 524–531.

Fromhage, L. and Schneider, J. M. (2005a). Safer sex with feeding females: sexual conflict in a cannibalistic spider. *Behavioral Ecology*, **16**, 377–382.

Fromhage, L. and Schneider, J. M. (2005b). Virgin doves and mated hawks: contest behaviour in a spider. *Animal Behaviour*, **70**, 1099–1104.

Fromhage, L. and Schneider, J. M. (2006). Emasculation to plug up females: the significance of pedipalp damage in *Nephila fenestrata*. *Behavioral Ecology*, **17**, 353–357.

Fromhage, L., Elgar, M. A. and Schneider, J. M. (2005). Faithful without care: the evolution of monogyny. *Evolution*, **59**, 1400–1405.

Gaskett, A. C. (2007). Spider sex pheromones: emission, reception, structures, and functions. *Biological Reviews*, **82**, 26–48.

Gaskett, A. C., Herberstein, M. E., Downes, B. J. and Elgar, M. A. (2004). Changes in male mate choice in a sexually cannibalistic orb-web spider (Araneae: Araneidae). *Behaviour*, **141**, 1197–1210.

Hack, M. A., Thompson, D. J. and Fernandes, D. M. (1997). Fighting in males of the autumn spider, *Metellina segmentata*: effects of relative body size, prior residency and female value on contest outcome and duration. *Ethology*, **103**, 488–498.

Hammer, O. (1941). Biological and ecological investigations on flies associated with pasturing cattle and their excrement. *Videnskabelige Meddelser Dansk Naturhistorisk Forening*, **105**, 1–257.

Hansen, L. S., Gonzalez, S. F., Toft, S. and Bilde, T. (2008). Thanatosis as an adaptive male mating strategy in the nuptial gift-giving spider *Pisaura mirabilis*. *Behavioral Ecology*, **19**, 546–551.

Harari, A., Ziv, M. and Lubin, Y. (2009). Conflict or cooperation in the courtship display of the white widow spider, *Latrodectus pallidus*. *Journal of Arachnology*, **37**, 254–260.

Hebets, E. A. (2003). Subadult experience influences adult mate choice in an arthropod: exposed female wolf spiders prefer males of a familiar phenotype. *Proceedings of the National Academy of Sciences of the USA*, **100**, 13 390–13 395.

Hebets, E. A. and Uetz, G. W. (2000). Leg ornamentation and the efficacy of courtship display in four species of wolf spider (Araneae: Lycosidae). *Behavioral Ecology and Sociobiology*, **47**, 280–286.

Hebets, E. A. and Vink, C. J. (2007). Experience leads to preference: experienced females prefer brush-legged males in a population of syntopic wolf spiders. *Behavioral Ecology*, **18**, 1010–1020.

Hebets, E. A., Elias, D. O., Mason, A. C., Miller, G. L. and Stratton, G. E. (2008a). Substrate-dependent signalling success in the wolf spider, *Schizocosa retrorsa*. *Animal Behaviour*, **75**, 605–615.

Hebets, E. A., Wesson, J. and Shamble, P. S. (2008b). Diet influences mate choice selectivity in adult female wolf spiders. *Animal Behaviour*, **76**, 355–363.

Hedrick, A. V. (1988). Female choice and the heritability of attractive male traits: an empirical study. *American Naturalist*, **132**, 267.

Herberstein, M. E., Barry, K. L., Turoczy, M. A., *et al.* (2005a). Post-copulation mate guarding in the sexually cannibalistic St Andrew's Cross spider (Araneae, Araneidae). *Ethology, Ecology and Evolution*, **17**, 17–26.

Herberstein, M. E., Gaskett, A. C., Schneider, J. M., *et al.* (2005b). Limits to male copulation frequency: sexual cannibalism and sterility in St Andrew's Cross spiders (Araneae, Araneidae). *Ethology*, **111**, 1050–1061.

Herberstein, M. E., Schneider, J. M. and Elgar, M. A. (2002). Costs of courtship and mating in a sexually cannibalistic orb-web spider: female mating strategies and their consequences for males. *Behavioral Ecology and Sociobiology*, **51**, 440–446.

Hoefler, C. D. (2002). Is contest experience a trump card? The interaction of residency status, experience, and body size on fighting success in *Misumenoides formosipes* (Araneae: Thomisidae). *Journal of Insect Behavior*, **15**, 779–790.

Hoefler, C. D. (2007). Male mate choice and size-assortative pairing in a jumping spider, *Phidippus clarus*. *Animal Behaviour*, **73**, 943–954.

Hoefler, C. D. (2008). The costs of male courtship and potential benefits of male choice for large mates in *Phidippus clarus* (Araneae, Salticidae). *Journal of Arachnology*, **36**, 210–212.

Hosken, D. J., Stockley, P., Tregenza, T. and Wedell, N. (2009). Monogamy and the battle of the sexes. *Annual Review of Entomology*, **54**, 361–378.

Hsu, Y. and Wolf, L. L. (2001). The winner and loser effect: what fighting behaviours are influenced? *Animal Behaviour*, **61**, 777–786.

Hsu, Y., Earley, R. L. and Wolf, L. L. (2006). Modulation of aggressive behaviour by fighting experience: mechanisms and contest outcomes. *Biological Reviews*, **81**, 33–74.

Huber, B. A. (2003). Rapid evolution and species-specificity of arthropod genitalia: fact or artifact? *Organisms Diversity and Evolution*, **3**, 63–71.

Huber, B. A. (2005). Sexual selection research on spiders: progress and biases. *Biological Reviews*, **80**, 363–385.

Huber, B. A. and Eberhard, W. G. (1997). Courtship, copulation, and genital mechanics in *Physocyclus globosus* (Araneae, Pholcidae). *Canadian Journal of Zoology*, **75**, 905–918.

Jackson, R. R. (1978). An analysis of alternative mating tactics of the jumping spider *Phidippus johnsoni* (Araneae, Salticidae). *Journal of Arachnology*, **5**, 185–230.

Jackson, R. R. (1981). Relationship between reproductive security and intersexual selection in a jumping spider *Phidippus johnsoni* (Araneae, Salticidae). *Evolution*, **35**, 601–604.

Jackson, R. R. (1983). The biology of *Mopsus mormon*, a jumping spider (Araneae: Salticidae) from Queensland: intraspecific interactions. *Australian Journal of Zoology*, **31**, 39–53.

Jackson, R. R. (1986). The display behaviour of *Cyllobelus rufopictus* (Simon) (Araneae, Salticidae), a jumping spider from Kenya. *New Zealand Journal of Zoology*, **13**, 27–43.

Jackson, R. R. (1997). Jumping spider mating strategies: sex among cannibals in and out of webs. In *Evolution of Mating Systems in Insects and Arachnids* (ed. J. Choe and B. Crespi). Cambridge, UK: Cambridge University Press.

Jackson, R. R. and Cooper, K. J. (1991). The influence of body size and prior residency on the outcome of male-male interactions of *Marpissa marina*, a New-Zealand jumping spider (Araneae, Salticidae). *Ethology, Ecology and Evolution*, **3**, 79–82.

Jackson, R. R. and Macnab, A. M. (1989a). Display behaviour of *Corythalia canosa*, an ant-eating jumping spider (Araneae: Salticidae) from Florida. *New Zealand Journal of Zoology*, **16**, 169–183.

Jackson, R. R. and Macnab, A. M. (1989b). Display, mating, and predatory behaviour of the jumping spider *Plexippus paykulli* (Araneae: Salticidae). *New Zealand Journal of Zoology*, **16**, 151–168.

Jackson, R. R. and Pollard, S. D. (1990). Intraspecific interactions and the function of courtship in mygalomorph spiders: a study of *Porrhothele antipodiana* (Araneae, Hexathelidae) and a literature-review. *New Zealand Journal of Zoology*, **17**, 499–526.

Jackson, R. R., Walker, M. W., Pollard, S. D. and Cross, F. R. (2006). Influence of seeing a female on the male-male interactions of a jumping spider, *Hypoblemum albovittatum*. *Journal of Ethology*, **24**, 231–238.

Jerhot, E., Stoltz, J. A., Andrade, M. C. B. and Schulz, S. (2010). Acylated serine derivatives: a unique class of arthropod pheromones of the Australian redback spider, *Latrodectus hasselti*. *Angewandte Chemie International Edition*, **49**, 1–5.

Jiao, X., Wu, J., Chen, Z., Chen, J. and Liu, F. (2009). Effects of temperature on courtship and copulatory behaviours of a wolf spider *Pardosa astrigera* (Araneae: Lycosidae). *Journal of Thermal Biology*, **34**, 348–352.

Johannesen, J. and Lubin, Y. (2001). Evidence for kin-structured group founding and limited juvenile dispersal in the sub-social spider *Stegodyphus lineatus* (Araneae, Eresidae). *Journal of Arachnology*, **29**, 413–422.

Johansson, B. G. and Jones, T. M. (2007). The role of chemical communication in mate choice. *Biological Reviews*, **82**, 265–289.

Johnson, J. C. (2005a). Cohabitation of juvenile females with mature males promotes sexual cannibalism in fishing spiders. *Behavioral Ecology*, **16**, 269–273.

Johnson, J. C. (2005b). The role of body size in mating interactions of the sexually cannibalistic fishing spider *Dolomedes triton*. *Ethology*, **111**, 51–61.

Johnson, J. C. and Sih, A. (2005). Precopulatory sexual cannibalism in fishing spiders (*Dolomedes triton*): a role for behavioral syndromes. *Behavioral Ecology and Sociobiology*, **58**, 390–396.

Johnson, J. C. and Sih, A. (2007). Fear, food, sex and parental care: a syndrome of boldness in the fishing spider, *Dolomedes triton*. *Animal Behaviour*, **74**, 1131–1138.

Johnson, S. A. and Jakob, E. M. (1999). Leg autotomy in a spider has minimal costs in competitive ability and development. *Animal Behaviour*, **57**, 957–965.

Jones, T. M. and Elgar, M. A. (2008). Male insemination decisions and sperm quality influence paternity in the golden orb-weaving spider. *Behavioral Ecology*, **19**, 285–291.

Kaston, B. J. (1970). Comparative biology of American black widow spiders. *Transactions of the San Diego Society of Natural History*, **16**, 33–82.

Kasumovic, M. M. and Andrade, M. C. B. (2004). Discrimination of airborne pheromones by mate-searching male western black widow spiders (*Latrodectus hesperus*): species- and population-specific responses. *Canadian Journal of Zoology*, **82**, 1027–1034.

Kasumovic, M. M. and Andrade, M. C. B. (2006). Male development tracks rapidly shifting sexual versus natural selection pressures. *Current Biology*, **16**, R242–R243.

Kasumovic, M. M. and Andrade, M. C. B. (2009). A change in competitive context reverses sexual selection on male size. *Journal of Evolutionary Biology*, **22**, 324–333.

Kasumovic, M. M., Bruce, M. J., Andrade, M. C. B. and Herberstein, M. E. (2008). Spatial and temporal demographic variation drives within-season fluctuations in sexual selection. *Evolution: International Journal of Organic Evolution*, **62**, 2316–2325.

Kasumovic, M. M., Elias, D. O., Punzalan, D., Mason, A. C. and Andrade, M. C. B. (2009). Experience affects the outcome of agonistic contests without affecting the selective advantage of size. *Animal Behaviour*, **77**, 1533–1538.

Kasumovic, M. M., Elias, D. O., Sivalinghem, S., Mason, A. C. and Andrade, M. C. B. (2010). Examination of prior contest experience and the retention of winner and loser effects. *Behavioral Ecology*, **21**, 404–409.

Kindle, T., Johnson, K., Ivy, T., Weddle, C. and Sakaluk, S. (2006). Female mating frequency increases with temperature in two cricket species, *Gryllodes sigillatus* and *Acheta domesticus* (Orthoptera: Gryllidae). *Canadian Journal of Zoology*, **84**, 1345–1350.

Knipling, E. F. (1955). Possibilities of insect control or eradication through the use of sexually sterile males. *Journal of Economic Entomology*, **48**, 459–462.

Knoflach, B. (1998). Mating in *Theridion varians* Hahn and related species (Araneae: Theridiidae). *Journal of Natural History*, **32**, 545–604.

Knoflach, B. and Benjamin, S. P. (2003). Mating without sexual cannibalism in *Tidarren sisyphoides* (Araneae, Theridiidae). *Journal of Arachnology*, **31**, 445–448.

Knoflach, B. and Van Harten, A. (2000). Palpal loss, single palp copulation and obligatory mate consumption in *Tidarren cuneolatum* (Tullgren, 1910) (Araneae, Theridiidae). *Journal of Natural History*, **34**, 1639–1659.

Kokko, H. and Jennions, M. D. (2008). Parental investment, sexual selection and sex ratios. *Journal of Evolutionary Biology*, **21**, 919–948.

Kotiaho, J., Alatalo, R. V., Mappes, J. and Parri, S. (1996). Sexual selection in a wolf spider: male drumming activity, body size, and viability. *Evolution*, **50**, 1977–1981.

Kotiaho, J. S. (2000). Testing the assumptions of conditional handicap theory: costs and condition dependence of a sexually selected trait. *Behavioral Ecology and Sociobiology*, **48**, 188–194.

Kotiaho, J. S. and Puurtinen, M. (2007). Mate choice for indirect genetic benefits: scrutiny of the current paradigm. *Functional Ecology*, **21**, 638–644.

Kotiaho, J. S., Alatalo, R. V., Mappes, J. and Parri, S. (1999a). Honesty of agonistic signalling and effects of size and motivation asymmetry in contests. *Acta Ethologica*, **2**, 0013–0021.

Kotiaho, J. S., Alatalo, R. V., Mappes, J. and Parri, S. (1999b). Sexual signalling and viability in a wolf spider (*Hygrolycosa rubrofasciata*): measurements under laboratory and field conditions. *Behavioral Ecology and Sociobiology*, **46**, 123–128.

Kotiaho, J. S., Alatalo, R. V., Mappes, J. and Parri, S. (2004). Adaptive significance of synchronous chorusing in an acoustically signalling wolf spider. *Proceedings of the Royal Society of London, B*, **271**, 1847–1850.

Kuntner, M., Coddington, J. A. and Hormiga, G. (2008). Phylogeny of extant nephilid orb-weaving spiders (Araneae, Nephilidae): testing morphological and ethological homologies. *Cladistics*, **24**, 147–217.

Kuntner, M., Coddington, J. A. and Schneider, J. M. (2009a). Intersexual arms race? Genital coevolution in nephilid spiders (Araneae, Nephilidae). *Evolution*, **63**, 1451–1463.

Kuntner, M., Kralj-Fiser, S., Schneider, J. M. and Li, D. (2009b). Mate plugging via genital mutilation in nephilid spiders: an evolutionary hypothesis. *Journal of Zoology*, **277**, 257–266.

Lang, A. (1996). Silk investment in gifts by males of the nuptial feeding spider *Pisaura mirabilis* (Araneae: Pisauridae). *Behaviour*, **133**, 697–716.

Leimar, O., Austad, S. and Enquist, M. (1991). A test of the sequential assessment game – fighting in the bowl and doily spider *Frontinella pyramitela*. *Evolution*, **45**, 862–874.

Li, D. and Kuan, J. Y. X. (2006). Natal dispersal and breeding dispersal of a subsocial spitting spider (*Scytodes pallida*) (Araneae: Scytodidae), from Singapore. *Journal of Zoology*, **268**, 121–126.

Linn, C. D., Molina, Y., Difatta, J. and Christenson, T. E. (2007). The adaptive advantage of prolonged mating: a test of alternative hypotheses. *Animal Behaviour*, **74**, 481–485.

Maddison, W. and Hedin, M. (2003). Phylogeny of *Habronattus* jumping spiders (Araneae: Salticidae), with consideration of genital and courtship evolution. *Systematic Entomology*, **28**, 1–21.

Maddison, W. P. and Stratton, G. E. (1988). Sound production and associated morphology in male jumping spiders of the *Habronattus agilis* species group (Araneae, Salticidae). *Journal of Arachnology*, **16**, 199–211.

Maklakov, A. A. and Lubin, Y. (2004). Sexual conflict over mating in a spider: increased fecundity does not compensate for the costs of polyandry. *Evolution*, **58**, 1135–1140.

Maklakov, A. A. and Lubin, Y. (2006). Indirect genetic benefits of polyandry in a spider with direct costs of mating. *Behavioral Ecology and Sociobiology*, **61**, 31–38.

Maklakov, A. A., Bilde, T. and Lubin, Y. (2003). Vibratory courtship in a web-building spider: signalling quality or stimulating the female? *Animal Behaviour*, **66**, 623–630.

Maklakov, A. A., Bilde, T. and Lubin, Y. (2004). Sexual selection for increased male body size and protandry in a spider. *Animal Behaviour*, **68**, 1041–1048.

Maklakov, A. A., Bilde, T. and Lubin, Y. (2005). Sexual conflict in the wild: elevated mating rate reduces female lifetime reproductive success. *American Naturalist*, **165**, S38–S45.

Mappes, J., Alatalo, R. V., Kotiaho, J. and Parri, S. (1996). Viability costs of condition-dependent sexual male display in a drumming wolf spider. *Proceedings of the Royal Society of London, B*, **263**, 785–789.

Mas, E., Ribera, C. and Moya-Larano, J. (2009). Resurrecting the differential mortality model of sexual size dimorphism. *Journal of Evolutionary Biology*, **22**, 1739–1749.

Masta, S. E. and Maddison, W. P. (2002). Sexual selection driving diversification in jumping spiders. *Proceedings of the National Academy of Sciences of the USA*, **99**, 4442–4447.

Meehan, C. J., Olson, E. J., Reudink, M. W., Kyser, T. K. and Curry, R. L. (2009). Herbivory in a spider through exploitation of an ant–plant mutualism. *Current Biology*, **19**, R892–R893.

Merrett, P. (1988). Notes on the biology of the neotropical pisaurid, *Ancylometes bogotensis* (Araneae: Pisauridae). *Bulletin of the British Arachnological Society*, **7**, 197–201.

Miller, J. A. (2007). Repeated evolution of male sacrifice behavior in spiders correlated with genital mutilation. *Evolution*, **61**, 1301–1315.

Miyatake, T., Katayama, K., Takeda, Y., *et al.* (2004). Is death-feigning adaptive? Heritable variation in fitness difference of death-feigning behaviour. *Proceedings of the Royal Society of London, B*, **271**, 2293–2296.

Mora, G. (1990). Paternal care in a neotropical harvestman, *Zygopachylus albomarginis* (Arachnida, Opiliones, Gonyleptidae). *Animal Behaviour*, **39**, 582–593.

Morse, D. H. (2007). Mating frequencies of male crab spiders, *Misumena vatia* (Araneae, Thomisidae). *Journal of Arachnology*, **35**, 84–88.

Morse, D. H. and Hu, H. H. (2004). Age affects the risk of sexual cannibalism in male crab spiders (*Misumena vatia*). *American Midland Naturalist*, **151**, 318–325.

Moya-Larano, J., Pascual, J. and Wise, D. H. (2003). Mating patterns in late-maturing female Mediterranean tarantulas may reflect the costs and benefits of sexual cannibalism. *Animal Behaviour*, **66**, 469–476.

Nessler, S., Uhl, G. and Schneider, J. (2009a). Sexual cannibalism facilitates genital damage in *Argiope lobata* (Araneae: Araneidae). *Behavioral Ecology and Sociobiology*, **63**, 355–362.

Nessler, S. H., Uhl, G. and Schneider, J. M. (2007). Genital damage in the orb-web spider *Argiope bruennichi* (Araneae: Araneidae) increases paternity success. *Behavioral Ecology*, **18**, 174–181.

Nessler, S. H., Uhl, G. and Schneider, J. M. (2009b). Scent of a woman: the effect of female presence on sexual cannibalism in an orb-weaving spider (Araneae: Araneidae). *Ethology*, **115**, 633–640.

Newman, J. A. and Elgar, M. A. (1991). Sexual cannibalism in orb-weaving spiders: an economic model. *American Naturalist*, **138**, 1372–1395.

Nishino, H. and Sakai, M. (1996). Behaviorally significant immobile state of so called thanatosis in the cricket *Gryllus bimaculatus* DeGeer: its characterization, sensory mechanism and function. *Journal of Comparative Physiology, A*, **179**, 613–624.

Norton, S. and Uetz, G. W. (2005). Mating frequency in *Schizocosa ocreata* (Hentz) wolf spiders: evidence for a mating system with female monandry and male polygyny. *Journal of Arachnology*, **33**, 16–24.

Papke, M. D., Riechert, S. E. and Schulz, S. (2001). An airborne female pheromone associated with male attraction and courtship in a desert spider. *Animal Behaviour*, **61**, 877–886.

Parker, G. A. (1970). Sperm competition and its evolutionary consequences in the insects. *Biological Reviews*, **45**, 525–567.

Parri, S., Alatalo, R. V., Kotiaho, J. and Mappes, J. (1997). Female choice for male drumming in the wolf spider *Hygrolycosa rubrofasciata*. *Animal Behaviour*, **53**, 305–312.

Parri, S., Alatalo, R. V., Kotiaho, J. S., Mappes, J. and Rivero, A. (2002). Sexual selection in the wolf spider *Hygrolycosa rubrofasciata*: female preference for drum duration and pulse rate. *Behavioral Ecology*, **13**, 615–621.

Perampaladas, K., Stoltz, J. A. and Andrade, M. C. B. (2008). Mated redback spider females re-advertise receptivity months after mating. *Ethology*, **114**, 589–598.

Peretti, A., Eberhard, W. G. and Briceno, R. D. (2006). Copulatory dialogue: female spiders sing during copulation to influence male genitalic movements. *Animal Behaviour*, **72**, 413–421.

Peretti, A. V. and Eberhard, W. G. (2010). Cryptic female choice via sperm dumping favours male copulatory courtship in a spider. *Journal of Evolutionary Biology*, **23**, 271–281.

Pérez-Miles, F., Postiglioni, R., Montes-De-Oca, L., Baruffaldi, L. and Costa, F. G. (2007). Mating system in the tarantula spider *Eupalaestrus weijenberghi* (Thorell, 1894): evidences of monandry and polygyny. *Zoology*, **110**, 253–260.

Persons, M. H. and Uetz, G. W. (2005). Sexual cannibalism and mate choice decisions in wolf spiders: influence of male size and secondary sexual characters. *Animal Behaviour*, **69**, 83–94.

Pitnick, S. and Brown, W. D. (2000). Criteria for demonstrating female sperm choice. *Evolution*, **54**, 1052–1056.

Prenter, J., Elwood, R. W. and Montgomery, W. I. (1994a). Assessments and decisions in *Metellina segmentata* (Araneae, Metidae): evidence of a pheromone involved in mate guarding. *Behavioral Ecology and Sociobiology*, **35**, 39–43.

Prenter, J., Elwood, R. W. and Montgomery, W. I. (1994b). Male exploitation of female predatory behavior reduces sexual cannibalism in male autumn spiders, *Metellina segmentata*. *Animal Behaviour*, **47**, 235–236.

Prenter, J., MacNeil, C. and Elwood, R. W. (2006). Sexual cannibalism and mate choice. *Animal Behaviour*, **71**, 481–490.

Prokop, P. (2006). Insemination does not affect female mate choice in a nuptial feeding spider. *Italian Journal of Zoology*, **73**, 197–201.

Pruden, A. J. and Uetz, G. W. (2004). Assessment of potential predation costs of male decoration and courtship display in wolf spiders using video digitization and playback. *Journal of Insect Behavior*, **17**, 67–80.

Pruitt, J. N. and Riechert, S. E. (2009). Male mating preference is associated with risk of pre-copulatory cannibalism in a socially polymorphic spider. *Behavioral Ecology and Sociobiology*, **63**, 1573–1580.

Pruitt, J. N., Riechert, S. E. and Jones, T. C. (2008). Behavioural syndromes and their fitness consequences in a socially polymorphic spider, *Anelosimus studiosus*. *Animal Behaviour*, **76**, 871–879.

Puurtinen, M., Ketolam, T. and Kotiaho, J. (2009). The good-genes and compatible-genes benefits of mate choice. *American Naturalist*, **174**, 741–752.

Quirici, V. and Costa, F. G. (2005). Seismic communication during courtship in two burrowing tarantula spiders: an experimental study on *Eupalaestrus weijenberghi* and *Acanthoscurria suina*. *Journal of Arachnology*, **33**, 159–166.

Ramos, M., Coddington, J. A., Christenson, T. E. and Irschick, D. J. (2005). Have male and female genitalia coevolved? A phylogenetic analysis of genitalic morphology and sexual size dimorphism in web-building spiders (Araneae: Araneoidea). *Evolution*, **59**, 1989–1999.

Real, L. (1990). Search theory and mate choice. I. Models of single-sex discrimination. *American Naturalist*, **136**, 376–405.

Riechert, S. E. (1988). The energetic costs of fighting. *American Zoologist*, **28**, 877–884.

Rivero, A., Alatalo, R. V., Kotiaho, J. S., Mappes, J. and Parri, S. (2000). Acoustic signalling in a wolf spider: can signal characteristics predict male quality? *Animal Behaviour*, **60**, 187–194.

Roberts, J. A. and Uetz, G. W. (2005). Information content of female chemical signals in the wolf spider, *Schizocosa ocreata*: male discrimination of reproductive state and receptivity. *Animal Behaviour*, **70**, 217–223.

Robinson, M. H. and Robinson, B. (1980). Comparative studies of the courtship and mating behaviour of tropical araneid spiders. *Pacific Insects Monograph*, **36**, 1–218.

Ross, K. and Smith, R. L. (1979). Aspects of the courtship behavior of the black widow spider, *Latrodectus hesperus* (Araneae: Theridiidae), with evidence for the existence of a contact sex pheromone. *Journal of Arachnology*, **7**, 69–77.

Rovner, J. S. (1968). Territoriality in the sheet-web spider *Linyphia triangularis* (Clerck) (Araneae, Linyphiidae). *Zeitschrift für Tierpsychologie*, **25**, 232–242.

Sasaki, T. and Iwahashi, O. (1995). Sexual cannibalism in an orb-weaving spider *Argiope aemula*. *Animal Behaviour*, **49**, 1119–1121.

Schaefer, D. and Uhl, G. (2003). Male competition over access to females in a spider with last-male sperm precedence. *Ethology*, **109**, 385–400.

Schaefer, M. A. and Uhl, G. (2002). Determinants of paternity success in the spider *Pholcus phalangioides* (Pholcidae: Araneae): the role of male and female mating behaviour. *Behavioral Ecology and Sociobiology*, **51**, 368–377.

Schaefer, M. A. and Uhl, G. (2005). Sequential mate encounters: female but not male body size influences female remating behavior. *Behavioral Ecology*, **16**, 461–466.

Schaefer, M. A., Misof, B. and Uhl, G. (2008). Effects of body size of both sexes and female mating history on male mating behaviour and paternity success in a spider. *Animal Behaviour*, **76**, 75–86.

Scheffer, S. J., Uetz, G. W. and Stratton, G. E. (1996). Sexual selection, male morphology, and the efficacy of courtship signalling in two wolf spiders (Araneae: Lycosidae). *Behavioral Ecology and Sociobiology*, **38**, 17–23.

Schmitt, A., Schuster, M. and Barth, F. G. (1992). Male competition in a wandering spider (*Cupiennius getazi*, Ctenidae). *Ethology*, **90**, 293–306.

Schmitt, A., Schuster, M. and Barth, F. G. (1994). Vibratory communication in a wandering spider, *Cupiennius getazi*: female and male preferences for features of the conspecific male's releaser. *Animal Behaviour*, **48**, 1155–1171.

Schmitt, M. (1992). Conjectures on the origins and functions of a bridal veil spun by the males of *Cupiennius coccineus* (Araneae, Ctenidae). *Journal of Arachnology*, **20**, 67–68.

Schneider, J. M. (1997). Timing of maturation and the mating system of the spider, *Stegodyphus lineatus* (Eresidae): how important is body size? *Biological Journal of the Linnean Society*, **60**, 517–525.

Schneider, J. M. (1999). Delayed oviposition: a female strategy to counter infanticide by males? *Behavioral Ecology*, **10**, 567–571.

Schneider, J. M. and Elgar, M. A. (2001). Sexual cannibalism and sperm competition in the golden orb-web spider *Nephila plumipes* (Araneoidea): female and male perspectives. *Behavioral Ecology*, **12**, 547–552.

Schneider, J. M. and Elgar, M. A. (2002). Sexual cannibalism in *Nephila plumipes* as a consequence of female life history strategies. *Journal of Evolutionary Biology*, **15**, 84–91.

Schneider, J. M. and Elgar, M. A. (2005). The combined effects of pre- and post-insemination sexual selection on extreme variation in male body size. *Evolutionary Ecology*, **19**, 419–433.

Schneider, J. M. and Lesmono, K. (2009). Courtship raises male fertilization success through post-mating sexual selection in a spider. *Proceedings of the Royal Society of London, B*, **276**, 3105–3111.

Schneider, J. M. and Lubin, Y. (1996). Infanticidal male eresid spiders. *Nature*, **381**, 655–656.

Schneider, J. M. and Lubin, Y. (1997a). Does high adult mortality explain semelparity in the spider *Stegodyphus lineatus* (Eresidae)? *Oikos*, **79**, 92–100.

Schneider, J. M. and Lubin, Y. (1997b). Infanticide by males in a spider with suicidal maternal care, *Stegodyphus lineatus* (Eresidae). *Animal Behaviour*, **54**, 305–312.

Schneider, J. M. and Lubin, Y. (1998). Intersexual conflict in spiders. *Oikos*, **83**, 496–506.

Schneider, J. M., Fromhage, L. and Uhl, G. (2005a). Copulation patterns in the golden orb-web spider *Nephila madagascariensis*. *Journal of Ethology*, **23**, 51–55.

Schneider, J. M., Fromhage, L. and Uhl, G. (2005b). Extremely short copulations do not affect hatching success in *Argiope bruennichi* (Araneae, Araneidae). *Journal of Arachnology*, **33**, 663–669.

Schneider, J. M., Gilberg, S., Fromhage, L. and Uhl, G. (2006). Sexual conflict over copulation duration in a cannibalistic spider. *Animal Behaviour*, **71**, 781–788.

Schneider, J. M., Herberstein, M. E., Bruce, M. J., *et al.* (2008). Male copulation frequency, sperm competition and genital damage in the golden orb-web spider (*Nephila plumipes*). *Australian Journal of Zoology*, **56**, 233–238.

Schneider, J. M., Herberstein, M. E., de Crespigny, F. E. C., Ramamurthy, S. and Elgar, M. A. (2000). Sperm competition and small size advantage for males of the golden orb-web spider *Nephila edulis*. *Journal of Evolutionary Biology*, **13**, 939–946.

Schneider, J. M., Thomas, M. L. and Elgar, M. A. (2001). Ectomised conductors in the golden orb-web spider, *Nephila plumipes* (Araneoidea): a male adaptation to sexual conflict? *Behavioral Ecology and Sociobiology*, **49**, 410–415.

Schüch, W. and Barth, F. G. (1990). Vibratory communication in a spider: female responses to synthetic male vibrations. *Journal of Comparative Physiology, A*, **166**, 817–826.

Schulz, S. (2004). Semiochemistry of spiders. In *Advances in Chemical Ecology* (ed. R. Carde and J. Millar). Cambridge, UK: Cambridge University Press.

Schulz, S. and Toft, S. (1993). Identification of a sex pheromone from a spider. *Science*, **260**, 1635–1637.

Schutz, D. and Taborsky, M. (2005). Mate choice and sexual conflict in the size dimorphic water spider *Argyroneta aquatica* (Araneae, Argyronetidae). *Journal of Arachnology*, **33**, 767–775.

Segoli, M., Arieli, R., Sierwald, P., Harari, A. R. and Lubin, Y. (2008a). Sexual cannibalism in the brown widow spider (*Latrodectus geometricus*). *Ethology*, **114**, 279–286.

Segoli, M., Lubin, Y. and Harari, A. R. (2008b). Frequency and consequences of damage to male copulatory organs in a widow spider. *Journal of Arachnology*, **36**, 533–537.

Singer, F. and Riechert, S. E. (1995). Mating system and mating success of the desert soldier *Agelenopsis aperta*. *Behavioral Ecology and Sociobiology*, **36**, 313–322.

Singer, F., Riechert, S. E., Xu, H. F., *et al.* (2000). Analysis of courtship success in the funnel-web spider *Agelenopsis aperta*. *Behaviour*, **137**, 93–117.

Snook, R. R. and Hosken, D. J. (2004). Sperm death and dumping in *Drosophila*. *Nature*, **428**, 939–941.

Snow, L. S. E. and Andrade, M. C. B. (2004). Pattern of sperm transfer in redback spiders: implications for sperm competition and male sacrifice. *Behavioral Ecology*, **15**, 785–792.

Snow, L. S. E. and Andrade, M. C. B. (2005). Multiple sperm storage organs facilitate female control of paternity. *Proceedings of the Royal Society of London, B*, **272**, 1139–1144.

Snow, L. S. E., Abdel-Mesih, A. and Andrade, M. C. B. (2006). Broken copulatory organs are low-cost adaptations to sperm competition in redback spiders. *Ethology*, **112**, 379–389.

Stalhandske, P. (2001). Nuptial gift in the spider *Pisaura mirabilis* maintained by sexual selection. *Behavioral Ecology*, **12**, 691–697.

Stalhandske, P. (2002). Nuptial gifts of male spiders function as sensory traps. *Proceedings of the Royal Society of London, B*, **269**, 905–908.

Stoltz, J. and Andrade, M. (2010). Female's courtship threshold allows intruding males to mate with reduced effort. *Proceedings of the Royal Society of London, B*, **277**, 585–592.

Stoltz, J. A., Elias, D. O. and Andrade, M. C. B. (2008). Females reward courtship by competing males in a cannibalistic spider. *Behavioral Ecology and Sociobiology*, **62**, 689–697.

Stoltz, J. A., Elias, D. O. and Andrade, M. C. B. (2009). Male courtship effort determines female response to competing rivals in redback spiders. *Animal Behaviour*, **77**, 79–85.

Stoltz, J. A., McNeil, J. N. and Andrade, M. C. B. (2007). Males assess chemical signals to discriminate just-mated females from virgins in redback spiders. *Animal Behaviour*, **74**, 1669–1674.

Stratton, G. E. (2005). Evolution of ornamentation and courtship behavior in *Schizocosa*: insights from a phylogeny based on morphology (Araneae, Lycosidae). *Journal of Arachnology*, **33**, 347–376.

Suhm, M., Thaler, K. and Alberti, G. (1996). Glands in the male palpal organ and the origin of the mating plug in *Amaurobius* species (Araneae: Amaurobiidae). *Zoologischer Anzeiger*, **234**, 191–199.

Taylor, P. W. and Elwood, R. W. (2003). The mismeasure of animal contests. *Animal Behaviour*, **65**, 1195–1202.

Taylor, P. W. and Jackson, R. R. (2003). Interacting effects of size and prior injury in jumping spider conflicts. *Animal Behaviour*, **65**, 787–794.

Taylor, P. W., Hasson, O. and Clark, D. L. (2001). Initiation and resolution of jumping spider contests: roles for size, proximity, and early detection of rivals. *Behavioral Ecology and Sociobiology*, **50**, 403–413.

Trivers, R. L. (1972). Parental investment and sexual selection. In *Sexual Selection and the Descent of Man* (ed. B. Campbell). London: Heinemann.

Uetz, G. W. and Norton, S. (2007). Preference for male traits in female wolf spiders varies with the choice of available males, female age and reproductive state. *Behavioral Ecology and Sociobiology*, **61**, 631–641.

Uhl, G. (2000). Female genital morphology and sperm priority patterns in spiders (Araneae). *European Arachnology*, 145–156.

Uhl, G., Nessler, S. H. and Schneider, J. (2007). Copulatory mechanism in a sexually cannibalistic spider with genital mutilation (Araneae: Araneidae: *Argiope bruennichi*). *Zoology*, **110**, 398–408.

Uhl, G., Nessler, S. H. and Schneider, J. (2010). Securing paternity in spiders? A review on occurrence and effects of mating plugs and male genital mutilation. *Genetica*, **138**, 75–104.

Uhl, G., Schmitt, S. and Schafer, M. (2005). Fitness benefits of multiple mating versus female mate choice in the cellar spider (*Pholcus phalangioides*). *Behavioral Ecology and Sociobiology*, **59**, 69–76.

Uhl, G. and Vollrath, F. (1998). Little evidence for size-selective sexual cannibalism in two species of *Nephila* (Araneae). *Zoology – Analysis of Complex Systems*, **101**, 101–106.

Venner, S., Bernstein, C., Dray, S. and Bel-Venner, M. (2010). Make love not war: when should less competitive males choose low-quality but defendable females? *American Naturalist*, **175**, 650–661.

Watson, P. J. (1986). Transmission of a female sex pheromone thwarted by males in the spider *Linyphia litigiose* (Linyphiidae). *Science*, 219–221.

Watson, P. J. (1990). Female-enhanced male competition determines the 1st mate and principal sire in the spider *Linyphia litigiosa* (Linyphiidae). *Behavioral Ecology and Sociobiology*, **26**, 77–90.

Watson, P. J. (1998). Multi-male mating and female choice increase offspring growth in the spider *Neriene litigiosa* (Linyphiidae). *Animal Behaviour*, **55**, 387–403.

Watson, P. J. and Lighton, J. R. B. (1994). Sexual selection and the energetics of copulatory courtship in the sierra dome spider, *Linyphia litigiosa*. *Animal Behaviour*, **48**, 615–626.

Welke, K. and Schneider, J. M. (2009). Inbreeding avoidance through cryptic female choice in the cannibalistic orb-web spider *Argiope lobata*. *Behavioural Ecology*, **20**, 1056–1062.

Wells, M. S. (1988). Effects of body size and resource value on fighting behaviour in a jumping spider. *Animal Behaviour*, **36**, 321–326.

West, H. P. and Toft, S. (1999). Last-male sperm priority and the mating system of the haplogyne spider *Tetragnatha extensa* (Araneae: Tetragnathidae). *Journal of Insect Behavior*, **12**, 433–450.

Whitehouse, M. E. A. (1991). To mate or fight: male–male competition and alternative mating strategies of *Argyrodes antipodiana* (Theridiidae, Araneae). *Behavioral Proceedings*, **23**, 163–172.

Whitehouse, M. E. A. (1997). Experience influences male-male contests in the spider *Argyrodes antipodiana* (Theridiidae: Araneae). *Animal Behaviour*, **53**, 913–923.

Wilder, S. M. and Rypstra, A. L. (2008a). Diet quality affects mating behaviour and egg production in a wolf spider. *Animal Behaviour*, **76**, 439–445.

Wilder, S. M. and Rypstra, A. L. (2008b). Prior encounters with the opposite sex affect male and female mating behavior in a wolf spider (Araneae, Lycosidae). *Behavioral Ecology and Sociobiology*, **62**, 1813–1820.

Wilder, S. M. and Rypstra, A. L. (2008c). Sexual size dimorphism mediates the occurrence of state-dependent sexual cannibalism in a wolf spider. *Animal Behaviour*, **76**, 447–454.

Wilder, S. M. and Rypstra, A. L. (2008d). Sexual size dimorphism predicts the frequency of sexual cannibalism within and among species of spiders. *American Naturalist*, **172**, 431–440.

Wilder, S. M., Rypstra, A. L. and Elgar, M. A. (2009). The importance of ecological and phylogenetic conditions for the occurrence and frequency of sexual cannibalism. *Annual Review of Ecology, Evolution, and Systematics*, **40**, 21–39.

Wilgers, D. J., Nicholas, A. C., Reed, D. H., Stratton, G. E. and Hebets, E. A. (2009). Condition-dependent alternative mating tactics in a sexually cannibalistic wolf spider. *Behavioral Ecology*, **20**, 891–900.

Wu, J., Jiao, X.-G., Chen, J., Peng, Y., Liu, F.-X. and Wang, Z.-H. (2007). Behavioral evidence for a sex pheromone in female wolf spiders *Pardosa astrigera*. *Acta Zoologica Sinica*, **53**, 994–999.

8

Group living in spiders: cooperative breeding and coloniality

TRINE BILDE AND YAEL LUBIN

Group living occurs in two different forms in spiders, cooperatively breeding social species and colonial species. The social species construct a communal nest and capture web, capture prey and feed together and cooperate in raising the young. Social spiders lack pre-mating dispersal, which results in regular inbreeding within colonies. Social species are thought to be derived from subsocial forms, which have lengthy maternal care and some cooperation among young, but pre-mating dispersal of juveniles limits inbreeding. There are currently only 25 known social species occurring in seven different families and representing perhaps 19 independent evolutionary transitions to sociality. Colonial group living is much more common and occurs in a wide range of forms, from short-lived or long-lived aggregations of web-building spiders to communal nesting of active hunting species. Colonial species generally do not cooperate in prey capture and feeding, though there are exceptions; they do not cooperate in brood care; they have pre-mating dispersal and are outbred. Coloniality is likely derived from aggregation at rich food sources or nesting sites. Cooperation in the colonial species takes the form of sharing silk structures such as frame threads and nesting sites. The benefits of close proximity include the capture of larger prey and reduced variance in prey amount per spider and early warning of the presence of predators or parasites. However, group living carries costs of greater visibility both to potential prey and to predators and parasites. These benefits and costs are similar in cooperative-breeding and colonial species, while the main differences between them lie in degree of cooperation and the mating and breeding systems.

Spider Behaviour: Flexibility and Versatility, ed. Marie Elisabeth Herberstein. Published by Cambridge University Press. © Cambridge University Press 2011.

8.1   Introducing group-living spiders

Spiders are predatory and cannibalistic, and are not generally known to be social. Of more than 41 000 species of spiders known to science, fewer than 80 species are group living (Lubin and Bilde, 2007). Nevertheless, group living has arisen independently in several spider families. Group living in spiders occurs in two fundamentally different forms: colonial and cooperative-breeding species (Figures 8.1, 8.2). Colonial spiders form groups consisting of interconnected

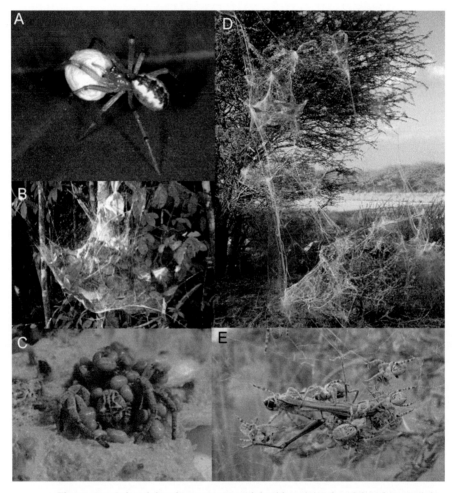

Figure 8.1 Subsocial and permanent social spiders. (A) Subsocial *Anelosimus akohi* female with egg sac. (B) Social *Anelosimus eximius* nest. (C) Subsocial *Stegodyphus lineatus* matriphagy; the young are feeding on the mother. (D) Social *Stegodyphus dumicola* nests with interconnected webs, on *Acacia* trees in Namibia. (E) Social *Stegodyphus dumicola* females capturing grasshopper in South Africa. (Photo credits: A and B: I. Agnarsson; C, D and E: T. Bilde.) See also colour plate.

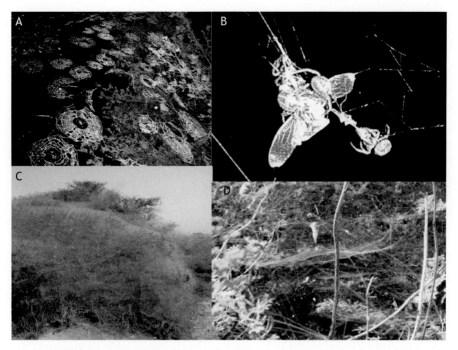

Figure 8.2 Colonial orb-web spiders (Araneidae). (A) *Parawixia bistriata* colony of
interconnected orb webs of different sizes. The spiders are active at night and hide
inside a communal retreat during the day. (B) *P. bistriata* individuals capturing a moth
together. (C) Layered, interconnected, horizontal orb webs of *Cyrtophora citricola* in an
Acacia tree. (D) A web of *C. citricola* with an egg-sac string above the drawn-up hub.
(Photo credits: A and B: F. Fernández Campón; C and D: Y. Lubin.) See also colour plate.

individual webs or, in non-web-building species, interacting individuals that nest
or feed in close proximity. In the web-building colonial species, spiders generally
forage individually and may exhibit competitive interactions over prey. They do
not cooperate in raising young. Colonies of interacting individuals may be temporary aggregations at rich food sources or, in some obligate colonial species, they are
long-lived groups lasting many generations (Lubin, 1974, Whitehouse and Lubin,
2005). Coloniality is thought to be derived from aggregations of individuals around
resources (the parasocial route to coloniality; Uetz and Hieber, 1997), but reduced
natal dispersal may play a role as well (see below). In contrast, cooperative spiders
– also referred to as social spiders – exhibit a range of social interactions: they
construct a communal web, capture prey and feed together, show cooperative
defensive behaviour against predators, and raise their young communally. The
social species likely evolved from subsocial forms that exhibit extended maternal
care of the young and where family groups arose from reduced juvenile dispersal
(Figure 8.1). This route to group living is well supported by phylogenetic studies

showing that social spiders arose from subsocial ancestors (Agnarsson *et al.*, 2007, Johannesen *et al.*, 2007). Spiders in both social systems benefit from catching larger prey than similar-sized solitary spiders, and derive better protection from predators through increased vigilance. The two social systems have fundamentally different breeding systems. Colonial species have pre-mating dispersal and are assumed to outbreed. In the social species, juvenile dispersal is lost and as a consequence they inbreed regularly. Another feature of the social spiders is the female-biased sex ratios that have also evolved repeatedly across different social species.

8.2   Subsocial spiders, and the subsocial route to cooperative sociality

Subsocial species are characterised by extended maternal care of the young, which includes egg-sac guarding, production of trophic eggs and regurgitation feeding of the young, and in some cases matriphagy, when the offspring kill and consume the mother (Evans *et al.*, 1995, Gundermann *et al.*, 1988, Jones and Parker, 2002, Kim and Horel, 1998, Kim and Roland, 2000, Marques *et al.*, 1998, Salomon *et al.*, 2005). Such extended maternal care usually results in a period of communal living and cooperation among siblings within the maternal nest. Juveniles disperse from the natal nest and subsequently live solitarily (Powers and Avilés, 2003). As with most web-building spiders, females are visited by roaming males in the mating season and thus generally outbreed. However, low dispersal ability may result in neighbourhoods of spiders with shared ancestry and hence an increased likelihood of mating among relatives (Bilde *et al.*, 2005). As a result, geographically restricted populations of subsocial spiders may be genetically structured (Johannesen and Lubin, 1999, 2001).

Extended maternal care and restricted dispersal ability are likely adaptations to ecological constraints such as a high risk of mortality during dispersal and establishment of new nest sites, or shortage of suitable habitat. Such adaptations are suggested to be the foundation for evolution of permanent sociality in the cooperative spiders, referred to as the subsocial pathway (Kullmann, 1972). The transition to permanent sociality thus involves at least three major shifts in behaviour: (a) from obligate pre-mating dispersal to post-mating dispersal, (b) from an outbreeding mating system to regular inbreeding, and (c) from maternal care of offspring to cooperative breeding. Once siblings are retained as family groups in subsocial species, the elimination of pre-mating dispersal sets the stage for mating among siblings and hence inbreeding. The shift to permanent group living could occur only if the benefits of group living outweigh the costs, as the transition to group living invariably also incurs increased competition among relatives and other costs (see also Section 8.3.5 on transition to sociality).

8.2.1   Phylogenetic relationships

Subsocial behaviour is known for at least one or a few species in at least 16 families, and these are scattered across the spider phylogeny (Agnarsson *et al.*, 2006). Social species are found in seven of these families (Table 8.1). In the genera *Anelosimus* (Theridiidae) and *Stegodyphus* (Eresidae), where phylogenies have been established, the social species are always nested within subsocial clades (Agnarsson, 2006, Agnarsson *et al.*, 2006, 2007, Johannesen *et al.*, 2007). Thus, these studies support a transition from subsociality to permanent sociality. Interestingly, of fewer than 25 known species of cooperative social spiders, as many as 19 are considered independent derivations of sociality, suggesting that common ecological conditions may favour cooperation and permanent sociality (Agnarsson *et al.*, 2006, Lubin and Bilde, 2007). Once sociality evolved, however, there was seemingly little further speciation, as social clades are almost always terminal. So while pre-adaptations in subsocial ancestors and ecological conditions are common factors shaping social evolution, there might also be common reasons why further diversification of social clades does not occur. This phenomenon also constitutes a major contrast to the social insects where the transition to eusociality has been overwhelmingly successful in terms of species richness, habitat occupancy and biomass (Wilson, 1971). What might be the factors that drive the transition to cooperation and permanent sociality? And why are the social spiders apparently so resistant to further diversification?

8.3   Cooperative social spiders

The permanent social spiders are characterised by sharing a nest and capture web, cooperative foraging and brood care, the elimination of pre-mating dispersal, and mating among individuals within the communal nest. The latter two traits result in regular inbreeding. The colony sex ratio is highly female biased, with males constituting less than 15% of the colony. Long-distance dispersal and foundation of new colonies may occur by gravid females after mating in the parent colony, such that new colonies are inbred from the start. This constellation of traits is typical of most of social species studied to date (Avilés, 1997, Lubin and Bilde, 2007). The social spiders are found in the following families: Agelenidae, Dictynidae, Eresidae, Oxyopidae, Theridiidae, Thomisidae and Sparassidae (see Table 8.1). Most social species are tropical in distribution, though some occur in semi-arid subtropical regions. The best studied species are *Anelosimus eximius* in South and Central America (Avilés, 1986, Avilés and Tufino, 1998, Yip *et al.*, 2008) and *Parasteatoda wau* in Papua New Guinea (Lubin, 1991, Lubin and Crozier, 1985) (both in the Theridiidae) and three social species of *Stegodyphus* (Eresidae) from subtropical eastern and

Table 8.1 *Social spiders (cooperative breeding and colonial): genera and the number of species known to exhibit cooperative breeding or colonial grouping organisation. Representative species are listed with their distribution and habitat*

Family	Genera (no. of known social or colonial species)	Specific example	Distribution	Species habitat (reference)
Social (cooperative breeding) species[a]				
Agelenidae	*Agelena* (2)	*A. consociata*	West Africa	Tropical rainforest understorey
Dictynidae	*Aebutina* (1)	*A. binotata*	South America	Tropical forest understorey
	Mallos (1)	*M. gregalis*	Central America	Subtropical savanna (Avilés, 1997)
Eresidae	*Stegodyphus* (3)	*S. dumicola*	Southern Africa	Semi-arid subtropical savanna
Oxyopidae	*Tapinillus* (1)	*Tapinillus* sp.	South America	Tropical forest
Theridiidae	*Parasteatoda* (3)	*P. wau*	New Guinea	Tropical montane forest edge
	Anelosimus (7)	*An. eximius*	Central and S. America	Tropical forest edge
	Theridion (1)	*T. nigroannulatum*	S. America	Tropical forest
Thomisidae	*Diaea* (2)	*D. socialis*	Australia	Eucalyptus woodland (Evans and Main, 1993)
Sparassidae[b]	*Delena* (1)	*D. cancerides*	Australia	Subtropical to temperate woodlands (Rowell and Avilés, 1995)
Colonial species[c]				
Araneidae	*Cyrtophora* (6)	*C. citricola*	Mediterranean, Africa	Semi-arid savanna
	Metepeira (4)	*M. incrassata*	Central America	Lowland tropical forest edge
	Parawixia (1)	*P. bistriata*	South America	Seasonal tropical forest
Desidae	*Phryganoporus* (1)	*P. candidus*	Australia	Subtropical, tropical woodland (Downes, 1994)
	Badumna (1)	*B. socialis*	Australia	Caves (Downes, 1995)
Dictynidae	*Dictyna* (2)	*D. albopilosa*	Western USA, Mexico	Subtropical (Jackson, 1978)
	Mexitla (1)	*M. trivittata*	Western USA	Semi-arid woodland (Jackson, 1978)

Table 8.1 (*cont.*)

Family	Genera (no. of known social or colonial species)	Specific example	Distribution	Species habitat (reference)
	Mallos (1)	*M. bryantae*	South-Western USA	Semi-arid woodland (Buskirk, 1981)
Diguetidae	*Diguetia* (1)	*D. canities*	Southern USA	Unknown (Buskirk, 1981)
Oecobiidae	*Oecobius* (2)	*O. civitas*	Mexico	Subtropical (Buskirk, 1981)
Pholcidae	*Holocnemus* (1)	*H. pluchei*[d]	Mediterranean, California	Semi-arid, sheltered habitats
Salticidae	*Myrmarachne* (2)	*M. assimilis*	Phillipines	Tropical trees near nests of *Oecophylla* ants (Nelson and Jackson, 2008)
	Portia (1)	*P. africana*	East Africa	Tropical, in colonial spider webs (Jackson *et al.*, 2008b)
	Bagheera (1)	*B. kiplingi*	Central America	Tropical, on ant-acacias (Meehan *et al.*, 2009)
Tetragnathidae	*Metabus* (1)	*M. ocellatus*	Central America	Over streams in montane tropical forest
	Nephila (4)	*N. clavipes*[d]	North and South America	Subtropical and tropical forest edge
	Tetragnatha (1)	*T. elongata*[d]	North America	Near water (Gillespie, 1987)
Theridiidae[e]	*Argyrodes* (12)	*A. antipodianus*	Australia and New Zealand	Kleptoparasite
	Faiditus (3)	*F. caudatus*	Americas	Kleptoparasite
	Neospintharus (1)	*N. syriacus*	Levant	Kleptoparasite
Uloboridae	*Philoponella* (5)	*P. republicana*	Central America	Seasonal rainforest understorey light gaps

[a] Data from Lubin and Bilde (2007), unless noted otherwise (last column).

[b] Sometimes considered as subsocial (Lubin and Bilde, 2007).

[c] Data from Whitehouse and Lubin (2005), unless noted otherwise (last column). Note that the list is far from complete as many group-living species have not been documented.

[d] Facultatively aggregating (Whitehouse and Lubin, 2005).

[e] Aggregating kleptoparasitic species, found in association with web-building spiders.

southern Africa and the Indian subcontinent (Bilde *et al.*, 2007, Crouch and Lubin, 2001, Kraus and Kraus, 1988, Seibt and Wickler, 1988a, 1988b). All of these species are web builders. The nests and communal webs of these species can be quite large, extending several metres in diameter, with populations of up to several hundred or even thousands of individuals. In some species, the nest is occupied for three to six generations, while in others the nests are more temporary. Non-web-building social crab spiders (*Diaea socialis*, Thomisidae) occur in Australia; these spiders live in communal nests, but forage individually (Evans, 2000, Evans and Main, 1993). *Delena cancerides* (Sparassidae) is a non-web-building bark-dwelling huntsman spider that differs from the other social species in having an outbred mating system and equal sex-ratio (Rowell and Avilés, 1995); this species has been redefined as subsocial by Lubin and Bilde (2007).

8.3.1   Cooperation and competition

In the social spiders, the nest and capture web are constructed and maintained cooperatively, and usually intercepted prey are captured and consumed communally. This, however, does not necessarily imply the existence of group-coordinated behaviour. Apparent coordination can develop as a consequence of similar responses of many individuals to a single cue, for example the web vibrations caused by a trapped insect (Vakanas and Krafft, 2001). Cooperation in social spider colonies is most evident in group rearing of the young, which is accomplished through sharing in caring for the egg sacs and in feeding the offspring (allomaternal care; see Section 8.3.3).

Unlike the eusocial insects, all individuals within a nest are totipotent, which implies they can take on all behavioural tasks and there is little evidence for behavioural or morphological castes and division of labour. Rather, tasks such as web construction, cleaning and prey capture are accrued by the young over time as they venture out of the protection of the nest. In *Theridion nigroannulatum* (Theridiidae), however, Avilés and co-workers found two distinct size classes of females and speculated that they may have different roles in the colony (Avilés *et al.*, 2006). Two behavioural morphs consisting of a cooperative type and a cheater type were found in the subsocial spider *Anelosimus studiosus* (Pruitt *et al.*, 2008, Riechert and Jones, 2008). These findings call for more detailed investigations of reproductive skew and task differentiation (see also Section 8.4.2).

Group living invariably incurs competition for resources. Whilst cooperative spiders are never aggressive to each other, competition during foraging was seen in several social species, for example when spiders jockey for the best feeding site on the prey (the thorax; Whitehouse and Lubin, 1999). Individuals placed at the most favourable foraging sites on a prey extract more mass and gain a growth advantage, which in turn provides advantages in scramble competition for monopolising the most nutritious feeding spots (Willey and Jackson, 1993). Competition for food thus leads to differential growth among group members. Those growing to maturity first are also those individuals that reproduce, while other subadult or immature group members become reproductive helpers and provide allomaternal care (Salomon *et al.*, 2008).

8.3.2   Dispersal and inbreeding

In the subsocial species, both sexes disperse before mating, thus ensuring some degree of outbreeding. There is considerable variation in the timing of dispersal and the duration of maternal care. Late instar juveniles of subsocial species often have highly philopatric dispersal, which results in the formation of clusters of related individuals. This population genetic structure could promote a mixed breeding system, with some matings occurring among close relatives and some between unrelated individuals. Such a breeding system is seen in the subsocial *Stegodyphus lineatus*, where juveniles are philopatric and males mate first with close neighbours before moving out of the natal patch in search of more females. There is no behavioural avoidance of mating with sibs and sib mating carries a relatively weak inbreeding cost (smaller body size at maturity), which suggests that the shift from outbreeding to inbreeding was not a strict limiting factor in the evolution of sociality in spiders (Bilde *et al.*, 2005). Assuming a predisposition to permanent inbreeding in the cooperative social spiders, the elimination of pre-mating dispersal as a major benefit of group living is likely driven by ecological constraints (Sections 8.2 and 8.3.5). The young that remain in the nest engage in cooperative prey capture and nest defence and contribute to enhanced group survival (Avilés and Tufino, 1998, Bilde *et al.*, 2007, Jones and Parker, 2002).

The transition to permanent group living and regular inbreeding, however, results in extremely subdivided populations consisting of inbred lineages, with little exchange of individuals among breeding units (Johannesen *et al.*, 2009a, Smith *et al.*, 2009). This combination of demographic traits results in a pattern of population dynamics observed in most of the social spider species, namely boom-and-bust cycles of establishment, growth and extinction of nest clusters. A scenario for such dynamics may be as follows (Lubin and Bilde, 2007): newly established nests grow rapidly owing to the female-biased sex ratio. As competition for resources in the nest increases, some individuals bud off and create subsidiary, daughter nests that are genetically identical to the mother nest. Large nests also produce long-distance dispersers in the form of single or small groups of mated females. The trigger for long-distance dispersal may be nest size per se, competition or parasites and pathogens. Parasites and pathogens could play an important role in population dynamics (Avilés *et al.*, 2006, Lubin and Bilde, 2007). As a nest or a cluster of nests grow, they increasingly become targets for parasites and pathogens, and the high level of inbreeding may lower their ability to withstand parasite and pathogen attacks. Thus, once a pathogen invades a nest, both the nest and its patch neighbours may be driven to extinction.

The rapid turnover of social spider nests may explain the phenomenon of long-distance dispersal by mated females that ensure the survival of social spider lineages. All species that have been studied so far have a distinct long-distance dispersal phase. In *Parasteatoda wau*, females construct a silk highway through the forest and settle out in small groups along the highway (Lubin and Robinson, 1982). *Stegodyphus dumicola* females disperse individually across the savanna by ballooning on broad bands of silk threads up to three metres long and a metre in width (Schneider *et al.*, 2001), while in *S. mimosarum*, swarms of individuals are blown by strong winds (Crouch *et al.*, 1998). *Aebutina binotata* (Dictynidae) undergoes a nomadic phase in the South American jungle, when it repeatedly shifts its entire nest over distances of several hundred metres (Avilés, 2000).

8.3.3   *Maternal care and cooperative breeding*

The evolution of cooperative breeding in social spiders required both behavioural and physiological transitions. In the ancestral subsocial species, each female cares for her own young. A possible transition stage is seen in the South American *Anelosimus jabaquara*, where several females breed in the communal nest, but are intolerant of one another and defend their individual egg sacs (Gonzaga and Vasconcellos-Netto, 2001, Marques *et al.*, 1998). Once the young are mobile, however, they mix in the nest and presumably derive benefits of protection and prey captured by females other than their mothers. The full transition to cooperative breeding implies that non-breeding and even juvenile females have acquired allomaternal traits. In the social *Stegodyphus dumicola*, non-breeding females (and even subadult females) provide regurgitated food to the young of other females. Matriphagy, where the young kill and consume their mother, occurs in all members of this genus; in *S. dumicola*, non-breeding females are also killed and consumed by the young. Experiments showed that young that were raised with non-breeding females as well as their mother had higher survival and grew larger than young that were raised by the mother alone (Salomon and Lubin, 2007). Thus, non-breeding females do indeed act cooperatively as helpers-at-the-nest. Owing to intragroup mating, relatedness among breeders and helpers is very high and this should ensure indirect kin-selected benefits to helping raise the young of other females (Koenig, 1997).

In the subsocial species *Stegodyphus lineatus*, Schneider (2002) demonstrated experimentally that subadult and virgin adult females and even mated females that have not yet reproduced, will not care for young of another female. Thus, allomaternal traits are clearly an adaptation acquired during social living, possibly requiring changes in hormone physiology as well as behaviour. During the transition to sociality, allomaternal care may have balanced the deleterious effects of inbreeding. This was suggested by Avilés and Bukowski (2006), who found that in the subsocial *Anelosimus arizona* inbreeding depression was evident in individually raised inbred young, but disappeared when the young were raised together.

Anelosimus studiosus is another possible transition species in which the advantage to multiple female nests may be driven by climatic factors. In this species, multiple-female nests occur in the more northern, colder parts of its range in south-eastern USA (Furey, 1998, Jones *et al.*, 2007), in contrast to the general association between sociality and both lower latitudes and altitudes (Avilés *et al.*, 2007). An explanation for this apparently anomalous distribution was that in a species with obligatory and extended maternal care, female mortality will be greater at higher latitudes owing to the short time available for development. Under such conditions, the young are more likely to survive to dispersal if they are raised by more than one female; if one female dies, another one will still be able to raise at least some of the brood (Jones *et al.*, 2007).

Collectively, evidence from these studies indicate that the transition to cooperative breeding and allomaternal care by non-reproducing females are adaptations that compensate for deleterious effects of inbreeding on the one hand, and for ecological constraints on individual breeding on the other. As non-reproducing helpers are extraordinarily highly related to reproducing females, they likely gain similar fitness returns as the reproducing females from allomaternal brood care.

8.3.4   Extraordinary sex ratios: the female bias and sociality

The social spiders are characterised by female-biased sex ratios with one to two males produced for seven to eight females (Lubin and Bilde, 2007). Such a marked departure from the Fisherian sex ratio of equal numbers of males and females in diplo-diploid species raises questions concerning both the mechanism of the sex ratio bias and the nature of the selective forces acting on the trait. Chromosomal studies of developing embryos in several species show that the female-biased sex ratio is caused by an overproduction of female embryos, resulting in a strong bias in the primary sex ratio (the sex ratio at the embryo stage). In *S. dumicola*, females appear to have control over the mean sex ratio – 17% males – but no direct control over the sex of individual offspring (Avilés *et al.*, 1999). In contrast, the neotropical spider *Anelosimus domingo* shows a precise sex ratio so as to guarantee at least one male per egg sac (Avilés *et al.*, 2000) indicating more control over the sex of individual offspring. Chromosomal studies of other social spiders have reported primary female-biased sex ratios with a proportion of males of 0.08 in *Anelosimus eximius* (Avilés and Maddison, 1991), 0.15 in *A. guacamayos* (Avilés *et al.*, 2007), and 0.28 in *Diaea socialis* (Rowell and Main, 1992). Under a heterogametic sex determination mechanism as in spiders, where females have two sets of X chromosomes ($X_1X_1X_2X_2$) and males have one set (X_1X_20) with males as the heterogametic sex, an equal number of sons and daughters is expected (White, 1973). The primary sex ratio bias therefore suggests a mechanism that allows some degree of control over the two types of sperm (X_1X_2 and 0) in order to attain relative precision in the proportion of sons and daughters produced in each clutch (Avilés *et al.*, 2000, Hurst and Vollrath, 1992). The specific mechanism responsible for the sex ratio bias in social spiders is not known.

Field data on the sex ratio among subadult and adult spiders in a nest reveal that a female bias is maintained throughout the colony life cycle. In the Australian crab spider *D. socialis*, Rowell and Main (1992) found a proportion of 0.19 males in adult and subadult colonies, suggesting an increased bias compared with the primary sex ratio (0.28). In contrast to this pattern, *P. wau* examined in Papua New Guinea had fewer female-biased sex ratios in colonies with adults than in colonies of juveniles (Lubin, 1991). Explanations for either pattern could be different rates of maturation or mortality among the sexes, or sex-biased emigration, for example the dispersal of gravid females after mating to establish new nests. Thus, the timing of sampling of the nest in relation to maturation of males and females could influence the effective or tertiary sex ratio; that is, the ratio of sexually mature (reproducing) females to mature males in the colony. Henschel *et al.* (1995) found strong female bias in the adult sex ratio – 12% adult males – in colonies of *S. dumicola*, but the sex ratio changed over the season and could be as high as 42% males. Lubin *et al.* (2009) showed that the proportion of males in *S. dumicola* colonies was low (7.9%) early in the mating season as females were beginning to mature, and increased to 13% towards the end of the season after dispersal of mated females. The tertiary sex ratio is also affected by competition for resources among females, which creates asymmetric growth. Thus, many females do not mature or mature only after the males have died (Henschel *et al.*, 1995, Salomon *et al.*, 2008, Ulbrich and Henschel, 1999). The late females do not reproduce and become potential helpers (see Section 8.3.3).

Hamilton's (1967) local mate competition (LMC) model for the evolution of female-biased sex ratios in structured populations is based in the argument that when mating occurs among the progeny of one or a few founders of a group, the best strategy is to produce exactly enough sons to fertilise all the daughters, which results in a departure from the sex ratio equilibrium proposed by Fisher

(1930). Inseminated females then disperse to colonise new resources. Frank (1987) pointed out that in structured populations, the interaction between cooperative effects that result in higher group productivity and genetic relatedness will favour a skewed sex ratio. The underlying process of sex ratio evolution may be adaptive parental control of the sex ratio (Nunney, 1985). Yet, in the social spiders, there is no evidence for adaptive changes in the sex ratio with increasing colony size (Henschel et al., 1995, Lubin, 1991). When colonies reach an optimal size, adaptive shifts of the sex ratio could be beneficial, for example by producing emigrating males; however, shifts in sex ratio have so far not been documented (Lubin et al., 2009). It may be that the social spiders are unable to alter the sex ratios of their offspring in response to environmental or genetic changes if they lack control over sex ratio determination (Hurst and Vollrath, 1992). The heterogametic sex determination system in spiders suggests that social spiders cannot adjust sex ratios as easily as seen in some haplo-diploid insect systems (Avilés et al., 1999, 2000, White, 1973).

8.3.5   Transitions to permanent sociality

The transition to permanent sociality is hypothesised to be rooted in predispositions of ancestral subsocial species, including philopatry, extended maternal care, reduced dispersal ability and kin-selected benefits of cooperation. Experimental evidence from the African social spider *Stegodyphus dumicola* showed that dramatic survival benefits to group living are a prominent benefit underlying the transition to permanent sociality. Within the group, the per-capita reproductive success of females decreases with increasing group size, probably owing to increased competition for food (Bilde et al., 2007). A similar result was found in the South American social spider *Anelosimus eximius* where increasing group size was associated with increased survival but decreased individual reproductive success (Avilés and Tufino, 1998). These studies suggest that ecological constraints on survival favour permanent sociality despite negative effects on individual reproductive success. Survival selection would also explain the evolution of female-biased sex ratios that result in rapid colony growth and enhanced colony survival (Avilés, 1986).

Cooperation in web building and prey capture would allow an expansion of the ecological niche to exploit larger prey, and thus facilitate group living while negating resource competition (Guevara and Avilés, 2007, Powers and Avilés, 2007). Recent ecological studies suggest that prey availability in tropical lowland facilitates permanent group living while fewer prey of large size could explain the absence of social spiders from higher latitudes and higher elevations (Yip et al., 2008).

As in most cases of group formation in cooperatively breeding birds, mammals and insects, sociality and cooperation in spiders evolved in family groups

with a high degree of relatedness. Despite much debate over the relative importance of relatedness in the evolution of cooperation, overwhelming empirical
evidence and recent theoretical work suggests a decisive role for kin selection in
the evolution of cooperation (e.g. Foster *et al.*, 2006). In the social spiders, group
living arises through delayed dispersal and cooperation among siblings, hence
fulfilling the criteria for kin cooperation and the potential for deriving indirect
benefits of cooperation (Hamilton, 1964). In a study on the subsocial spider
S. lineatus, genetic relatedness was shown to decrease the costs of communal
foraging (Schneider and Bilde, 2008). This provides a solution to a common
problem facing cooperating groups, where selfishness pays off and may lead
to the breakdown of the social structure, a phenomenon also known as the
'tragedy of the commons'. Kin selection provides a solution to this dilemma, as
an increased cost of selfishness includes the cost to relatives, which prevents the
invasion of cheater mutants (Schneider and Bilde, 2008). In another subsocial
spider, *S. tentoriicola*, a similar result was found as groups of kin performed better
during communal foraging than groups of non-kin (Ruch *et al.*, 2009). Evidence
for kin recognition to facilitate cooperation with genetic kin is accumulating
within different families of social/subsocial spiders (Beavis *et al.*, 2007, Bilde and
Lubin, 2001, Evans, 1999, Yip *et al.*, 2009).

Kin selection is likely to also play an important role in the evolution of
cooperative breeding and allomaternal care among non-reproducing helpers.
While the role of kin selection in the transition to sociality needs further study
in the cooperative social spiders, it seems plausible that it is a major driving
force, since sociality evolves in family groups characterised by high relatedness.
Hence cooperation evolves among genetically related individuals providing
indirect benefits to those performing cooperative acts (Hamilton, 1964), a situation similar to that found in cooperative-breeding birds and mammals and in
the social insects (Foster *et al.*, 2006, Griffin and West, 2003).

8.4   Conclusions and outlook – social spiders

8.4.1   *Why is inbred sociality so rare in spiders?*

Permanent group living, cooperation and regular inbreeding have
evolved repeatedly across the spider phylogeny. Phylogenetic constraints are
an unlikely explanation, as the social species are scattered across the spider
phylogeny and do not occur in social clades (Agnarsson *et al.*, 2006, 2007). The
closest relatives to the social species are subsocial and transitional species, and
even these presumed transition species share only a few of the traits typical
of the inbred social species. The scarcity of transition forms and the rarity of
inbred sociality among spiders suggest that the barriers to evolving the social

syndrome are not easily overcome and furthermore, once attained, the social syndrome is resistant to further change. And yet, at least some of the social species are very successful: *A. eximius* has a geographic distribution from Central to South America, and *S. mimosarum* stretches from East Africa and Madagascar to southern Africa. Some lineages, such as the three social *Stegodyphus* species, are relatively old, suggesting either a stable lifestyle or one that adapts readily to local conditions (Johannesen *et al.*, 2007, 2009b).

What makes the inbred social syndrome so different from most other cooperative breeding and social taxa? An interesting hypothesis is that the social spiders are locked into a syndrome of correlated traits from which they cannot escape. Or, another way of expressing this is that they have reached a narrow adaptive peak and any move away from this peak will result in an extreme loss of fitness leading to extinction. The social syndrome includes the loss of juvenile dispersal, inbreeding, a female-biased sex ratio, and a post-mating long-distance dispersal stage. The female-biased sex ratio enables the colony to grow rapidly in the initial stages and reach a size that is safe from predators and that will be able to produce long-distance dispersers. The larger the colony, the more propagules it will produce and the higher the reproductive rate, the faster it will be able to put out new propagules. Inbreeding ensures reproduction by eliminating the waiting time and uncertainty of male arrival and – once inbreeding depression is overcome – perpetuates successful, co-adapted gene complexes.

The cost of this successful strategy may be an inherent instability of the colony over time. First, competition for food will increase rapidly because colony population size increases at a steeper rate than web size. Second, disease pathogens or parasites will build up, causing local extinctions, and the only escape method that will perpetuate the lineage is long-distance dispersal of mated females. The role of disease dynamics in selecting for dispersal in inbred social species was suggested in 1967 by W. D. Hamilton and the organisms he had in mind were social aphids, which are clonal. Hamilton also proposed occasional outbreeding as an alternative escape strategy. Outbreeding generations do occur in the social aphids, but seem less likely in social spiders. Outbreeding would require male dispersal, which would favour an unbiased sex ratio (Lubin *et al.*, 2009), and thus would be selected against at the group level. Occasional outbreeding could occur when colonies of different genetic lineages fuse, but the frequency of occurrence of such an event is probably low (but see Lubin and Crozier, 1985). Thus, social spiders indeed may be locked into a particular social syndrome dictated largely by group-level selection for rapid nest growth and high productivity.

The above ideas are in need of rigorous testing at many levels. First, the effects and consequences of inbreeding versus outbreeding in the social spiders are quite unknown. Second, dispersal and population-genetic structure need to be investigated at the level of the local population to determine the extent of movement between colonies and the possibility of gene exchange among lineages. Third, the ecology of congeneric subsocial and social species should be studied to obtain insights into selection for sociality via ecological benefits or constraints (e.g. Powers and Avilés, 2007, Yip *et al.*, 2008). And finally, as the study of social spiders both in the field and in captivity is notoriously difficult, alternative genomic methods will provide insights into phylogenetic relationships and the age and persistence of social lineages, and the consequences of the shift to an inbreeding mating system on population genetics, while modelling can help to detect which factors are likely to play an important role in maintaining the social syndrome.

8.4.2   *A new perspective on reproductive skew and task differentiation*

Eusocial organisms are characterised by extreme reproductive skew where reproduction is monopolised by a single or a few individuals within a colony, and true division of labour where worker casts can even be sterile. Studies on social spiders so far have not identified reproductive morphs; however, reproductive skew with less than half of the females in a colony reproducing has been observed in both *Anelosimus eximius* and *Stegodyphus dumicola* (Rypstra, 1993, Salomon *et al.*, 2008). The occurrence of two behavioural morphs was recently shown in the subsocial spider *Anelosimus studiosus*, consisting of social (cooperative) and asocial (cheater) phenotypes (Pruitt *et al.*, 2008, Riechert and Jones, 2008). Studies on foraging success indicated that the asocial phenotype experienced negative frequency-dependent foraging success, as they outperformed the social phenotype when the asocial type was in relatively low proportion (Pruitt and Riechert, 2009). In accordance with these findings, mixed colonies were frequent in nature, containing on average 58% social and 42% asocial individuals.

We have virtually no information on what determines reproductive skew and whether it is genetically or environmentally predisposed, or determined by stochastic ecological factors. Nor do we have much information on whether there are more subtle patterns of division of labour, for example determined by life history stage or age as seen in the social insects. Future studies on potential task allocation and reproductive division will provide a valuable source of insight into the functioning of spider societies.

8.5   Colonial spiders

Colonial (sometimes referred to as 'communal') spiders are an interesting contrast to cooperative social spiders. While the degree of cooperation is lower in the colonial species, they are more diverse in their social organisation and in the types of interactions, and they are much more numerous than the cooperative social spiders (Table 8.1; Figure 8.2). Colonial spiders generally defend individual foraging territories and do not cooperate in care of the offspring. What creates the colony is the sharing of a common foraging or nesting site. In the colonial web-building species, individual capture webs are interconnected and share common frame threads (Uetz and Hieber, 1997, Whitehouse and Lubin, 2005). Group sizes are quite variable, ranging from a few individuals to several thousands, and colonies may be short lived (less than a generation) or persist for many generations at the same site. Many colonial species belong to families that construct an orb web: Araneidae, Tetragnathidae, Nephilidae and Uloboridae. Some non-web-building species are also colonial. These include some jumping spiders (Salticidae), which aggregate around rich food resources such as nests of social insects (Jackson et al., 2008a), or share nest sites and even feed together on large prey. Some kleptoparasitic species (Argyrodes, Faiditus and Neospintharus, Theridiidae) are arguably colonial, as they aggregate in the web of a host spider and feed together on prey captured by the larger host spider (Whitehouse and Jackson, 1994). Colonial spiders were likened by Rypstra (1979) to foraging flocks of birds: while individuals generally hunt and capture prey alone, each individual on average benefits from foraging in company of others. While this is a good analogy for web-building colonial species, colonial nesting, such as occurs in many seabirds, might be a better analogy for many non-web-building species. For example, for the colonially nesting salticids the main benefit may be protection of the broods from predators and parasitoids (Nelson and Jackson, 2008).

8.5.1   *Ecology and social organisation*

Only a few colonial species have been investigated in any detail (reviewed by Uetz and Hieber, 1997). These are mainly in the orb-web genera *Metabus* (Tetragnathidae), *Metepeira*, *Cyrtophora* and *Parawixia* (all in the Araneidae), and *Philoponella* (Uloboridae) and a sheet-web spider *Holocnemus pluchei* (Pholcidae). Colonial jumping spiders (Salticidae) of several genera and aggregations of kleptoparasites (*Argyrodes* and *Faiditus*, Theridiidae) are still poorly studied (Whitehouse and Lubin, 2005). Colonial spiders vary in the levels of aggressive versus cooperative interactions, in the way the colonies are established and in their persistence. Colony organisation ranges from temporary aggregations with little or no cooperation to long-lived groups lasting for many generations and with reduced intraspecific aggression and indirect cooperation. There is no clear demarcation among different types of colony organisation; rather it seems that the differences reflect the different species' habitats and life history constraints.

Temporary aggregations can result from philopatric dispersal of young or aggregation of unrelated individuals at a rich and persistent food source, or both. Species in tropical orb-web nephilid and tetragnathid families are usually solitary, but can form transient aggregations on telephone and electricity wires or forest-edge vegetation (e.g. *Nephila clavipes*), on tree trunks and houses (e.g. *Nephilengys* spp.) or above water (*Tetragnatha* spp.). *Nephila* and other normally solitary web builders may also build webs in association with obligate colonial species such as *Metepeira incrassata* in Mexico (Hodge and Uetz, 1992, 1996). Rypstra (1985) found that aggregations of *Nephila clavipes* occurred only where prey were abundant, and when prey were removed experimentally the groups rapidly disbanded. Species with more persistent colonies also vary colony structure and size as a function of prey availability. Average colony size in the Mexican orb-web spider *Metepeira spinipes* (Araneidae) decreased with elevation, and was correlated with availability of potential prey (Uetz, 2001). Likewise, in the hyperarid Arava desert of Israel, large colonies of *Cyrtophora citricola* (Araneidae) occur only at oases and artificial sources of prey enrichment (e.g. compost dumps) while in dry sites the spiders occur solitarily or in small groups (Rao and Lubin, 2010, Lubin, personal observations).

An exceptional species is the orb-web spider *Parawixia bistriata* (Araneidae), which constructs a communal daytime retreat and at night creates a sheet of interconnected orb webs (Fowler and Diehl, 1978). Unlike other colonial species that lack group feeding, *P. bistriata* individuals capture large prey together (up to nine individuals) and feed together (sometimes more than 20 individuals). Fernández Campón (2007) found that spiders in semi-arid sites in Argentina tended to engage in group capture and group feeding more than those in mesic sites and the numbers of individuals feeding together was also greater. Interestingly, spiders from arid-habitat populations showed greater plasticity in group-foraging behaviour than ones from mesic populations. When transplanted to a mesic habitat, arid-habitat spiders shifted to foraging alone with a higher frequency (Fernández Campón, 2008), but individuals from mesic habitats did not change their generally solitary foraging behaviour when transplanted to an arid habitat. This pattern contrasts with other studies showing that aggregations are more frequent in prey-rich habitats (see above). The social (cooperative) species also tend to occur in prey-rich habitats where large insects are available, while their subsocial congeners occur in habitats with smaller potential prey (Guevara and Avilés, 2007, Powers and Avilés, 2007). However, plasticity in group-foraging tendencies may be related to factors other than prey size and quantity, such as availability of supporting structures, or presence of predators or parasites (Fernández Campón, 2008).

The distribution and arrangement of webs within a colony is determined by the outcome of interactions among individuals. *Metabus ocellatus* (Tetragnathidae) connects its orb webs to span streams in montane forests of Costa Rica. The colonies occupied fixed locations along the stream banks, but spiders frequently changed location within colonies. Buskirk (1975a) found that individuals defend a space larger than that of their individual webs, and aggressive interactions occurred mainly during web building. Web location within the colony determined the individual's prey capture success. Spiders that built near the centre of the colony above the stream caught the greatest number of insects, while spiders near the periphery received less prey, but also suffered less interference and completed their webs more quickly (Buskirk, 1975a, 1975b). Similar location effects influence the level of aggression and web defence in other colonial spiders. The horizontal, non-sticky orb webs of *Cyrtophora citricola* in West Africa occur on trees, where several layers of webs extend from the interior of the tree to the outer branch tips. Prey capture was maximised in the intermediate layers, and aggressive interactions were greatest in this layer (Rypstra, 1979).

In some species colonies are established by groups of juveniles from the same egg sac or from a few egg sacs in close proximity. Spiderlings of *Holocnemus pluchei* build group webs, often within the frame threads of the mother's web (Jakob, 1991, 1994). As they grow, the young move away and construct their own webs, but individuals of all ages remain clustered in suitable habitat, suggesting that colony clusters are composed of related individuals. Colonies of *Philoponella republicana* (Uloboridae) are established by cohorts of spiderlings that disperse together. The colonies occur in small light gaps in tropical forest understorey and the entire colony moves with the changing configuration of the gaps. The young mature and adult females reproduce in the colony, placing their egg sacs in a tangle of threads in the centre of the colony and surrounded by interconnected individual orb webs (Lubin, 1980). Colonies of *P. republicana* usually last for a generation or less. By comparison, *Cyrtophora moluccensis* (Araneidae) colonies in Papua New Guinea were recorded at the same sites for more than ten generations. *Cyrtophora* colonies are established by offspring of one or more females, or by a cohort of young that disperse from an established colony, and as the colony grows, more juvenile cohorts are added (Lubin, 1980).

Colonial salticids do not build prey-capture webs, but construct nests that are attached to one another. *Portia africana*, a jumping spider that specialises on feeding on other spiders, forms clusters of a few individuals in the webs of potential prey species, which are mostly colonial web-building spiders (Jackson *et al.*, 2008a). They have been observed feeding together on a prey. Jackson (1986) recorded up to 120 nests (commonly 40–50) of three species of salticids found together in multispecies clusters in Kenya, in association with silk of colonial orb-web spiders such as *Cyrtophora* and *Nephila*. The clusters contained all age classes of individuals. One of the grouping salticid species in Kenya,

Myrmarachne melanotarsa, is a Batesian mimic of a species of the ant *Crematogaster* and may derive protection owing to the combination of mimicry, coloniality and the proximity of trails or nests of these aggressive ants (Jackson *et al.*, 2008a). Similarly, *Myrmarachne assimilis* mimics the aggressive Asian weaver ant *Oecophylla smaragdina* and constructs small clusters of nests on leaves in the same habitat as the ant model (Nelson and Jackson, 2008). These colonies have a primarily defensive function and thus colonial *Myrmarachne* may fit the colonial-nesting bird model (see above). An unusual neotropical salticid, *Bagheera kiplingi*, is found in large numbers on specific ant-acacias, where they feed primarily on Beltian bodies produced by the plant. These spiders have evolved a specialised foraging strategy that takes advantage of the ant–plant mutualism (Meehan *et al.*, 2009). Group living in this species is clearly related to the utilisation of a spatially limited resource, but may have originated from associating defensively with highly aggressive swollen-thorn acacia ants.

8.5.2   Benefits and costs of foraging in groups

Whitehouse and Lubin (2005) referred to colonial spiders as foraging societies, and suggested that for these species group living provides mainly a foraging benefit. Colonial web builders share common frame threads when constructing their webs, resulting in a three-dimensional maze of threads in which individual webs are embedded. Young spiders often fit their small webs between those of larger individuals. Sharing frame threads can save energy, both in silk production, which is largely composed of proteins and therefore costly to synthesise, and in the time needed to construct the web. Young of the sheet-web spider *Holocnemus pluchei* (Pholcidae) save energy by utilising the frame threads of adult spiders (Jakob, 1991) and *Cyrtophora citricola* (Araneidae) young built webs more rapidly in the proximity of an adult's web, whether or not the adult's web was occupied (Rao and Lubin, 2010). The energetic gain in silk may be offset, however, by an increase in the frequency of aggressive encounters during web building, especially when moving to a new web site within the colony (Jakob *et al.*, 2001). The amount of time spent in aggressive interactions differed among group members depending on their size and the size of the group: small spiders rarely engaged in encounters, while medium and large size individuals spent more time in encounters in larger groups (Jakob *et al.*, 2000). In Costa Rican *Metabus ocellatus*, such interactions resulted in larger individuals occupying favoured foraging sites, while smaller ones built webs on the edges and were subject to frequent disturbance (Buskirk, 1975a).

By attaching their webs, colonial spiders can span gaps between trees (e.g. colonial *Cyrtophora*, *Metepeira* and *Parawixia*), build over streams (*Metabus ocellatus*) or in openings in the forest understorey (*Philoponella*). Such habitats serve as insect fly-ways and are rich in potential prey, and they are generally less accessible to solitary web builders. The foraging benefits of group living were demonstrated in *Metepeira incrassata* in Mexico (Uetz and Hieber, 1997). Spiders in peripheral webs in a colony received more insect strikes than those in webs closer to the centre of the colony, but an insect that was not stopped by the first web it struck was often captured in the second or later web encountered. This 'ricochet effect' increased the size of prey that could be captured, as well as the probability of capture for each individual in the colony. Furthermore, the variance in per-capita prey capture was correlated negatively with colony size, which led Uetz to suggest that group living in spiders is a risk-averse foraging strategy (reviewed in Uetz and Hieber, 1997). A risk-averse strategy is expected when resource abundance is variable, but the average per-capita resource availability in the habitat is above the minimum required for maintenance.

The risk-sensitive foraging hypothesis leads to the prediction that group living should occur mainly in habitats with high prey availability. For example, the highly colonial *M. incrassata* occurs in prey-rich lowland tropical habitats, and is replaced in grassland–desert habitats by *M. atascadero*, a species that is more often solitary or lives in small temporary colonies. Similarly, colony-living jumping spiders (Salticidae) are associated with social insect colonies (ants, termites) or with other species of colonial spiders (Jackson, 1986, Nelson and Jackson, 2008, Whitehouse and Lubin, 2005), and groups of kleptoparasitic spiders (*Argyrodes*) are often found in colonial webs, all of which provide a reliable and abundant food source. An exception to this general rule seems to be the colonial orb-web spider *P. bistriata*, where spiders in arid-habitat populations are more likely to exhibit group foraging than those in mesic populations (see above, Fernández Campón, 2008). In this species, group foraging may be a 'scrounger' strategy, whereby the web owner is unable to defend a large resource (large prey) against invaders (scroungers). The potential benefit to an invading individual is large, particularly in a prey-poor habitat, and reduced aggression allows individuals to create a large web complex that will trap more prey per individual. The diversity of foraging tactics described for colonial species suggests that local conditions may play an important role in determining the degree of cooperation. Phylogenetic effects, however, remain to be investigated in these taxa.

8.5.3   *Predators, parasites and defence*

Spider colonies are attacked by a range of predators, parasites and kleptoparasites. Large colonies are often more conspicuous to predators, and persistent colonies can acquire a heavy load of parasites and parasitoids. Counteracting these disadvantages might be increased defence capabilities of grouped individuals. Both costs and benefits have been demonstrated in a range of colonial spider species.

Colonial females of *Philoponella oweni* suffered significantly greater losses of eggs to parasitoid wasps than did solitary individuals (Smith, 1982). By contrast, single nests of the ant-mimicking jumping spider *Myrmarachne assimilis* (Salticidae) had a higher percentage of egg loss to predators than did nest sites shared by several females (Nelson and Jackson, 2008). *Argyrodes* and *Faiditus* are specialised, obligate kleptoparasites and predators of web-building spiders. Some *Argyrodes* species are egg predators as well, and were shown to significantly reduce the hatching success of egg sacs in colonies of *Cyrtophora citricola* (Pasquet *et al.*, 1997). In *Metepeira incrassata*, the abundance of *Argyrodes* was correlated positively with colony size and with the number of individuals of other species of web-building spiders occurring in the colony (colony associates). Nevertheless, both *M. incrassata* and some of its colony associates benefited by having fewer *Argyrodes* per web when in a group (McCrate and Uetz, 2010).

Wasps and flies of several species parasitise the broods of colonial orb-web spiders, and females guard their egg sacs by shaking the web and encircling the egg sacs with their legs to prevent the parasitoid from landing on them (e.g. tachinid flies in colonies of *Cyrtophora moluccensis*; Lubin, 1974). The relationship between group size and rate of brood parasitism or predation may be complex. Uetz and colleagues investigated mechanisms of attack abatement in *Metepeira incrassata*, both at the colony and the individual level. While the frequency of wasp encounters with colonies increased with colony size, the rate of increase was lower than would be predicted by the rate of encounter of a single web multiplied by the number of colony members (Uetz *et al.*, 2002). This decrease in the marginal rate of encounter with increasing group size may be due to geometry: colony diameter (and thus its size as a visual target) increases at a lower rate than colony volume. Once a wasp encountered a colony, the rate of attack of egg-sac clusters decreased with increasing colony size and, for an individual wasp, with the number of spiders it attacked sequentially. This group benefit derives from the network of interconnected webs: when one spider is alerted to the presence of a wasp, its web vibrations and movements alerted nearby individuals, which then responded more quickly to the wasp. The early warning effect benefited individuals in the centre of the colony in particular, perhaps balancing the relative prey-capture disadvantage of interior positions (Rayor and Uetz, 1990). Other web-building species associated with *M. incrassata* colonies also received early warning of predator incursions and responded to predators from a greater distance than did solitary individuals (Hodge and Uetz, 1992).

8.5.4   What drives group living in colonial spiders?

Colonial organisation is widespread in spiders; it occurs in numerous genera of web-building spiders and in some non-web-builders (Whitehouse and Lubin, 2005). In addition, some genera have multiple colonial species, suggesting that there has been a diversification of colony-forming lineages. The genera *Metepeira*, *Cyrtophora* and *Philoponella*, for example, have multiple colonial species while many other orb-web spider genera found in the same habitats never aggregate. Several tetragnathids aggregate and a few have more permanent colony organisation. *Metepeira* and *Cyrtophora* have three-dimensional, long-lived webs, as do pholcids (Pholcidae), and this may enhance the ability to intersperse webs within a common framework of threads, providing the benefit of reduced silk costs. This is not a trait that is common to all colonial species, however. Natal philopatry or group dispersal of cohorts of juveniles may contribute to colony formation (e.g. *Cyrtophora*, *Philoponella*, *Parawixia*), but we have too little knowledge of the biology of most colonial species to know if this is a shared trait. Some colonial species have wide geographic distributions and are found in a variety of habitats, while others seem restricted to special habitats. For example *Cyrtophora citricola* ranges in the Old World from hyperarid deserts to tropical grassland and forest edge habitats; by contrast, *Metabus ocellatus* and other colonial species of *Tetragnatha* (personal observations) are found only near water.

Most colonial species are tropical or subtropical in distribution, in climatic regions that afford adequate prey supply and perhaps a distribution of prey sizes or types that will favour colonial foraging. Guevara and Avilés (2007) suggested a similar argument to explain the distribution of cooperative social spiders. Colony size is clearly related to prey availability, and the largest colonies always occur where there is an abundance of prey. Thus, as a foraging strategy, group living appears to be particularly successful in conditions of abundant and predictable food supply. In the case of jumping spiders, a rich and persistent food supply is undoubtedly the underlying condition of group living, although the potential benefits remain unknown. Successful foraging may also explain the presence of numerous kleptoparasitic species, as well as normally solitary web-building species, living in association with colonial spiders. Prey abundance alone, however, is insufficient to explain the evolution of group living, as solitary spiders should be just as able to take advantage of a rich food source. Rather it is likely the combination of abundant prey and the specialised habitats that require a measure of cooperation in order to take advantage of them. Both features are necessary to induce juveniles to remain in the colony, acting against natal dispersal typical of non-group-living species.

Defence against predators or parasites is often suggested as a driving force behind the association of individuals in groups (Bertram, 1978). However, specialised group defences against predators and parasites could arise only after the appearance of group living. Increased predator and parasite pressure, along with competition for prey and web sites, are costs of group living that may influence colony size and habitat distribution of colonies and ultimately the species' geographic range. Kin-selected benefits of cooperation, either direct or indirect, can favour grouping among related individuals. We know surprisingly little, however, about the population genetic structure and demography of colonial spiders. *Cyrtophora moluccensis* colonies in Papua New Guinea were founded either by groups of small juveniles that may have been dispersing cohorts, or by one or a few females and their offspring. Similarly, new colonies of *Philoponella republicana* in a Panama forest understorey were established by groups of dispersing young (Lubin, 1980). In both cases, some kin structuring is likely. Allozyme studies of *C. citricola* indicate that the spiders outbreed, but that there is also some differentiation among colonies (J. Wennmann and J. Johannesen, personal communication). Colonial species may have a population structure similar to that of some subsocial species, namely natal philopatry combined with male mating-dispersal (Johannesen and Lubin, 1999, 2001). Pending further studies of population structure, there is little further that can be said about the role of kin selection in the evolution of group living in colonial spiders.

8.6   Conclusions and outlook – colonial spiders

8.6.1   *Whither colonial spider research?*

Researchers have used a few species of colonial spiders as model systems to investigate the costs and benefits of group living and some of the ways that interactions within a colony can determine the fitness of individuals. They have shown foraging benefits as measured by per-capita prey capture, size of prey and reduced variance in prey intake. They have also shown the important role of risk of predation and parasitism as part of the balance between costs and benefits of group living. The structuring of colonies, however, in terms of interactions among individuals should be examined in more detail. For example, what are the fitness consequences of aggressive or cooperative interactions? As pointed out by Jakob (2000), only a small fraction of an individual's time budget is taken up in aggressive encounters. What is their impact on fitness? Finally, the possible influence of relatedness on these interactions has barely been addressed in the colonial species. Are kin-structure colonies (if kin structuring exists) more cooperative than open colonies?

Future work on colonial spiders especially needs to address questions about their breeding systems and population genetic structure. In their review of 1997, Uetz and Hieber pointed out our lack of knowledge of population genetic structure; little has been done to remedy this so far. Especially, it is important to broaden the range of species studied. The colonial jumping spiders in particular offer a wealth of behavioural and life-history adaptations that need to be examined in the light of current ideas about the evolution of group living.

Finally, phylogenies are now available for some of the families in which colonial species occur. As yet, these have not been incorporated into any of the studies of the distribution across taxa of traits associated with colonial group living. A phylogenetic perspective will surely shed light on the question of why group living is so common in some genera and nearly absent in others.

Acknowledgements

We are very grateful to Ingi Agnarsson and Marie Herberstein for thoughtful and insightful comments on this chapter. This is publication number 695 of the Mitrani Department of Desert Ecology.

References

Agnarsson, I. (2006). A revision of the New World *eximius* lineage of *Anelosimus* (Araneae, Theridiidae) and a phylogenetic analysis using worldwide exemplars. *Zoological Journal of the Linnean Society*, **146**, 453–593.

Agnarsson, I., Avilés, L., Coddington, J. A. and Maddison, W. P. (2006). Sociality in theridiid spiders: repeated origins of an evolutionary dead end. *Evolution*, **60**, 2342–2351.

Agnarsson, I., Maddison, W. P. and Avilés, L. (2007). The phylogeny of the social *Anelosmus* spiders (Araneae: Theridiidae) inferred from six molecular loci and morphology. *Molecular Phylogenetics and Evolution*, **43**, 833–851.

Avilés, L. (1986). Sex-ratio bias and possible group selection in the social spider *Anelosimus eximius*. *American Naturalist*, **128**, 1–12.

Avilés, L. (1997). Causes and consequences of cooperation and permanent-sociality in spiders. In *The Evolution of Social Behavior in Insects and Arachnids* (ed. B. Crespi and J. Choe). Cambridge, UK: Cambridge University Press, pp. 476–498.

Avilés, L. (2000). Nomadic behaviour and colony fission in a cooperative spider: life history evolution at the level of the colony? *Biological Journal of the Linnean Society*, **70**, 325–339.

Avilés, L. and Bukowski, T. (2006). Group living and inbreeding depression in a subsocial spider. *Proceedings of the Royal Society of London, B*, **270**, 157–163.

Avilés, L. and Maddison, W. (1991). When is the sex ratio biased in social spiders? Chromosome studies of embryos and male meiosis in *Anelosimus* species. *Journal of Arachnology*, **19**, 126–135.

Avilés, L. and Tufino, P. (1998). Colony size and individual fitness in the social spider *Anelosimus eximius*. *American Naturalist*, **152**, 403–418.

Avilés, L., Agnarsson, I., Salazar, A., *et al.* (2007). Altitudinal patterns of spider sociality and the biology of a new midelevation social *Anelosimus* species in Ecuador. *American Naturalist*, **170**, 783–792.

Avilés, L., Maddison, W. P. and Agnarsson, I. (2006). A new independently derived social spider with explosive colony proliferation and a female size dimorphism. *Biotropica*, **38**, 743–753.

Avilés, L., McCormack, J., Cutter, A. and Bukowski, T. (2000). Precise, highly female-biased sex ratios in a social spider. *Proceedings of the Royal Society of London, B*, **267**, 1445–1449.

Avilés, L., Varas, C. and Dyreson, E. (1999). Does the African social spider *Stegodyphus dumicola* control the sex of individual offspring? *Behavioral Ecology and Sociobiology*, **46**, 237–243.

Beavis, A. S., Rowell, D. M. and Evans, T. (2007). Cannibalism and kin recognition in *Delena cancerides* (Araneae: Sparassidae), a social huntsman spider. *Journal of Zoology*, **271**, 233–237.

Bertram, B. C. R. (1978). Living in groups: predators and prey. In *Behavioural Ecology: An Evolutionary Approach* (ed. J. R. Krebs and N. B. Davies). Oxford, UK: Blackwell.

Bilde, T. and Lubin, Y. (2001). Kin recognition and cannibalism in a subsocial spider. *Journal of Evolutionary Biology*, **14**, 959–966.

Bilde, T., Coates, K., Birkhofer, K., Bird, T., *et al.* (2007). Survival benefits select for group living despite reproductive costs in a social spider. *Journal of Evolutionary Biology*, **20**, 2412–2426.

Bilde, T., Lubin, Y., Smith, D., Schneider, J. and Maklakov, A. A. (2005). The transition to social inbred mating systems in spiders: role of inbreeding tolerance in a subsocial predecessor. *Evolution*, **59**, 160–174.

Buskirk, R. E. (1975a). Aggressive display and orb defense in a colonial spider, *Metabus gravidus*. *Animal Behaviour*, **23**, 560–567.

Buskirk, R. E. (1975b). Coloniality, activity patterns and feeding in a tropical orb-weaving spider. *Ecology*, **56**, 1314–1328.

Buskirk, R. E. (1981). Sociality in the Arachnida. In *Social Insects*, Vol. 2 (ed. H. Hermann). London: Academic Press, pp. 281–367.

Crouch, T. and Lubin, Y. (2001). Population stability and extinction in a social spider *Stegodyphus mimosarum* (Araneae: Eresidae). *Biological Journal of the Linnean Society*, **72**, 409–417.

Crouch, T., Lubin, Y. and Bodasing, M. (1998). Dispersal in the social spider *Stegodyphus mimosarum* Pavesi 1883 (Araneae: Eresidae). *Durban Museum Novitates*, **23**, 52–55.

Downes, M. F. (1994). The nest of the social spider *Phryganoporus candidus* (Araneae: Desidae): structure, annual growth cycle and host plant relationships. *Australian Journal of Zoology*, **42**, 237–259.

Downes, M. F. (1995). Australasian social spiders: what is meant by 'social'? *Records of the Western Australian Museum, Supplement*, **52**, 25–32.

Evans, T. A. (1999). Kin recognition in a social spider. *Proceedings of the Royal Society of London, B*, **266**, 287–292.

Evans, T. A. (2000). Male work and sex ratio in social crab spiders. *Insectes Sociaux*, **47**, 285–288.

Evans, T. A. and Main, B. Y. (1993). Attraction between social crab spider: silk pheromones in *Diaea socialis*. *Behavioral Ecology*, **4**, 99–105.

Evans, T. A., Wallis, W. E. J. and Elgar, M. A. (1995). Making a meal of mother. *Nature*, **376**, 299.

Fernández Campón, F. (2007). Group foraging in the colonial spider *Parawixia bistriata* (Araneidae): an effect of resource levels and prey size. *Animal Behaviour*, **74**, 1551–1562.

Fernández Campón, F. (2008) More sharing when there is less: insights on spider sociality from an orb-weaver's perspective. *Animal Behaviour*, **75**, 1063–1073.

Fisher, R. A. (1930). *The Genetical Theory of Natural Selection*. Oxford, UK: Clarendon Press.

Foster, K. R., Wenseleers, T. and Ratnieks, F. L. W. (2006). Kin selection is the key to altruism. *Trends in Ecology and Evolution*, **21**, 57–60.

Fowler, H. G. and Diehl, J. (1978). Biology of a Paraguayan colonial orb-weaver, *Eriophora bistriata* (Rengger) (Araneae, Araneidae). *Bulletin of the British Arachnological Society*, **4**, 241–250.

Frank, S. A. (1987). Demography and sex ratio in social spiders. *Evolution*, **41**, 1267–1281.

Furey, R. E. (1998). Two cooperatively social populations of the theridiid spider *Anelosimus studiosus* in a temperate region. *Animal Behaviour*, **55**, 727–735.

Gillespie, R. G. (1987). The role of prey availability in aggregative behavior of the orb weaving spider *Tetragnatha elongata*. *Animal Behaviour*, **35**, 675–681.

Gonzaga, M. O. and Vasconcellos-Netto, J. (2001). Female body size, fecundity parameters and foundation of new colonies in *Anelosimus jabaquara* (Araneae, Theridiidae). *Insectes Sociaux*, **48**, 94–100.

Griffin, A. S. and West, S. A. (2003). Kin discrimination and the benefit of helping in cooperatively breeding vertebrates. *Science*, **302**, 634–636.

Guevara, J. and Avilés, L. (2007). Multiple techniques confirm elevational differences in insect size that may influence spider sociality. *Ecology*, **88**, 2015–2023.

Gundermann, J. L., Horel, A. and Krafft, B. (1988). Maternal food-supply activity and its regulation in *Coelotes terrestris* (Araneae: Agelenidae). *Behaviour*, **107**, 278–296.

Hamilton, W. D. (1964). The genetical evolution of social behaviour. I and II. *Journal of Theoretical Biology*, **7**, 1–16, 17–52.

Hamilton, W. D. (1967). Extraordinary sex ratios. *Science*, **156**, 477–488.

Henschel, J. R., Lubin, Y. and Schneider, J. (1995). Sexual competition in an inbreeding social spider, *Stegodyphus dumicola* (Araneae: Eresidae). *Insectes Sociaux*, **42**, 419–426.

Hodge, M. A. and Uetz, G. W. (1992). Antipredator benefits of single- and mixed-species grouping by *Nephila clavipes* L. (Araneae, Tetragnathidae). *Journal of Arachnology*, **20**, 212–216.

Hodge, M. A. and Uetz, G. W. (1996). Foraging advantages of mixed-species association between solitary and colonial orb-weaving spiders. *Oecologia*, **107**, 578–587.

Hurst, L. D. and Vollrath, F. (1992). Sex-ratio adjustment in solitary and social spiders. *Trends in Ecology and Evolution*, **7**, 326–327.

Jackson, R. R. (1978). Comparative studies of *Dictyna* and *Mallos* (Araneae, Dictynidae). I. Social organization. *Revue Arachnologique*, **1**, 133–164.

Jackson, R. R. (1986). Communal jumping spiders (Araneae: Salticidae) from Kenya: interspecific nest complexes, cohabitation with web-building spiders, and intraspecific interactions. *New Zealand Journal of Zoology*, **13**, 13–26.

Jackson, R. R., Nelson, X. J. and Salm, K. (2008a). The natural history of *Myrmarachne melanotarsa*, a social ant mimicking jumping spider. *New Zealand Journal of Zoology*, **35**, 225–235.

Jackson, R. R., Pollard, S. D. and Salm, K. (2008b). Observations of *Portia africana*, an araneophagic jumping spider, living together and sharing prey. *New Zealand Journal of Zoology*, **35**, 237–243.

Jakob, E. M. (1991). Costs and benefits of group living for pholcid spiderlings: losing food, saving silk. *Animal Behaviour*, **41**, 711–722.

Jakob, E. M. (1994). Contests over prey by group-living pholcids. *Journal of Arachnology*, **22**, 39–45.

Jakob, E. M., Blanchong, J. A., Popsen, M. A., Sedey, K. A. and Summerfield, M. S. (2000). Ontogenetic shifts in the costs of living in groups: focal observations of a pholcid spider (*Holocnemus pluchei*). *American Midland Naturalist*, **143**, 405–413.

Jakob, E. M., Porter, A. H. and Uetz, G. W. (2001). Site fidelity and the costs of movement among territories: an example from colonial web-building spiders. *Canadian Journal of Zoology*, **79**, 2094–2100.

Johannesen, J. and Lubin, Y., (1999). Group founding and breeding structure in the subsocial spider *Stegodyphus lineatus* (Eresidae). *Heredity*, **82**, 677–686.

Johannesen, J. and Lubin, Y. (2001). Evidence for kin structured group founding and limited juvenile dispersal in the sub-social spider *Stegodyphus lineatus* (Araneae, Eresidae). *Journal of Arachnology*, **29**, 413–422.

Johannesen, J., Lubin Y., Bilde, T. Smith, D. R. and Schneider, J. M. (2007). The age and evolution of sociality in *Stegodyphus* spiders: a molecular phylogenetic approach. *Proceedings of the Royal Society of London, B*, **274**, 231–237.

Johannesen, J., Moritz, R. F. A., Simunek, H., Seibt, U. and Wickler, W. (2009a). Species cohesion despite extreme inbreeding in a social spider. *Journal of Evolutionary Biology*, **22**, 1137–1142.

Johannesen, J., Wickler, W., Seibt, U. and Moritz, R. F. A. (2009b). Population history in social spiders repeated: colony structure and lineage evolution in *Stegodyphus mimosarum* (Eresidae). *Molecular Ecology*, **18**, 2812–2818.

Jones, T. C. and Parker, P. G. (2002). Delayed juvenile dispersal benefits both mother and offspring in the cooperative spider *Anelosimus studiosus* (Araneae: Theridiidae). *Behavioral Ecology*, **13**, 142–148.

Jones, T. C., Riechert, S. E., Dalrymple, S. E. and Parker, P. G. (2007). Fostering model explains variation in levels of sociality in spider system. *Animal Behaviour*, **73**, 195–204.

Kim, K.-W. and Horel, A. (1998). Matriphagy in the spider *Amaurobius ferox* (Araneae, Amaurobiidae): an example of mother-offspring interactions. *Ethology*, **104**, 1021–1037.

Kim, K.-W. and Roland, C. (2000). Trophic egg laying in the spider, *Amaurobius ferox*: mother-offspring interactions and functional value. *Behavioural Processes*, **50**, 31–42.

Koenig, B. (1997). Cooperative care of young in mammals. *Naturwissenschaften*, **84**, 95–104.

Kraus, O. and Kraus, M. (1988). The genus *Stegodyphus* (Arachnida, Araneae) sibling species, species groups, and parallel evolution of social living. *Verhandlungen des Naturwissenschaftlichen Vereins Hamburg*, **30**, 151–254.

Kullmann, E. J. (1972). Evolution of social behavior in spiders (Araneae, Eresidae and Theridiidae). *American Zoologist*, **12**, 419–426.

Lubin, Y. D. (1974). Adaptive advantages and evolution of colony formation in *Cyrtophora* (Araneae, Araneidae). *Zoological Journal of the Linnean Society*, **54**, 321–339.

Lubin, Y. D. (1980). Population studies of two colonial orb-weaving spiders. *Zoological Journal of the Linnean Society*, **70**, 265–287.

Lubin, Y. D. (1991). Patterns of variation in female-biased colony sex ratios in a social spider. *Biological Journal of the Linnean Society*, **43**, 297–311.

Lubin, Y. and Bilde, T. (2007). The evolution of sociality in spiders. *Advances in the Study of Behavior*, **37**, 83–145.

Lubin, Y. D. and Crozier, R. H. (1985). Electrophoretic evidence for population differentiation in a social spider, *Achaearanea wau* Levi (Theridiidae). *Insectes Sociaux*, **32**, 297–304.

Lubin, Y. D. and Robinson, M. H. (1982). Dispersal by swarming in social spiders. *Science*, **216**, 319–321.

Lubin, Y., Birkhofer, K., Berger-Tal, R. and Bilde, T. (2009). Limited male dispersal in a social spider with extreme inbreeding. *Biological Journal of the Linnean Society*, **97**, 227–234.

Marques, E. S. A., Vasconcellos-Netto, J. and de Mello, M. B. (1998). Life history and social behavior of *Anelosimus jabaquara* and *Anelosimus dubiosus* (Araneae, Theridiidae). *Journal of Arachnology*, **26**, 227–237.

McCrate, A. T. and Uetz, G. W. (2009). Kleptoparasites: a twofold cost of group living for the colonial spider, *Metepeira incrassata* (Araneae, Araneidae). *Behavioural Ecology and Sociobiolog*, **64**, 389–399.

Meehan, C. J., Olsen, E. J., Reudnick, M. W., Kyser, T. K. and Curry, R. L. (2009). Herbivory in a spider through exploitation of an ant-plant mutualism. *Current Biology*, **19**, R892.

Nelson, X. J. and Jackson, R. R. (2008). Anti-predator crèches and aggregations of ant-mimicking jumping spiders (Araneae: Salticidae). *Biological Journal of the Linnean Society*, **94**, 475–481.

Nunney, L. (1985). Female-biased sex ratios: individual or group selection. *Evolution*, **39**, 349–361.

Pasquet, A., Leborgne, R. and Cantarella, T. (1997). Opportunistic egg-feeding in the kleptoparasitic spider *Argyrodes gibbosus*. *Ethology*, **103**, 160–170.

Powers, K. S. and Avilés, L. (2003). Natal dispersal patterns of a subsocial spider *Anelosimus* cf. *jucundus* (Theridiidae). *Ethology*, **109**, 725–737.

Powers, K. S. and Avilés, L. (2007). The role of prey size and abundance in the geographical distribution of spider sociality. *Journal of Animal Ecology*, **76**, 995–1003.

Pruitt, J. N. and Riechert, S. E. (2009). Frequency-dependent success of cheaters during foraging bouts might limit their spread within colonies of a socially polymorphic spider. *Evolution*, **63**, 2966–2973.

Pruitt, J. N., Riechert, S. E. and Jones, T. C. (2008). Behavioural syndromes and their fitness consequences in a socially polymorphic spider, *Anelosimus studiosus*. *Animal Behaviour*, **76**, 871–879.

Rao, D. and Lubin, Y. (2010). Conditions favouring group living in web-building spiders in an extreme desert environment. *Israel Journal of Ecology and Evolution* (in press).

Rayor, L. S. and Uetz, G. W. (1990). Trade-offs in foraging success and predation risk with spatial position in colonial spiders. *Behavioral Ecology and Sociobiology*, **27**, 77–85.

Riechert, S. E. and Jones, T. C. (2008). Phenotypic variation in the social behaviour of the spider *Anelosimus studiosus* along a latitudinal gradient. *Animal Behaviour*, **75**, 1893–1902.

Rowell, D. M. and Avilés, L. (1995). Sociality in a bark-dwelling huntsman spider from Australia, *Delena cancerides* Walckenaer (Araneae: Sparassidae). *Insectes Sociaux*, **42**, 287–302.

Rowell, D. M. and Main, B. Y. (1992). Sex ratio in the social spider *Diaea socialis* (Araneae: Thomisidae). *Journal of Arachnology*, **20**, 200–206.

Ruch, J., Heinrich, L., Bilde, T. and Schneider, J. M. (2009). Relatedness facilitates cooperation in the subsocial spider, *Stegodyphus tentoriicola*. *BMC Evolutionary Biology*, **9**, 257.

Rypstra, A. L. (1979). Foraging flocks in spiders: a study of aggregate behaviour in *Cyrtophora citricola* Forskaal (Araneae: Araneidae) in West Africa. *Behavioral Ecology and Sociobiology*, **5**, 291–300.

Rypstra, A. L. (1985). Aggregations of *Nephila clavipes* (L.) (Araneae, Araneidae) in relation to prey availability. *Journal of Arachnology*, **13**, 71–78.

Rypstra, A. L. (1993). Prey size, social competition, and the development of reproductive division-of-labor in social spider groups. *American Naturalist*, **142**, 868–880.

Salomon, M. and Lubin, Y. (2007). Cooperative breeding increases reproductive success in the social spider *Stegodyphus dumicola* (Araneae, Eresidae). *Behavioral Ecology and Sociobiology*, **61**, 1743–1750.

Salomon, M., Mayntz, D. and Lubin, Y. (2008). Colony nutrition skews reproduction in a social spider. *Behavioral Ecology*, **19**, 605–611.

Salomon, M., Schneider, J. and Lubin, Y. (2005). Maternal investment in a spider with suicidal maternal care, *Stegodyphus lineatus* (Araneae, Eresidae). *Oikos*, **109**, 614–622.

Schneider, J. M. (2002). Reproductive state and care giving in *Stegodyphus* (Araneae: Eresidae) and the implications for the evolution of sociality. *Animal Behaviour*, **63**, 649–658.

Schneider, J. M. and Bilde, T. (2008). Benefits of cooperation with genetic kin in a subsocial spider. *Behavioral Ecology and Sociobiology*, **105**, 10 843–10 846.

Schneider, J. M., Roos, J., Lubin, Y. and Henschel, J. R. (2001). Dispersal of *Stegodyphus dumicola*: they do balloon after all! *Journal of Arachnology*, **29**, 114–116.

Seibt, U. and Wickler, W. (1988a). Bionomics and social structure of 'family spiders' of the genus *Stegodyphus*, with special reference to the African species *S. dumicola* and *S. mimosarum* (Araneae, Eresidae). *Verhandlungen des Naturwissenschaftlichen Vereins in Hamburg*, **30**, 255–303.

Seibt, U. and Wickler, W. (1988b). Why do 'family spiders,' *Stegodyphus* (Eresidae) live in colonies? *Journal of Arachnology*, **16**, 193–198.

Smith, D. R. (1982). Reproductive success of solitary and communal *Philoponella oweni* (Araneae: Uloboridae). *Behavioral Ecology and Sociobiology*, **11**, 149–154.

Smith, D., van Rijn, S., Henschel, J., Bilde, T. and Lubin, Y. (2009). Amplified fragment length polymorphism fingerprints support limited gene flow among social spider populations. *Biological Journal of the Linnean Society*, **97**, 235–246.

Uetz, G. W. (2001). Understanding the evolution of social behavior in colonial web-building spiders. In *Model Systems in Behavioral Ecology: Integrating Empirical, Theoretical and Conceptual Approaches* (ed. L. A. Dugatkin). Monographs in Behavior and Ecology. Princeton, NJ: Princeton University Press, pp. 110–130.

Uetz, G. W. and Hieber, C. S. (1997). Colonial web-building spiders: balancing the costs and benefits of group living. In *The Evolution of Social Behavior in Insects and Arachnids* (ed. J. Choe and B. Crespi). Cambridge, UK: Cambridge University Press, pp. 458–475.

Uetz, G. W., Boyle, J., Hieber, C. S. and Wilcox, R. S. (2002). Antipredator benefits of group living in colonial web-building spiders: the 'early warning' effect. *Animal Behaviour*, **63**, 445–452.

Ulbrich, K. and Henschel, J. R. (1999). Intraspecific competition in a social spider. *Ecological Modelling*, **115**, 243–251.

Vakanas, G. and Krafft, B. (2001). Coordination of behavioral sequences between individuals during prey capture in a social spider, *Anelosimus eximius*. *Journal of Insect Behavior*, **14**, 777–798.

White, M. J. D. (1973). *Animal Cytology and Evolution*. Cambridge, UK: Cambridge University Press.

Whitehouse, M. A. E. and Jackson, R. R. (1994). Group structure and time budgets of *Argyrodes antipodiana* (Araneae, Theridiidae), a kleptoparasitic spider from New Zealand. *New Zealand Journal of Zoology*, **20**, 201–206.

Whitehouse, M. A. E. and Lubin, Y. (1999). Strategic interference competition by individuals in social spider foraging groups. *Animal Behaviour*, **58**, 677–688.

Whitehouse, M. E. A. and Lubin, Y. (2005). The function of societies and the evolution of group living: spider societies as a test case. *Biological Reviews*, **80**, 347–361.

Willey, M. B. and Jackson, R. R. (1993). Predatory behavior of a social spider, *Stegodyphus sarasinorum* (Araneae, Eresidae): why attack first? *Canadian Journal of Zoology*, **71**, 2220–2223.

Wilson, E. O. (1971). *The Insect Societies*. Cambridge, MA: Harvard University Press.

Yip, E. C., Clarke, S. and Rayor, L. S. (2009). Aliens among us: nestmate recognition in the huntsman spider, *Delena cancerides. Insectes Sociaux*, **56**, 223–231.

Yip, E. C., Powers, K. S. and Avilés, L. (2008). Cooperative capture of large prey solves scaling challenge faced by spider societies. *Proceedings of the National Academy of Sciences of the USA*, **105**, 11 818–11 822.

9

Plasticity, learning and cognition

ELIZABETH JAKOB, CHRISTA SKOW AND SKYE LONG

As is becoming increasingly clear, spiders are not entirely instinct driven and inflexible in their behaviour. Here we review evidence for behavioural plasticity, learning and other cognitive processes such as attentional priming and memory. We first examine these attributes in several natural contexts: predation, interactions with conspecifics and potential predators, and spatial navigation. Next we examine two somewhat more artificial experimental approaches, heat aversion and rearing in enriched versus impoverished environments. We briefly describe the neurobiological underpinnings of these behaviours. Finally, we point to areas where our knowledge gaps are greatest, and we offer advice for researchers beginning their own studies of spider learning.

9.1   Overview

The history of the study of spider learning parallels that of insect learning, but lags well behind. At the start of the twentieth century, the general view was that insect learning was generally guided by instinct, but a steady accumulation of data has transformed our view of the importance of learning in their daily lives (reviewed in Dukas, 2008). In spite of their tiny brains, insects are capable of learning a multitude of tasks related to foraging, anti-predatory behaviour, aggression, social interactions, courtship and mate choice (Dukas, 2008). The study of spider behaviour is undergoing a similar transformation. Beginning over a century ago, researchers have periodically delved into the question of whether spider behaviour is primarily instinctual or can be modified with experience. For example, Peckham and Peckham (1887) reported that

Spider Behaviour: Flexibility and Versatility, ed. Marie Elisabeth Herberstein. Published by Cambridge University Press. © Cambridge University Press 2011.

spiders initially dropped out of their webs when approached by a ringing tuning fork, but after repeated presentations they disregarded it. Despite that early beginning, spider learning and cognition was generally neglected until the last several decades, when it began to be addressed more systematically and with well-controlled experiments. Unfortunately, these are still far fewer in number than those on insects.

As there is some variation in how different authors use terminology, we begin by defining our terms. *Cognition* includes the processes by which animals acquire, store, process and act upon information from the environment. Thus, cognition encompasses processes such as attention and priming, perception, information processing and decision making, in addition to learning and memory (Shettleworth, 2001). *Learning* is a sustained change in behavioural performance resulting from a change in the cognitive representation of relationships between cues (Domjan, 2006). The terms cognition and learning do not require us to infer any level of consciousness (Shettleworth, 2001). We define *behavioural plasticity* as a change in an animal's behaviour over time or under different circumstances. Plasticity alone is not sufficient evidence of learning or any other cognitive process, as behaviours may change because of a variety of non-cognitive processes, including satiation (e.g. Bilde *et al.*, 2002, Chmiel *et al.*, 2000, Li, 2000), maturational differences (Edwards and Jackson, 1994, Kreiter and Wise, 1996), reproductive condition (Cross *et al.*, 2007a), or temporal shifts in the environment (Chien and Morse, 1998). Without experiments, it is generally difficult, if not impossible, to distinguish plasticity from learning. The spider literature offers numerous examples of behavioural plasticity where the underlying mechanism has not been identified, whereas in other cases learning has been clearly demonstrated.

In selecting studies for review, we omit those in which there is evidence of choice but not of behavioural plasticity (e.g. male spiders select larger over smaller females; Hoefler, 2008). We also omit studies in which plasticity has been documented but is very unlikely to have a cognitive component, such as the cessation of feeding prior to moult or the halt in the production of prey-capture webs when a male matures. At the risk of overlap with other chapters in this volume, we briefly describe studies where cognition seems likely to play a role in plasticity but has not yet been experimentally addressed, as these suggest promising areas for future research.

9.2   Predation

Of all the types of behavioural plasticity we review, plasticity in predatory behaviour is the most commonly studied. Successful prey capture is a complex feat for spiders, regardless of whether they rely on webs or actively hunt. Prey quality and availability vary across time and space, so there is a clear selective advantage for animals that are capable of distinguishing between relevant and irrelevant information. Here we focus on how spiders select and capture prey, choose web or foraging sites, and modify their web designs. Predatory plasticity is addressed in more detail in Chapter 3 of this volume.

9.2.1   Prey choice and capture strategies

Most spider species consume a wide variety of prey, limited primarily by their ability to subdue it. Nonetheless, a number of species change their predatory behaviour over time or under specific circumstances.

Prey choice

Prey choice in spiders often appears to be based on simple rules of thumb that may vary across species. Spiders may distinguish prey from non-prey, or one type of prey from another, based on very particular cues (e.g. Harland and Jackson, 2000, 2001, 2002). Preference for prey may be based on cues such as size, quality and species of prey. For example, in choice tests, the web-building spider *Micrathena sagittata* (Araneidae) consistently prefers larger over smaller prey (Diaz-Fleischer, 2005). Conversely, the wandering spider *Loxosceles reclusa*, though rarely a scavenger in nature, prefers smaller dead prey over larger live prey, thereby minimising predation risk (Cramer, 2008).

Some species have innate preferences for particular prey types, but these preferences are sometimes malleable. For example, some species prefer ants and exhibit an ant-specific predatory behaviour, independent of previous experience (reviewed in Huseynov et al., 2005). Although the jumping spider *Aelurillus muganicus* exhibits an innate ant preference in laboratory choice tests, the frequency of ant encounters in the field is limited, so ants only account for 20% of their natural diet (Huseynov et al., 2005). The salticid *Aelurillus m-nigrum* expresses its innate ant preference only when the laboratory environment closely mimics its native sandy habitat (Huysenov et al., 2008). Prey preferences may also disappear with food deprivation. For example, three myrmecophagic species of *Aelurillus* shift from attacking only ants to accepting both ants and insects (Li et al., 1999), although three species of *Zenodorus* continue to prefer ants even after 21 days without feeding (Jackson and Li, 2001). Similarly, the preference of araneophagic spiders for spiders over insect prey also disappears as they grow hungrier (Jackson and Li, 1998, Li, 2000, Li et al., 1997). Preference may also vary based on venom availability. When offered a choice between two types of cockroaches that differed in venom sensitivity, the hunting spider *Cupiennius salei* chooses the more vulnerable prey when its venom glands are depleted, but expresses no preference when glands are full (Wullschleger and Nentwig, 2002).

In the examples above, we generally do not know whether experience affects plasticity. In other cases, we have direct evidence of the role of experience. The wolf spider *Hogna helluo* (Lycosidae) does not exhibit an a-priori prey preference, but preference can be induced after regular feeding of a single prey type (Persons and Rypstra, 2000). When fed either crickets or a smaller wolf spider (*Pardosa milvina*) twice per week for one month, *H. helluo* spends more time on substrates with chemical cues from familiar prey. Prey preference has also been induced in *Oxyopes salticus* (Oxyopidae) spiderlings (Punzo, 2002a, 2002b) and *Hogna carolinensis* spiderlings (Punzo and Preshkar, 2002), and this preference persists even after subsequent feedings on alternative prey. By maintaining a preference for prey based on positive recent experiences, spiders can minimise the risk of the unknown, particularly when there is a chance that novel prey may be poorer quality or even toxic (Toft, 1999).

Spiders can learn to associate a new odour with food (Patt and Pfannenstiel, 2008). The nectarivorous spider *Hibana futilis* (Anyphaenidae) does not normally respond to the odour of vanilla. When spiders were offered vanilla (in the terminology of classical conditioning, the conditioned stimulus) along with sugar solution (the unconditioned stimulus) in an artificial nectary, they learned to associate the vanilla scent with the reward in a single trial and retained this association for several hours.

Several species are capable of developing aversions to toxic and/or distasteful prey. One of the earliest reports of a thorough experiment on spider learning is from Bays (1962), who reported that five orb-web spiders (*Araneus diadematus*, Araneidae) were trained to associate prey quality with frequencies of a ringing tuning fork. First, a dead fly dipped in an aversive quinine solution was thrown in the web and made to vibrate with a tuning fork. Five minutes later, a glucose-dipped fly was presented, along with a tuning fork of a different frequency. After 15 trials, all five spiders 'regularly' bit the glucose fly but not the quinine fly. After further training, flies were replaced by tasteless glass, and all spiders bit the beads only when they were vibrated with the frequency associated with glucose-dipped prey. Although this work was based on a small sample size and the report omits some procedural details, the results are intriguing. To our knowledge, this study has not been replicated.

Typically, the stronger an aversive stimulus, the longer that avoidance learning persists and the more likely it will generalise to similar stimuli across different contexts (Domjan, 2006). Not surprisingly, naive wolf spiders (*Pardosa prativaga*, Lycosidae) fed on one low-quality aphid species develop generalised aversions to other aphid species after only a few trials, and the aversion persists for several hours (Toft, 1997). In contrast, the wolf spider *Hogna carolinensis* (Lycosidae) generally avoids unpalatable buckeye caterpillars, but there is no evidence that their avoidance behaviour improves with learning (Theodoratus and Bowers, 1999).

As has been well documented in the psychology literature, animals may learn not only the primary association, such as between the appearance or odour of prey and its bad taste, but also the context in which the association occurs (Pearce and Bouton, 2001). The jumping spider *Phidippus princeps* (Salticidae) learns to decrease its attacks on unpalatable milkweed bugs over eight successive trials (Skow and Jakob, 2006). Spiders are more likely to retain their aversion when background cues, also called contextual cues, remain identical to those present during learning. When contextual cues change, spiders do not generalise their aversion and are more likely to resume attacking milkweed bugs (Figure 9.1). Perhaps the lack of generalisation occurs because the cost of making a mistake is small: spiders release the bugs before ingesting toxic chemicals. In a different experiment, *P. princeps* did not avoid vegetation cues that had been previously paired with unpalatable milkweed bugs, but did avoid those same cues when they had been paired with a stronger aversive stimulus of mild electrical shock (Skow, 2007).

Hunting animals may become more likely to detect prey species with which they have had experience. In some cases, this phenomenon is due to Pavlovian conditioning: the predator's repeated experiences with prey lead to an association between the prey's characteristics and a food reward (Hollis, 1982). In other cases, another cognitive process may be involved, that of selective attention. Animals are capable of perceiving a wide range of stimuli in different sensory modes, but at any given moment only a subset of these stimuli are relevant. Attention is the mechanism by which animals select what to respond to from moment to moment (Shettleworth, 1998). Attention can be primed by experience. For example, the araneophagic spider *Portia labiata* is more likely to find a prey spider in a testing arena after a single experience with a prey of the same type (Jackson and Li, 2004). The fact that the behavioural change comes after only a single experience suggests that *P. labiata* has formed a search image for particular optical cues (Jackson and Li, 2004).

An even more compelling case for a role for selective attention comes from cross-modal priming, where experience with one cue heightens the response to another cue. The salticid *Evarcha culicivora* prefers to feed upon mosquitoes that have had a blood meal. Cross and Jackson (2009a) tested whether the presence of the odour of blood-carrying mosquitoes primes spiders to detect mosquitoes using visual cues. Test spiders were reared on lake flies and had never encountered a mosquito or its odour. Mosquito lures were made by mounting a dead

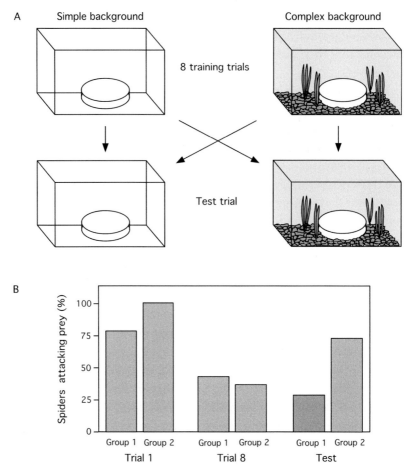

Figure 9.1 (A) Experimental design to test for the role of contextual cues (different visual backgrounds) in learning to avoid toxic prey. (B) After learning not to attack distasteful prey, spiders tested with a new background resumed attacking prey, but spiders tested with a familiar background did not attack prey. (From Skow and Jakob, 2006, with kind permission from Oxford University Press.)

mosquito on a cork and spraying it with plastic adhesive to remove odour cues. When mosquito lures were conspicuous, spiders primed with odour were no more successful at detecting lures than were spiders that were not primed. However, when mosquito lures were made cryptic by including distractors and by covering the lures with nylon netting, spiders were more likely to find the lure when they were exposed to the scent of a blood-carrying mosquito. These results suggest that the odour had 'called up' an innate search image for the prey (Cross and Jackson, 2009a). Similarly, *Portia fimbriata* more quickly detected optical cues from its prey, the salticid *Jacksonoides queenslandicus*, after exposure to chemicals in its dragline, even though *P. fimbriata* had no experience in capturing the prey (Jackson *et al.*, 2002a). For a complete discussion of attention, search images, and priming in spiders, see Cross and Jackson (2006).

Capture strategies

Attack strategies may also be plastic. Some strategies change with age and size: for example, in the myrmecophagic spider *Aphantochilus rogersi* (Thomisidae), smaller spiders can only get a grip on an ant's petiole if they attack from the front, whereas older, larger spiders shift to attacking from behind (Castanho and Oliveira, 1997). Spiders may improve their prey-capture technique with experience. Several studies have shown that the attack success of spiderlings increases over repeated trials (Edwards and Jackson, 1994, Forster, 1977). With experience, crab spiders (*Misumena vatia*, Thomisidae) change the location of their strikes on prey (Morse, 1991), and orient to prey more rapidly (Morse, 2000a). Finally, naive *Nephila clavipes* (Nephilidae) are more likely to throw silk at a novel prey (stingless bees), but with repeated experience use a biting attack (Higgins, 2008).

Attack strategies may also change with energy state. For example, in the kleptoparasitic spider *Argyrodes flavescens* (Theridiidae), invaders use a host's web for prey capture, but the size of prey stolen from the web depends upon hunger levels (Koh and Li, 2003). Hungry invaders are more likely to either steal small prey or co-feed with the host on a larger prey item caught by the host, whereas well-fed invaders prefer to feed independently from the host.

The best-known work on flexible attack strategies comes from araneophagic salticids. Four genera (*Brettus*, *Cocalus*, *Cyrba* and *Portia*) all engage in 'cognitive smokescreen' behaviour during web invasions (Cerveira *et al.*, 2003). *Portia fimbriata* produces a series of signals, ranging from accurate mimicry of trapped insects to larger random disturbances in an effort to conceal its approach towards the host spider (Clark and Jackson, 2000, Tarsitano *et al.*, 2000). *Portia* can also take advantage of vibrations produced when the host spider is capturing prey to stealthily mask its own advances (Jackson *et al.*, 2002b). Initially, the invading *Portia* broadcasts a wide array of signals, but narrows its signal over time based on the behaviour of the host spider. This change in behaviour is evidence of trial-and-error learning (or operant conditioning) during web invasion (Jackson, 2002, Jackson and Wilcox, 1993a). Reliance on trial-and-error learning varies across lab-reared spiders derived from different populations of *P. labiata*, suggesting local adaptation to specific habitats. Spiders from areas with lower prey diversity exhibited far less reliance on trial-and-error learning than those from areas of higher prey diversity (Jackson and Carter, 2001). This pattern across populations supports the argument that innate predatory behaviour (resulting in streamlined informational processing of specific stimuli) is favoured when environments remain stable over evolutionary time whereas learning is more advantageous in unpredictable environments (Japyassu and Caires, 2008, Japyassu and Viera, 2002).

Retaining information about captured prey

Finally, spiders have also been shown to change their behaviour based on the prey they have already captured and stored. Web-building spiders can face concurrent feeding opportunities if prey items are snared simultaneously. *Zygiella x-notata* (Araneidae) gain more energy from shorter feedings on multiple prey versus prolonged feeding on one prey item (Sebrier and Krafft, 1993). If *Zygiella x-notata* captures two prey items, it reduces its feeding duration on the first prey, even if the second prey is removed from the web. This behavioural change suggests that spiders retain information about the capture of the second prey. Similar behaviour is demonstrated by the araneid *Argiope argentata* (Ades, 1982).

9.2.2   Selection of web and foraging sites

Instead of actively searching for prey, many spiders wait for prey to come to them. If foraging site quality is temporally autocorrelated and thus good sites are likely to remain good over time, the ability to select good sites is likely to increase fitness. Foraging success correlates with growth and egg production in many species (e.g. Fritz and Morse, 1985, Vollrath, 1987). Sites may also differ in other characteristics, such as the availability of web supports and the presence of predators.

A sit-and-wait predator has two decision points: the initial selection of a hunting site, and the decision to abandon the site in search of a better one. Both have been studied extensively, especially in web-building spiders. Webs can be costly to produce. They are made of protein, which is frequently limited in spiders' diets (reviewed in Blamires *et al.*, 2009). Web construction can divert resources away from growth and development (Jakob, 1991). Even orb-web spiders, which consume their webs and thus can recycle much of the raw material (Peakall, 1971), must expend energy in the complicated movements needed to construct a web (Venner *et al.*, 2003). All spiders, even those that do not build webs, may incur lost-opportunity costs during a move (time spent moving is time lost foraging; e.g. Morse and Fritz, 1982). Spiders may be more vulnerable to predators during and after relocation (reviewed in Smith, 2009). Thus, selecting a good foraging site prior to settlement should be advantageous.

Spiders can sometimes directly assess cues that indicate a high-quality site, as a large literature attests. For example, web-building spiders select sites with adequate space and anchorage points for webs (e.g. Lubin *et al.*, 1993), initiate web building more quickly when in the presence of conspecifics (Salomon, 2007), or build webs near artificial lights that also attract prey (Adams, 2000). Some species avoid chemical signatures left by predators (e.g. Persons and Uetz, 1996a, Rypstra *et al.*, 2007). Some can also detect prey cues. For example, in laboratory experiments, wolf spiders (*Schizocosa ocreata*) stay longer in patches that have chemical or visual cues of prey, even without food rewards (Persons and Uetz, 1996b, 1998). *Agelenopsis aperta* (Agelenidae) can choose web sites based on airborne vibrations generated by flies or by artificial means (Riechert, 1985). Crab spiders (*Misumena vatia*) wait for prey on flowers and attend to a variety of cues, including plant species, the quality of the bloom, and the presence of prey, even if they do not capture it (e.g. Chien and Morse 1998, Morse, 1988, 1993, 2000a).

Learning may modify the level of response to site quality cues. For example, Punzo (1997) compared the amount of time that wolf spiders (*Schizocosa avida*) spend on plain filter paper and filter paper that had come in contact with a scorpion, a voracious predator. Control spiders spent equivalent amounts of time on each substrate, whereas spiders that had escaped from a scorpion by autotomising a leg avoid the scorpion-scented paper. The behaviour of spiders with legs autotomised by the experimenter did not differ from control spiders.

Immediate cues of site quality may not always be available (e.g. Hoefler *et al.*, 2002), and spiders must instead sample a site in order to estimate its quality. Because of the stochastic nature of prey arrival, it would seem beneficial for a spider to remember its foraging experiences at a particular site. Indeed, Nakata *et al.* (2003) modelled the effect of memory on fitness, and predicted that spiders that have a longer memory window for their prey capture success in a particular site will make more accurate decisions about whether to abandon the site or stay. The effects of different costs of memory were not explored.

Although there are exceptions (e.g. Vollrath and Houston, 1986), numerous studies have shown that recent prey capture success influences a spider's decision to stay in a site. Many species apparently follow the rule of 'Win, stay; lose, shift', remaining in a site where they have captured prey, and moving on when they have not (reviewed in Jakob, 2004, Nakata *et al.*, 2003). However, although there may be a correlation between a spider's selection of a foraging site and its recent experience, it does not necessarily follow that a spider remembers its experience. Instead, it could be basing its decisions on its current hunger state. Nonetheless, some spiders do appear to have a short-term memory of prey capture: when experimenters stole captured prey from the webs of *Argiope argentata* (Araneidae), *Nephila clavipes* (Nephilidae) and *Neriene peltata* (Linyphiidae), spiders searched for the prey by walking around and pulling on the web threads (Rodríguez and Gamboa, 2000). Spiders did not perform searching behaviour in response to artificial disturbance, nor did they home in on prey that were moved to a new section of the web. However, they did search longer for larger prey, suggesting that spiders were indeed looking for remembered prey.

We can get more insight into what a spider has learned about a site by experimentally manipulating a spider's foraging experience. For example, in the field, adult *Holocnemus pluchei* (Pholcidae) stay in webs longer when additional prey are added to the webs. A possible explanation is that spiders associate the presence of prey with a particular web site. However, a laboratory experiment demonstrated that this is not the case. When fed and starved spiders are moved to a new web, their decisions to leave or stay are based on their condition, even without the opportunity to sample prey availability at the new site (Jakob, 2004). Of course, when there is no experimental intervention, a spider's condition is likely to be correlated with its experience in a particular web, and thus condition can be a reliable indicator of site quality.

In another species, the effect of prey removal depended on how long spiders were in a site. Nakata and Ushimaru (1999) removed prey every three minutes throughout the foraging day from the orb webs of *Cyclosa argenteoalba* (Araneidae), wresting it out of the spiders' jaws when necessary. Spiders undergoing prey removal were more likely to move their webs the next day. This effect was particularly pronounced for spiders that had spent only a single day at the experimental site, suggesting that spiders incorporated both recent and earlier experience to determine whether to abandon a site. In contrast, neither prey capture nor prey cues experienced at a particular site influence subsequent visits to that site by the wolf spider *Schizocosa ocreata*, and Persons and Uetz (1997) suggest that learning is not important for this species in site selection.

Crab spiders (Thomisidae) select flowering plants on which to wait for prey. Morse's (2007) long-term studies of the foraging decisions of *Misumena vatia* suggest that the role of experience in site assessment increases as spiders grow. Spiderlings appear to have innate preferences for particular substrates, but older spiders show greater flexibility (Morse, 2000b, 2007). Older spiders select substrates similar to their immediately previous ones more frequently than expected by chance. Site fidelity is particularly strong if a spider moults on a particular flower type (Morse, 1999). Spiders that are shifted from milkweed, a good site, to rose, a poorer site, are more likely to leave the new site than were those moved to another plant of their accustomed species, suggesting that spiders remember their previous site from two days earlier and judge the new one accordingly (Morse, 2000c).

Another site characteristic that cannot be easily assessed prior to settlement is the possibility of web damage. When web damage is predictable, such as along paths used by mammals, relocation in response to damage will be beneficial. When the orb webs of *Argiope keyserlingi* (Araneidae) were experimentally damaged, spiders built new webs away from the direction of the damage (Chmiel *et al.*, 2000).

9.2.3   Web design

Spider web architecture varies not only across species, but across webs spun by a particular individual (see also Chapter 3). Sometimes, variation results from purely mechanistic constraints, such as available space, weather and spider growth (reviewed in Heiling and Herberstein, 2000). Some spiders vary their webs in response to more unusual environmental cues: for example, *Nephila clavipes* (Nephilidae) spiders change the colour of their silk in response to the spectral quality and light intensity in their environment, producing yellower webs when foraging in high light environments and thereby attracting bees (Craig *et al.*, 1996).

In some species, web size or structure depends on energy state. Orb-web spiders generally reduce investment in web building when satiated (reviewed in Venner *et al.*, 2000). In sheet-web spiders, the situation is more complicated because webs generally require more energy to construct and a starved spider may not have enough energy to build a web. In the linyphiid *Frontinellina* cf. *frutetorum*, spiders in better condition build larger webs, the opposite of most orb-web spiders. Western black widow spiders (*Latrodectus hesperus*, Theridiidae) modify both the amount of silk (Salomon, 2007) and the shape (Zevenbergen *et al.*, 2008) of their three-dimensional cob webs based on body condition. Webs built by starved western black widows are more effective traps because they contain more sticky gumfooted threads (Zevenbergen *et al.*, 2008).

As in the studies of choice of foraging site, it can be difficult to ascertain whether spiders with different feeding experiences build webs of different structures because of a memory of prey availability or simply because of internal cues about hunger state. Several experimenters have separated the effects of different aspects of the predation sequence on subsequent behaviour. For example, different groups of *Zygiella x-notata* (Araneidae) spiders were allowed to (a) detect prey that was then removed before the spider touched it; (b) capture prey and transport it to the retreat but not consume it; (c) complete the predation sequence; or (d) to feed on prey that they had not subdued themselves. Control spiders (e) were given no prey. The webs were then destroyed. During the next nocturnal period, spiders that had completed the entire predation sequence built smaller webs. Spiders that captured prey without feeding built webs similar to those of spiders that had completed the predation sequence. There was no effect of prey detection alone on web construction. Spiders that were fed prey by hand delayed web building but did not modify the characteristics of their web. Thus, spiders used information gained during the act of prey capture to change the size and structure of the next web (Venner *et al.*, 2000).

Similarly, Nakata (2007) separated the experience of detecting prey from that of feeding on it by luring orb-web spiders *Cyclosa octotuberculata* with syrphid flies, but pulling the flies away before they were captured. Spiders that only sensed prey increased the total thread length and capture area of their webs relative to controls, but not as much as fed spiders, suggesting that both sensing and capturing prey provide information. In another study, only airborne vibrations of various types and density of prey were available to *Argiope keyserlingi* (Araneidae). Spiders were more likely to build webs when prey were present, but did not alter either the web size or mesh height of their orb (Herberstein *et al.*, 2000).

Orb webs are often asymmetrical, with the hub generally above the centre point. This design is thought to improve prey capture because the spider generally rests at the hub facing downward. Heiling and Herberstein (1999) noted that webs of older *Argiope keyserlingi* and *Larinioides sclopetarius* are more asymmetrical than those of juveniles. By depriving some spiders of the experience of building webs but controlling food intake by hand feeding, they found that spiders that are experienced with web building build more asymmetrical webs than those without experience. In addition, asymmetry increases when the lower portion of the web caught the most prey.

Besides amount of prey, the species of prey influences web structure in some species. *Parawixia bistriata* (Araneidae) build webs of fine mesh at sunset, capturing mainly small dipterans, but build webs of wide mesh during seasonal diurnal termite swarms (Sandoval, 1994). However, this behaviour is exhibited by spiderlings during their first encounter with termites, suggesting that it is not learned. *Parasteatoda tepidariorum* spin thicker and stronger threads when they had previously been fed crickets instead of less feisty pillbugs (Boutry and Blackledge, 2008).

Web architecture sometimes changes in the presence of predator cues. *Argiope versicolor*, like many other orb-web spiders, sometimes includes thick bands of silk called decorations or stabilimenta in its web. A number of functions have been proposed for stabilimenta, including prey attraction and predator defence. In *A. versicolor*, the stabilimentum has the unwanted side effect of attracting a visually hunting predatory spider, *Portia labiata* (Salticidae; Seah and Li, 2001). When exposed to odour cues from *P. labiata*, *A. versicolor* reduced stabilimentum area compared with groups exposed to no odour or the odour of a non-predatory spider, *Lecauge decorata* (Araneidae; Li and Lee, 2004). In contrast, the odour of a praying mantid did not affect web-building behaviour in *Argiope keyserlingi* (Bruce and Herberstein, 2006). The role of learning in building decorations remains unknown.

9.3   Interactions with other animals

Here, we address behavioural plasticity in the contexts of agonistic, social and mating interactions, as well as anti-predator interactions. Spider communication is well studied and we touch on only a few highlights.

9.3.1   Agonistic behaviour

Spider contests can be costly, especially because losers are sometimes cannibalised. Thus, spiders that can adjust their fighting behaviour to behave more cautiously when warranted are likely to have a selective advantage. In spiders, contest duration, intensity and outcome are influenced by relative size of the combatants (e.g. Jakob, 1994, Taylor and Jackson, 2003), a cue that indicates the presence of a valuable resource (e.g. Cross and Jackson, 2009b, Cross *et al.*, 2006, 2007b, Jackson *et al.*, 2006, Wells, 1988), ownership of a resource (e.g. Hoefler 2002), and prior injury (e.g. Taylor and Jackson, 2003). Of particular interest to us is the role of experience in influencing contests. Whitehouse (1997) was first to document in a well-controlled experiment that previous experience influences spider contests. Male *Argyrodes antipodianus* of average size were paired. One spider was then repeatedly paired with larger combatants, and thus had the experience of losing. The other was similarly trained with smaller combatants, and thus trained to be a winner. Members of each pair were then matched against one another for the first time. Spiders trained as winners were more likely to continue to win. Similar effects of fighting experience have been found in other spider species, including crab spiders (Dodson and Schwaab, 2001, Hoefler, 2002) and jumping spiders (Kasumovic *et al.*, 2009).

Combatants may assess their chances of winning a fight by mutual assessment – that is, by assessing their own fighting ability relative to that of their opponent – or self-assessment, in which they determine only their own ability and fighting reserves. These two types of assessment generate different predictions about contest dynamics (Taylor and Elwood, 2003), so it is sometimes possible to distinguish between assessment modes (reviewed in Elias *et al.*, 2008). In an analysis of repeated contests with the same opponent in the jumping spider *Phidippus clarus*, Elias *et al.* (2008) suggest that contest duration is primarily driven by self-assessment, with a secondary role for mutual assessment. As in other species, losing males decrease aggression in subsequent fights.

While the physiological underpinnings of aggressive behaviour in insects are now becoming better understood (e.g. Hoyer *et al.*, 2008, Johnson *et al.*, 2009), only a little is known about the physiological response to aggression in spiders (see Section 9.7). However, the jumping spider *Portia labiata* can distinguish between the draglines of conspecifics that have lost fights versus those that have won fights (Clark *et al.*, 1999), implying that a physiological change brought on by fighting leads to chemical differences in their silk.

9.3.2   Social behaviour

Less than 1% of described spider species show some level of sociality (Uetz and Hieber, 1997). In a number of species, the tendency to form groups varies across populations, generally in those that face different ecological conditions. Common-garden experiments in which individuals from different populations are exposed to the same conditions enable us to ascertain whether the tendency to exhibit social behaviour is predominantly influenced by genetics (e.g. Cangialosi and Uetz, 1987) or the environment. For example, populations of *Parawixia bistriata* from dry habitats show plasticity for group capture of prey, whereas populations from wet habitats did not (Fernández Campón, 2008).

Variation in social behaviour can exist within a population, and even within a social group. For example, *Anelosimus studiosus* (Theridiidae) show two different behavioural phenotypes. 'Social' female spiders cooperate with other adult females in multifemale nests, react less aggressively to predatory cues and prey, and are less active. 'Asocial' females defend their nests against intrusions by adult conspecifics, and are more aggressive and active in other contexts as well (reviews in Pruitt and Riechert, 2009, Pruitt *et al.*, 2008). However, the role of experience in these two behavioural syndromes appears to be minimal (S. Riechert, personal communication). *Holocnemus pluchei*, the pholcid described in Section 9.2.2, joins and leaves groups depending on its size relative to other spiders in the group and on its energy state (Jakob, 1991, 2004), but whether its decisions are influenced by learning is unknown. In another species, the role of experience is clearer. Pourié and Trabalon (2001) forced a normally solitary agelenid, *Tegenaria atrica*, to live in groups after the period when they would normally disperse. Spiders in groups kept with few prey were likely to eat each other, but when prey was abundant, spiders built a communal prey-capture web and foraged in the same area. Thus, in social spiders there is ample evidence for variation in social tendencies, but the role of learning in influencing these tendencies is understudied.

9.3.3   *Mating behaviour*

Although many models of sexual selection assume that a female's preference is consistent (Andersson, 1994), female preference for male traits may in fact be plastic over the female's reproductive period. In spiders, female mating behaviour is influenced by female age (Uetz and Norton, 2007), female diet (Hebets *et al.*, 2008, Wilder and Rypstra, 2008a), and mating history (e.g. Cross *et al.*, 2007a). Male animals may also be choosy, especially when mating is rare and females vary in quality (Bonduriansky, 2001, Hoefler, 2008). In spiders, male choosiness may also change after mating (Gaskett *et al.*, 2004).

The role of experience with members of the opposite sex, separate from the physical act of mating, has been explicitly examined in several species. Several studies have shown that mating behaviours are influenced by what individuals experienced as juveniles. Fishing spider (*Dolomedes triton*, Pisauridae) females exposed, as juveniles, to a series of males were more likely to exhibit pre-copulatory cannibalism than were females that were not exposed to males. This may be because the exposure gives females a way to assess future mate availability, and thus alters the cost of sexual cannibalism (Johnson, 2005). Similarly, the mating behaviour of both male and female *Hogna helluo* (Lycosidae) depends on previous exposure to potential mates (Wilder and Rypstra, 2008b). Females exposed to males without mating were more likely to mate in a subsequent trial, whereas males showed the opposite pattern. Male choice may be acting in this species, so differences between the sexes may be due to the spiders' perceptions of mate availability and willingness to mate (Wilder and Rypstra, 2008b).

Juvenile experience also influences mate choice in *Schizocosa uetzi* (Lycosidae). In a single population, males vary in the amount of black pigmentation on the tibia of their forelegs. Hebets (2003) exposed penultimate females to males of a given phenotype, with forelegs painted either black or brown to mimic the extremes of the natural phenotypic spectrum. After maturity, females were then paired with males of either a familiar or unfamiliar phenotype. Females were more likely to mate with males of a familiar phenotype, and more likely to cannibalise males of an unfamiliar phenotype. This finding is especially interesting given that females were tested at least 11 days after their exposure treatment, and after they had undergone a moult, suggesting very long-term memory.

A different pattern is seen in another species. Hebets and Vink (2007) also examined *Schizocosa* from a mixed population composed of *S. ocreata*, in which males have forelegs ornamented with brushes, and *S. rovneri*, which are not ornamented. Here, females experienced with either brush-legged or non-ornamented males are more likely to mate with brush-legged males upon maturity. Inexperienced females show no preference. Hebets and Vink suggest that experience with males may influence a female's perception of the availability and quality of potential mates, or possibly the female's perception of her own attractiveness.

There are limits to the effects of juvenile experience on mating preferences. Hebets (2007) examined whether subadult female experience with a sympatric heterospecific male could change mating preferences. Regardless of their exposure as juveniles, *Schizocosa uetzi* (Lycosidae) females were more likely to mate with conspecifics rather than *S. stridulans*, implying that species-specific cues override juvenile experience.

9.3.4   Anti-predator behaviour

Spiders respond to cues of their predators. We described in Section 9.2.3 how web architecture may change in the presence of predator cues. Hunting spiders also respond to cues from predators. A number of studies have examined the response of wolf spiders to chemical cues. The wolf spider *Pardosa milvina* reduces activity in the presence of chemical cues from a larger species, *Hogna helluo* (Persons and Rypstra, 2001), especially when the cues come from *Hogna* that had fed on *Pardosa* (Persons et al., 2001). In these studies, field-caught *Pardosa* were used, so the role of learning cannot be evaluated. In another study, naive *Rabidosa rabida* wolf spiders that are exposed to chemical cues to a larger *Pardosa milvina* show more effective anti-predator responses to a live *Pardosa* (Eiben and Persons, 2007). The authors suggest that chemical cues may prime *Rabidosa* to be more attentive towards the predator, and that the response to chemical cues is unlikely to be learned. In contrast, as described in Section 9.2.2, an unpleasant encounter with a scorpion is necessary before *Schizocosa avida* avoids scorpion odour (Punzo, 1997). Thus, within this single family, we see a range in responses to chemical cues from innate to learned.

Courting animals are often at particular risk from predators. The araneophagic salticid *Portia fimbriata* is a predator of the salticid *Jacksonoides queenslandicus*, and prefers to eat females over males. Su and Li (2006) separated members of male and female pairs of *J. queenslandicus* with a clear barrier so that a male could court, but not reach, the female. Members of the pair then were exposed separately to a view of a predatory *Portia*. Male courtship frequency and duration was reduced when females could see the predator, but not when males could see it. Thus, the female's perception of risk most likely led to reduced responsiveness to the male, which in turn reduced his courtship effort (Su and Li, 2006).

9.4   Spatial learning and navigation

Spiders frequently face the challenge of finding their way back to a place they have been before, such as the location where they have left captured prey or the location of a prospective mate. In some cases, spiders can simply follow their own dragline back, but in a complex environment or over a long distance, this option is not available.

Navigation has been most extensively studied in wandering spiders that construct some sort of a retreat, such as a nest or a burrow. They then behave as central-place foragers, leaving the retreat on expeditions to find food or mates and then returning. Retreats are often very valuable resources, offering shelter during the night, in inclement weather, and when moulting, mating, ovipositing and guarding young (Jackson, 1979). They may be energetically expensive to construct, requiring an investment of both time and energy in the form of calorically rich silk or in digging out a suitable hole. Suitable places to construct retreats may also be difficult to find, and even if new sites are available, remaining in an area may bring benefits such as familiarity with the location of resources. For example, when the retreats of the salticid *Paraphidippus aurantius* were destroyed, spiders constructed new nests in the same locations as the old nests even though alternative sites appeared to be available (Mooney and Haloin, 2006). If spiders generally leave the immediate vicinity of their retreat, out of range of proximal cues emanating from it, then some form of memory must be used in order to locate it again. Web-building spiders may face similar problems, albeit over a smaller area. In the absence of odour or vibration cues, spiders might need to remember the location of a retreat or captured and quiescent prey.

Navigating animals may make use of local cues, such as landmarks or beacons, that indicate the location of the goal; the use of global cues, such as celestial or gravitational information, that indicate direction; or path integration, in which an animal keeps track of the direction and distance it has travelled from its starting point (reviewed in Healy, 1998, Wehner and Srinivasan, 2003). These mechanisms are not mutually exclusive (see Cheng *et al.*, 2009, for an example in which multiple strategies are employed). For instance, an animal may use path integration to return to the vicinity of its home, and then rely on local environmental cues for precise location. The use of a particular cue can often be demonstrated experimentally. For example, the araneid *Zygiella x-notata* captures prey on an orb web, and then returns to a nearby retreat to feed. If the web and retreat are flipped upside down when the spider is capturing prey, the spider initially runs in the original direction, and can only find its retreat after exploration (LeGuelte, 1969), suggesting that it uses gravity as a cue.

9.4.1   Landmarks and beacons

Animals may learn that some features of the environment, such as trees or rocks, may indicate the location of their retreat. Environmental features that are close to a goal are called beacons, while those that are further from the goal are landmarks. Intuitively, use of beacons is computationally less demanding than use of landmarks (Shettleworth, 1998).

The use of landmarks and beacons is relatively easy to confirm through experimental manipulation, as was famously demonstrated by Tinbergen and Kruyt's (1938) successful efforts to confuse digger wasps about the location of their nests by moving the surrounding pine cones. Hoefler and Jakob (2006) studied beacon use by the jumping spider *Phidippus clarus* in an overgrown field. By establishing a grid of potential retreat sites (plastic tubes) and individually marking spiders with bee tags, they demonstrated that spiders departed their retreats during the day and then returned to them at night. The role of beacon colour as a cue in locating retreats was then tested by placing nest tubes on dowels of different colours. Spiders colonised the tubes and constructed nests. Spiders were then captured from tubes, and released from a vial placed near a beacon. The first experiment tested three groups: naive spiders that were collected from a nest that did not have a nearby beacon; spiders collected from a nest on a beacon and released near that same familiar beacon; and spiders collected from a nest on a beacon and released near an unfamiliar beacon of the same colour but in a different location. The latter two groups were significantly more likely to approach the beacon than the naive spiders, but did not differ from each other. In a second experiment, all spiders were experienced with beacons, and were tested with a new beacon that was either the same colour as the beacon their nest had been on, or a beacon of a different colour. Spiders were significantly more likely to approach the beacon if it was the same colour as their own, even though other potential cues, such as the surrounding vegetation and the direction of the sun, were not available. Möller (2002) points out that picking out distinctive cues is the first step in landmark navigation, and these brightly coloured beacons against the green vegetation may have been noticeable to the spiders. Spiders in this genus are attracted to tall objects and are willing to cross gaps in order to reach them (Baker *et al.*, 2009), so they may have been predisposed to attend to these beacons.

Another spider that uses local cues to find its nest is *Leucorchestris arenicola* (Araneae, Sparassidae), a large species endemic to the Namib Desert, where it digs burrows into the sand. Because of lethal daytime temperatures on the sand's surface, these spiders are active only at night. Over long distances, these spiders most likely use path-integration mechanisms, as described below, but use local cues when in the vicinity of their nests. Nørgaard *et al.* (2007) captured spiders foraging away from their burrows and displaced them by several metres, a distance too small for spiders to make reliable use of celestial cues. Ten of 12 spiders returned to their burrows. In contrast, when burrows themselves were displaced while spiders were away from them, only three of 15 spiders succeeded in finding them. Thus, spiders are not using odour cues emanating from the burrows, but rather may be using visual cues of the burrow's surroundings.

The jumping spider *Phidippus princeps* can also use beacons to find prey (Jakob *et al.*, 2007). Spiders were given a choice in a T-maze between a red and a blue cube. In training trials, a prey was secured behind a cube of a particular colour. Each spider was given four training trials followed by a probe trial with no prey present, and then a second set of four training trials followed by a probe trial. During the training trials, cubes were randomly assigned to different sides of the T-maze, so that only beacon colour but not its location indicated the location of prey. Spiders were allowed to explore the T-maze for an hour, but not all spiders successfully captured prey during the training trials. During probe trials, the first block chosen by the spider was scored. During the first probe trial (after four training trials) there was no evidence of learning. During the second probe trial (after eight training trials), there was a positive relationship between the number of successful training trials a spider had completed and its ability to correctly choose a block. This task was more difficult than situations that spiders are likely to encounter in nature, given that only colour and not location indicated the correct choice and that spiders were given only one trial per day.

9.4.2   Path integration

An animal using path integration (also known as dead reckoning) is able to take a circuitous outbound journey and then return directly to its starting point without retracing its path (reviewed in Wehner and Srinivasan, 2003). In order to do so, the animal continually updates its estimate of its position by monitoring the direction and distance of its travel and the angles of its turns. In spite of the apparent computational difficulty of this task, a number of arthropods, especially desert ants, are well known to be masters of path integration (e.g. Müller and Wehner 1988). While web-building spiders have also been shown to use path integration (e.g. Moller and Görner, 1994), here we focus on wandering spiders.

A typical test for the use of path integration is to capture an animal that is about to start a return journey to its home location and displace it to a new location. An animal that is using path integration will search for its home location in a spot that is displaced by the same distance and in the same direction as the animal was from the location at which it was captured, whereas an animal that is relying on cues emanating from the home location should be able to find it again, as long as the displacement is not too large.

The wandering spider *Cupiennius salei* (Ctenidae) uses path integration to return to the site of captured prey after being chased away (Seyfarth *et al.*, 1982). To accomplish this task, *Cupiennius* uses idiothetic cues: it monitors its own body movements on the outbound path in order to keep an estimate of its location. Spiders gather information about their body position via lyriform organs, each consisting of a group of parallel slits in the exoskeleton that acts like a strain gauge: deformations in the slits when the animal moves excite nerve cells (Barth, 2002). The role of the lyriform organs in path integration was nicely demonstrated through ablation experiments (Seyfarth and Barth, 1972). Control spiders with intact lyriform organs were able to return to their nests, often in a straight line, whereas manipulated spiders with ablated lyriform organs were not.

The wolf spider *Lycosa tarantula* uses several sources of information during path integration. To measure turn angles, the spiders require visual input acquired through the anterior lateral eyes (Ortega-Escobar, 2006, and references therein). To measure distance travelled, *Lycosa tarantula* uses proprioceptive information (Reyes-Alcubilla *et al.*, 2009). Spiders that are chased away from their burrows can find them again, but those displaced passively in a clear container search near their release point, suggesting that active locomotion is necessary for spiders to estimate distances.

Path integration based solely on idiothetic (animal-centred) cues works only over short distances, because small errors quickly compound to make navigation imprecise (Benhamou *et al.*, 1990, Nørgaard, 2005). Over longer distances, accurate path integration must incorporate external cues for directional information, such as landmarks, celestial cues or magnetism. The desert spider *Leucorchestris arenicola* (Sparassidae), whose use of landmarks was described in the previous section, makes long journeys from the burrow (Henschel, 2002, Nørgaard, 2005), travelling a path as long as 810 m in a single night (Nørgaard, 2005). By masking different eyes with paint, Nørgaard *et al.* (2008) found that vision is necessary for navigation, even though these spiders are active only in darkness. Calculations reveal that the eyes are likely to employ spatial and temporal pooling in order to gain enough resolution to detect landscape structures. In lycosids and gnaphosids, the secondary eyes have evolved different mechanisms to detect the orientation of polarised light (Dacke *et al.*, 1999, 2001), a potential navigational cue.

9.4.3   *Detours and confinement tests*

Detouring is the ability to identify an alternative route to a reward when the direct route is blocked. The araneophagic salticid *Portia* can recognise prey on the basis of visual cues from as far as 30 cm away (Jackson and Blest, 1982), and is able to take long (>1 m) circuitous routes to reach potential prey in a web (Jackson and Wilcox, 1993b). These can be 'reverse-route' detours (Tarsitano and Jackson, 1994), in which the spider must turn away from the prey in order to reach it, and thus must hold a memory of the prey's location when the prey is out of sight. In the laboratory, *Portia* was presented with a prey lure visible from its starting platform, and a choice of routes that either led to the prey or did not. *Portia* can correctly select routes that required walking about 180° away from the lure and walking past where the incorrect route began (Tarsitano and Jackson, 1997), and can select complete routes over those with a gap (Tarsitano and Andrew, 1999; Figure 9.2). *Portia* appears to make its determination of which route to choose by following a simple set of rules: beginning at the lure, visually scan a potential route away from the lure along a horizontal feature, and if the potential route ends, turn back to the lure (Tarsitano and Andrew, 1999). When beginning in an open arena rather than a starting platform, *Portia* performs similarly, initially visually inspecting isolated objects but then switching to objects that are connected to the lure (Tarsitano, 2006). In these experiments, spiders were tested once, and did not learn to solve a problem through trial and error.

The detour behaviour of *Portia* can be flexible depending on the risk imposed by their prey. Spitting spiders in the genus *Scytodes* (Scytodidae) can spit sticky gum from their fangs. *Scytodes* and *Portia* co-occur only in some habitats (Jackson *et al.*, 1998). Because *Scytodes* are dangerous prey, *Portia* will detour around to attack them from the rear. However, *Scytodes* carrying eggs are less dangerous – they are reluctant to drop their eggs but cannot spit when they are holding them, and *Portia* prefer them (Li and Jackson, 2003). When presented with an option to attack a scytodid by leaping directly at it or by taking a time-consuming but safer detour, *Portia* from populations that co-occur with scytodids adjust their predatory strategy based on whether the scytodid is holding eggs. *Portia* spiders chose a direct leap more often when the scytodid is holding eggs and presents less of a risk, and they detour more often when stalking eggless scytodids. In contrast, *Portia* from a population that does not co-occur with scytodids did not vary their approach (Jackson *et al.*, 2002c).

In another design, Jackson *et al.* (2001) tested the role of trial-and-error learning in the ability of *Portia fimbriata* to solve a confinement problem: how to escape from an island surrounded by water. Two options were available: to leap

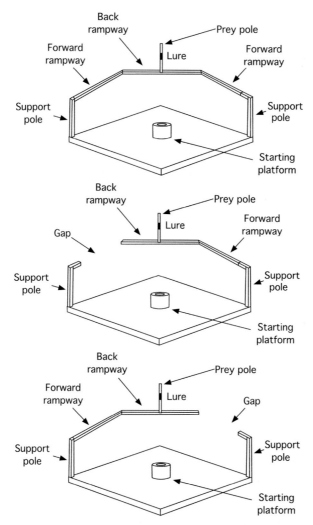

Figure 9.2 Spiders can select the complete route before setting out. (From Tarsitano and Andrew, 1999, with kind permission from Elsevier.)

from the island towards an atoll (Figure 9.3), or to swim. The experimenters could reward either option by making small waves to push the spider towards the atoll, or could instead make waves to push the spider back towards the island. Once on the atoll or back on the island, the spider could make a second choice. From the atoll, it could choose to either swim or leap to reach the edge of the tray. From the island, it could choose again to either swim or leap to reach the atoll. Thus, the relationship between the success of the first choice and the second choice could be determined. Spiders that leaped first and were successful always leaped again. Spiders that leaped first but were preventing from reaching

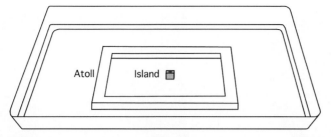

Figure 9.3 Apparatus for testing the ability of salticids to solve a confinement problem. Spiders could leap or swim to reach the atoll from the island, and then leap or swim to reach the wall from the atoll. Spiders were more likely to use a strategy in their second choice if it was successful in their first choice. (From Jackson *et al.*, 2001.)

the atoll usually switched to swimming. Similarly, successful swimmers usually swam again in their second choice, and swimmers that failed in the first trial usually switched to leaping.

9.5   Heat aversion

Several groups of researchers have successfully trained jumping spiders to associate particular colours with an aversive level of heat. Nakamura and Yamashita (2000) were primarily interested in the ability of *Hasarius adansoni* to distinguish particular sets of colours. Spiders were placed in a small cylindrical arena, with floor and sides divided into two semicircles with different colours of papers. During training, half of the arena was heated from below. Spiders were given three three-minute sessions in the arena: no heat (control session), with heat, and again with no heat (test session). Immediately after training, spiders consistently avoided the colour associated with the heat during the test session (Figure 9.4). One day after training, spiders no longer discriminated between the two colours, suggesting that their memory of the association was lost.

VanderSal and Hebets (2007) used a similar procedure, but with a twist: they added a cross-modal cue. Spiders were exposed to a heat stimulus, as above. Some spiders, however, were simultaneously exposed to a seismic cue: a mini-shaker vibrated the arena during all trials. Other spiders were trained with only the heat stimulus. In a test trial with no heat, seismic-group spiders were more likely to avoid the previously heated colour than were non-seismic spiders. The authors suggest that the seismic stimulus may have increased the spiders' arousal or enhanced their attention to the visual cue.

In spite of their somewhat artificial nature, the simplicity of these experimental designs may offer a good tool for comparative studies of salticid abilities.

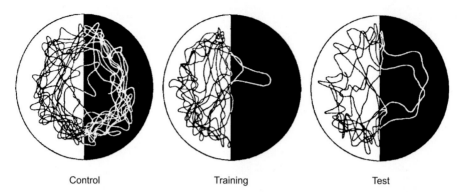

Control   Training   Test

Figure 9.4 Path of a spider in control, training and test trials. In the control trial, the arena (60 mm in diameter) was unheated. In the training trial, the dark side was heated from the bottom. The test trial was in a new, unheated arena. Trials lasted for 3 minutes. (From Nakamura and Yamashita, 2000, with kind permission from Springer.)

For example, our research group (unpublished data) has not been able to replicate the Nakamura and Yamashita (2000) results with several species of *Phidippus*, even though we used colours that we know these spiders can distinguish. Further exploration of species-specific differences is warranted.

9.6   Environmental enrichment

To our knowledge, there are only two studies that show the effect of rearing conditions on the behaviour of spiders. Salticids (*Phidippus audax*) that were laboratory reared were less active in an open-field test, completed less of a reversed-route detour test, and were less likely to respond to videos of prey than were field-caught spiders. Behaviour was also affected by cage size and whether a green stick was provided in the cage (Carducci and Jakob, 2000). Wolf spiderlings (*Hogna carolinensis*) allowed to ride on their mothers' backs, as is normal, for 3 or 5 days were quicker to enter a novel arena than those that did not have this experience (Punzo and Alvarez, 2002). As described in the next section, in wolf spiders these differences are reflected in brain development.

9.7   The neurobiological basis of learning

We begin with a brief overview of the central nervous system (CNS) of spiders. A spider's CNS is divided into two regions, the suboesophageal and supraoesophageal masses, named for their position relative to the oesophagus (Barth, 2002, Foelix, 1996). The suboesophageal region is associated with the nerves of the pedipalps and legs, the viscera, and non-visual sensory systems (Barth, 2002, Foelix, 1996). The supraoesophageal region comprises the cheliceral ganglia, which are associated with the chelicerae, fangs, and poison glands, as well as the protocerebrum (Barth, 2002, Foelix, 1996). For a discussion of the development and organisation of the neuromeres that compose these regions, as well as a comparison with other arthropods, see Scholtz and Edgecombe (2006). Within the protocerebrum, the third optic neuropils of the spider's eyes merge with other nerve tissue to form the visual-association centres (Barth, 2002). As far as is known, the protocerebrum receives direct sensory information only from the visual system, while the suboesophageal region receives direct information from all other sensory systems (Barth, 2002, Foelix, 1996). The protocerebrum and suboesophageal region are connected by longitudinal nerve tracts (Barth, 2002). While a major function of the protocerebrum is visual processing, connections between it and sensory and motor neurons in the suboesophageal mass raise interesting questions about its role in sensory integration and behaviour. In the context of learning and cognition, it is the area of most interest (Barth, 2002, Foelix, 1996).

Much of what we know about the neurobiology of spiders comes from the wandering spider *Cupiennius salei* (Barth, 2002). In *C. salei*, the protocerebrum is divided into two visual association centres, the mushroom bodies and the central body. The paired mushroom bodies accept visual input only from the secondary eyes, while the central body accepts input from both the secondary and principal eyes. In essence, then, visual information from the different eyes undergoes separate but parallel processing (Barth, 2002, Strausfeld and Barth, 1993, Strausfeld *et al.*, 1993).

The names for the mushroom bodies and the central body come from their superficial similarity to structures found in insects, crustaceans, myriapods and onychophorans (Strausfeld, 2009, Strausfeld and Barth, 1993, Strausfeld *et al.*, 1993, 1998), and indeed the structures in spiders were once thought to be homologous (reviewed in Barth, 2002). That hypothesis was challenged by comparative studies suggesting that the chelicerate protocerebrum is not homologous to its insect counterpart (Strausfeld and Barth, 1993, Strausfeld *et al.*, 1993, 2006), but additional studies at the level of gene expression are required.

Experimental manipulations of spider experience and its effect on brain structure have proved informative. For example, wolf spiderlings (*Hogna carolinensis*) allowed to remain with their mother and ride on her back with their siblings have larger protocerebrums, are able to capture prey more efficiently, and learn a maze task more easily than spiderlings raised in isolation (Punzo and Ludwig, 2002). These data indicate that spider brains are affected by the environment and continue to develop after hatching, and suggest that the protocerebrum links to hunting ability, spatial learning and memory (Punzo and Ludwig, 2002), although other regions may also be involved in these behaviours.

Along with structural changes, neurochemical changes have also been linked to spider behaviour. Tarantulas (*Aphonopelma chalcodes*, Theraphosidae) that are trained to raise their legs to avoid a shock show decreased acetylcholinesterase (AchE) activity in their supraoesophageal region (Punzo, 1988a). Punzo (1983) suggests that decreases in AchE might be associated with memory consolidation. The spiders also showed significant increases in RNA and protein synthesis in both the central body and the mushroom bodies (Punzo, 1988a). RNA activity and protein synthesis has been shown to increase in the CNS of grasshoppers, *Schistocerca americana*, when they are subjected to a training regime similar to that of the tarantulas (Punzo, 1980). Tarantulas injected with cycloheximide, which inhibits protein synthesis, show impaired learning (Punzo, 1988a).

Neurochemical changes related to behaviour have also been studied in the tarantula *Aphonopelma hentzi* (Punzo and Punzo, 2001). Males exposed to antagonistic interactions with other males show decreased serotonin and octopamine in their supraoesophageal region compared with control males. The losers of fights show significantly lower levels of both serotonin and octopamine than do winners. Serotonin levels are depressed for up to 24 hours after the fight, while octopamine levels return to normal more rapidly. The complex role played by octopamine in arthropod aggression is still not well understood, and in *Drosophila*, its actions appear to be context dependent (reviewed in Hoyer *et al.*, 2008). Other neurochemicals have been found in the brains of spiders, and much more work needs to be done to identify how these chemicals affect behaviour (Barth, 2002, Punzo, 1988b).

Many mysteries remain in our understanding of the function of the different brain regions and their relationship to behaviour. Arachnologists are somewhat limited in their experimental approaches because the hydrostatic pressure of spiders makes in vivo nerve recording or lesioning extremely difficult (but see Gronenberg, 1989, 1990). However, a large-scale, phylogenetically informed comparative study of brain region interconnectivity, neuronal density and neurochemistry may reveal correlations between behaviour and the brain and offer insights about the general patterns of brain organisation (as in Breidbach *et al.*, 1995). Finally, additional experimental studies in which experience is manipulated and then brain morphology and biochemistry are examined would shed light on the neurological correlates of learning (as in Punzo, 1988a, Punzo and Ludwig, 2002, Punzo and Punzo, 2001). It would be particularly interesting to examine araneomorph spiders, as most manipulative neurochemical work has been done in mygalomorphs.

9.8   Conclusions and outlook

This volume illustrates the value of spiders as excellent organisms for the study of many larger questions in behaviour. This is especially the case for the study of learning and other cognitive processes, a field that offers many opportunities. The following areas are particularly ripe for exploration, and include both proximate and ultimate levels of analysis.

(1) *Neurobiological bases of behaviour.* Neurobiologists are not yet certain about which regions of the central nervous systems of spiders and insects are homologous or independently evolved. We should thus be particularly cautious about assuming that what we learn about the neurobiological basis of learning and cognition in insects applies to spiders. Mapping brain functions and additional studies of the neurochemical changes that underlie behavioural change are the next steps.

(2) *Characterising learning and memory.* Comparative psychologists have developed a battery of methods designed to test different aspects of learning and cognition (e.g. Shettleworth, 2009). Few studies of learning in spiders have explicitly examined fundamental properties of learning, such as how long spiders can remember tasks, and whether learning one task blocks the learning of another task. These questions are especially interesting to study in animals with small brains, as the extent to which brain size restricts the capacity to learn is unclear (e.g. Dukas, 2008).

(3) *Attention and priming.* Of current interest is how animals filter sensory information or are primed to attend to particular stimuli (e.g. Dukas, 2004a). Recent studies suggest that priming, even across sensory modalities (e.g. Cross and Jackson, 2006, 2010), might be a way that spiders direct their attention to what is important in their environment.

(4) *Fitness consequences of learning and cognition.* Throughout this review, we have tried to make it clear why learning or other cognitive processes might be beneficial in a particular context. However, few studies explicitly measure fitness benefits or costs of learning. Although by necessity many studies of learning and cognition must be carried out under controlled conditions, we should not lose sight of the selective forces acting on individuals in nature. Also neglected to date is a thorough investigation of individual differences in learning abilities and cognition (see Dukas, 2004b, for review). Recent work with *Drosophila* (reviewed in Kawecki, 2010) documents how quickly learning

may change in a population when genetic variation is present, and how the evolution of learning may have trade-offs. The presence of interpopulation variation in some of the behaviours we have described (e.g. Jackson *et al.*, 2002c) suggests that this will be a fruitful area of research.

(5) *Comparative studies.* The value of comparative studies in cognition have been amply demonstrated over the last 15 years or so, such as by exploring the correlation between the abilities of corvid species on learning tasks and their dependence on stored seeds (e.g. Balda and Kamil, 1998). The great diversity of spiders – from active hunters to web builders, from salticids with highly acute vision to those taxa that are essentially blind – offers opportunities for comparative studies of learning and cognition that have only begun to be explored. For example, there is tremendous variation even within families. The unusual araneophagic habits and complex environment of *Portia*, for example, may have led to its remarkable cognitive abilities (see Chapter 2). Carducci and Jakob (2000) tested detour behaviour in a much more typical salticid, *Phidippus audax*, with the same apparatus and experimental design that Tarsitano and Jackson (1994) used for *Portia*. Whereas *Portia* easily completed the detour, *P. audax* did not. Although these experiments were done at different times and in different labs and thus comparisons must be drawn with caution, the differences are intriguing. Coupling large-scale comparative analyses of behaviour with neurobiological studies may prove especially fruitful. Perhaps in a decade we will see advances as impressive as in the studies of mushroom bodies of insects (Farris, 2005).

We end our chapter with advice for researchers who may wish to study cognition and learning. Conversation with other arachnologists about their unpublished data, as well as our own experiences, suggests that there are many common experimental methods in animal learning that are very difficult to get to work with spiders. Careful experimental tests of learning require a negative or positive stimulus that can be consistently offered. In many learning studies, particularly in rodents, small bits of food are the usual reward in experiments using positive reinforcement. Selecting an appropriate food reward for spiders generates several difficulties as spiders are famously resistant to starvation (Foelix, 1996). However, even moderately food-deprived spiders can be enthusiastic predators. Spiders offered prey that are small relative to their body size made up to eight consecutive successful predatory attacks on different prey items (Skow and Jakob, 2006).

A second difficulty with food rewards is that many spider species do not detect, or refuse to eat, dead or immobile prey. Using live prey can be problematic because common experimental designs require a certain number of presentations of prey, and an uncooperative insect can mean discarding hard-won data. The use of small arenas, such as petri dishes, can mitigate this problem, but of course this means sacrificing a realistic environment. Where spatial location of the prey is important, it is sometimes possible to tether prey in place so that it can still make small movements (e.g. Jakob *et al.*, 2007). For spiders with good vision, such as lycosids and salticids, videotaped or computer-generated prey can provide a consistent stimulus (Clark and Uetz, 1990, Harland and Jackson, 2002). Of course, video prey do not provide any direct reward, but we have found that spiders persistently attack video images even in the absence of reward. Spiders can be motivated to escape from confinement (Jackson *et al.*, 2001). Finally, heat (e.g. Nakamura and Yamashita, 2000) or low-level foot shock (e.g. Skow, 2007) can be effective aversive stimuli. No method is foolproof or transferable to all species, so when embarking on research with a new spider species, it is essential to allow time for preliminary work in order to devise an appropriate training protocol.

Acknowledgements

We are grateful to Karen Hollis, Fiona Cross, Dan Papaj, Adam Porter, and Marie Herberstein for their thoughtful critiques of earlier drafts. Robert Jackson provided helpful correspondence on several points. We thank Nicholas Strausfeld for sharing his expertise and commenting on a draft of our final sections.

References

Adams, M. R. (2000). Choosing hunting sites: web site preferences of the orb weaver spider, *Neosconsa crucifera*, relative to light cues. *Journal of Insect Behavior*, **13**, 299–305.

Ades, C. (1982). Immediate stimulation and recent experiences as controlling factors in the predatory sequence of the spider *Argiope argentata (Fabricius)*. *Interamerican Journal of Psychology*, **16**, 57–63.

Andersson, M. A. (1994). *Sexual Selection*. Princeton, NJ: Princeton University Press.

Baker, L., Kelty, E. C. and Jakob, E. M. (2009). The effect of visual features on jumping spider movements across gaps. *Journal of Insect Behavior*, **22**, 350–361.

Balda, R. P. and Kamil, A. C. (1998). The ecology and evolution of southwestern seed caching corvids: the perplexing pinyon jay. In *Animal Cognition in Nature* (ed. R. P. Balda, I. Pepperberg and A. C. Kamil). San Diego, CA: Academic Press, pp. 29–64.

Barth, F. G. (2002). *A Spider's World: Senses and Behavior*. Berlin: Springer.

Bays, S. (1962). A study of the training possibilities of *Araneus diadematus* Cl. *Experientia*, **18**, 423–424.

Benhamou, S., Sauvé, J. P. and Bovet, P. (1990). Spatial memory in large scale movements: efficiency and limitation of the egocentric coding process. *Journal of Theoretical Biology*, **145**, 1–12.

Bilde, T., Maklakov, A. A., Taylor, P. W. and Lubin, Y. (2002). State-dependent decisions in nest site selection by a web-building spider. *Animal Behaviour*, **64**, 447–452.

Blamires, S. J., Hochuli, D. F. and Thompson, M. B. (2009). Prey protein influences growth and decoration building in the orb spider *Argiope keyserlingi*. *Ecological Entomology*, **34**, 545–550.

Bonduriansky, R. (2001). The evolution of male mate choice in insects: a synthesis of ideas and evidence. *Biological Reviews*, **76**, 305–339.

Boutry, C. and Blackledge, T. (2008). The common house spider alters the material and mechanical properties of cobweb silk in response to different prey. *Journal of Experimental Zoology*, **309A**, 542–552.

Breidbach, O., Dircksen, H. and Wegerhoff, R. (1995). Common general morphological pattern of peptidergic neurons in the arachnid brain: crustacean cardioactive peptide-immunoreactive neurons in the protocerebrum of 7 arachnid species. *Cell and Tissue Research*, **279**, 183–197.

Bruce, M. J. and Herberstein, M. E. (2006). The influence of predator cues on orb-web spider foraging behavior. *Ethology, Ecology and Evolution*, **18**, 91–98.

Cangialosi, K. R. and Uetz, G. W. (1987). Spacing in colonial spiders: effects of environment and experience. *Ethology*, **76**, 236–246.

Carducci, J. P. and Jakob, E. M. (2000). Rearing environment affects behaviour of jumping spiders. *Animal Behaviour*, **59**, 39–46.

Castanho, L. M. and Oliveira, P. S. (1997). Biology and behaviour of the neotropical ant-mimicking spider *Aphantochilus rogersi* (Araneae: Aphantochilidae): nesting, maternal care and ontogeny of ant-hunting techniques. *Journal of Zoology*, **242**, 643–650.

Cerveira, A. M., Jackson, R. R. and Guseinov, E. F. (2003). Stalking decisions of web-invading araneophagic jumping spiders from Australia, Azerbaijan, Israel, Kenya, Portugal, and Sri Lanka: the opportunistic smokescreen tactics of *Brettus*, *Cocalus*, *Cyrba*, and *Portia*. *New Zealand Journal of Zoology*, **30**, 21–30.

Cheng, K., Narenda, A., Sommer, S. and Wehner, R. (2009). Traveling in clutter: navigation in the Central Australian desert ant *Melophorus bagoti*. *Behavioral Processes*, **80**, 261–268.

Chien, S. A. and Morse, D. H. (1998). The roles of prey and flower quality in the choice of hunting sites by adult male crab spiders *Misumena vatia* (Araneae, Thomisidae). *Journal of Arachnology*, **26**, 238–243.

Chmiel, K., Herberstein, M. E. and Elgar, M. A. (2000). Web damage and feeding experience influence web site tenacity in the orb-web spider *Argiope keyserlingi* Karsch. *Animal Behaviour*, **60**, 821–826.

Clark, D. L. and Uetz, G. W. (1990). Video image recognition by the jumping spider *Maevia inclemens* (Araneae, Salticidae). *Animal Behaviour*, **40**, 884–890.

Clark, R. J. and Jackson, R. R. (2000). Web use during predatory encounters between *Portia fimbriata*, an araneophagic jumping spider, and its preferred prey, other jumping spiders. *New Zealand Journal of Zoology*, **27**, 129–136.

Clark, R. J., Jackson, R. R. and Waas, J. R. (1999). Draglines and assessment of fighting ability in cannibalistic jumping spiders. *Journal of Insect Behavior*, **12**, 753–766.

Craig, C. L., Weber, R. S. and Bernard, G. D. (1996). Evolution of predator-prey systems: spider foraging plasticity in response to the visual ecology of prey. *American Naturalist*, **147**, 205–229.

Cramer, K. L. (2008). Are brown recluse spiders, *Loxosceles reclusa* (Araneae, Sicariidae) scavengers? The influence of predator satiation, prey size, and prey quality. *Journal of Arachnology*, **36**, 140–144.

Cross, F. R. and Jackson, R. R. (2006). From eight-legged automatons to thinking spiders. In *Diversity of Cognition* (ed. K. Fujita and S. Itakura). Kyoto, Japan: Kyoto University Press, pp. 188–215.

Cross, F. R. and Jackson, R. R. (2009a). Cross-modality priming of visual and olfactory selective attention by a spider that feeds indirectly on vertebrate blood. *Journal of Experimental Biology*, **212**, 1869–1875.

Cross, F. R. and Jackson, R. R. (2009b). How cross-modality effects during intraspecific interactions of jumping spiders differ depending on whether a female-choice or mutual-choice mating system is adopted. *Behavioural Processes*, **80**, 162–168.

Cross, F. R. and Jackson, R. R. (2010). The attentive spider: search-image use by a mosquito-eating predator. *Ethology*, **116**, 1–8.

Cross, F. R., Jackson, R. R. and Pollard, S. D. (2007a). Male and female mate-choice decisions by *Evarcha culicivora*, an East African jumping spider. *Ethology*, **113**, 901–908.

Cross, F. R., Jackson, R. R., Pollard, S. D. and Walker, M. W. (2006). Influence of optical cues from conspecific females on escalation decisions during male-male interactions of jumping spiders. *Behavioral Processes*, **73**, 136–141.

Cross, F. R., Jackson, R. R., Pollard, S. D and Walker, M. W. (2007b). Cross-modality effects during male-male interactions of jumping spiders. *Behavioural Processes*, **75**, 290–296.

Dacke, M., Doan, T. A. and O'Carroll, D. C. (2001). Polarized light detection in spiders. *Journal of Experimental Biology*, **204**, 2481–2490.

Dacke, M., Nilsson, D.-E., Warrant, E. J., Blest, A. D. and Land, M. F. (1999). Built-in polarizers form part of a compass organ in spiders. *Nature*, **401**, 470–473.

Diaz-Fleischer, F. (2005). Predatory behavior and prey-capture decision-making by the web-weaving spider *Microthena sagittata*. *Canadian Journal of Zoology*, **83**, 268–273.

Dodson, G. N. and Schwaab, A. T. (2001). Body size, leg autotomy, and prior experience as factors in the fighting success of male crab spiders, *Misumenoides formosipes*. *Journal of Insect Behavior*, **14**, 841–855.

Domjan, M. (2006). *The Principles of Learning and Behavior: Active Learning Edition*, 5th edn. Belmont, CA: Thomson Wadsworth.

Dukas, R. (2004a). Causes and consequences of limited attention. *Brain, Behavior and Evolution*, **63**, 197–210.

Dukas, R. (2004b). Evolutionary biology of animal cognition. *Annual Review of Ecology, Evolution and Systematics*, **35**, 347–374.

Dukas, R. (2008). Evolutionary biology of insect learning. *Annual Review of Entomology*, **53**, 145–60.

Edwards, G. B. and Jackson, R. R. (1994). The role of experience in the development of predatory behaviour in *Phidippus regius*, a jumping spider (Araneae, Salticidae) from Florida. *New Zealand Journal of Zoology*, **21**, 269–277.

Eiben, B. and Persons, M. (2007). The effect of prior exposure to predator cues on chemically-mediated defensive behavior and survival in the wolf spider *Rabidosa rabida* (Araneae: Lycosidae). *Behaviour*, **144**, 889–906.

Elias, D. O., Kasumovic, M. M., Punzalan, D., Andrade, M. C. B. and Mason, A. (2008). Assessment during aggressive contests between male jumping spiders. *Animal Behaviour*, **76**, 901–910.

Farris, S. M. (2005). Evolution of insect mushroom bodies: old clues, new insights. *Arthropod Structure and Development*, **34**, 211–234.

Fernández Campón F. (2008). More sharing when there is less: insights on spider sociality from an orb-weaver's perspective. *Animal Behaviour*, **75**, 1063–1073.

Foelix, R. F. (1996). *Biology of Spiders*, 2nd edn. New York: Oxford University Press.

Forster, L. M. (1977). Some factors affecting feeding behaviour in jumping spiders (Araneae: Salticidae). *New Zealand Journal of Zoology*, **4**, 435–443.

Fritz, R. S. and Morse, D. H. (1985). Reproductive success, growth rate and foraging decisions of the crab spider *Misumena vatia*. *Oecologia*, **65**, 194–200.

Gaskett, A. C., Herberstein, M. E., Downes, B. J. and Elgar, M. A. (2004). Changes in male mate choice in a sexually cannibalistic orb-web spider (Araneae: Araneidae). *Behaviour*, **141**, 1197–1210.

Gronenberg, W. (1989). Anatomical and physiological observations on the organization of mechanoreceptors and local interneurons in the central nervous-system of the wandering spider *Cupiennius salei*. *Cell and Tissue Research*, **258**, 163–175.

Gronenberg, W. (1990). The organization of plurisegmental mechanosensitive interneurons in the central nervous system of the wandering spider *Cupiennius salei*. *Cell and Tissue Research*, **260**, 49–61.

Harland, D. P. and Jackson, R. R. (2000). Cues by which *Portia fimbriata*, an araneophagic jumping spider, distinguishes jumping-spider prey from other prey. *Journal of Experimental Biology*, **203**, 3485–3494.

Harland, D. P. and Jackson, R. R. (2001). Prey classification by *Portia fimbriata*, a salticid spider that specializes at preying on other salticids: species that elicit cryptic stalking. *Journal of Zoology*, **255**, 445–460.

Harland, D. P. and Jackson, R. R. (2002). Influence of cues from the anterior medial eyes of virtual prey on *Portia fimbriata*, an araneophagic jumping spider. *Journal of Experimental Biology*, **205**, 1861–1868.

Healy, S. (1998). *Spatial Representation in Animals*. Oxford, UK: Oxford University Press.

Hebets, E. A. (2003). Subadult experience influences adult mate choice in an arthropod: exposed female wolf spiders prefer males of a familiar phenotype. *Proceedings of the National Academy of Sciences of the USA*, **100**, 13 390–13 395.

Hebets, E. A. (2007). Subadult female experience does not influence species recognition in the wolf spider *Schizocosa uetzi* Stratton 1997. *Journal of Arachnology*, **35**, 1–10.

Hebets, E. A. and Vink, C. J. (2007). Experience leads to preference: experienced females prefer brush-legged males in a population of syntopic wolf spiders. *Behavioral Ecology*, **18**, 1010–1020.

Hebets, E. A., Wesson, J. and Shamble, P. S. (2008). Diet influences mate choice selectivity in adult female wolf spiders. *Animal Behaviour*, **76**, 355–363.

Heiling, A. M. and Herberstein, M. E. (1999). The role of experience in web-building spiders (Araneae). *Animal Cognition*, **2**, 171–177.

Heiling, A. M. and Herberstein, M. E. (2000). Interpretations of orb-web variability: a review of past and current ideas. *Ekológia (Bratislava)*, **19**, 97–106.

Henschel, J. R. (2002). Long-distance wandering and mating by the dancing white lady spider (*Leucorchestris arenicola*) (Araneae, Sparassidae) across Namib dunes. *Journal of Arachnology*, **30**, 321–330.

Herberstein, M. E., Gaskett, A. C., Glenross, D., *et al.* (2000). Does the presence of potential prey affect web design in *Argiope keyserlingi* (Araneae, Araneidae)? *Journal of Arachnology*, **28**, 346–350.

Higgins, L. (2008). Juvenile *Nephila* (Araneae, Nephilidae) use various attack strategies for novel prey. *Journal of Arachnology*, **35**, 530–534.

Hoefler, C. D. (2002). Is contest experience a trump card? The interaction of residency status, experience, and body size on fighting success in *Misumenoides formosipes* (Araneae: Thomisidae). *Journal of Insect Behavior*, **15**, 779–790.

Hoefler, C. D. (2008). The costs of male courtship and potential benefits of male choice for large mates in *Phidippus clarus* (Araneae, Salticidae). *Journal of Arachnology*, **36**, 210–212.

Hoefler, C. D. and Jakob, E. M. (2006). Jumping spiders in space: movement patterns, nest site fidelity and the use of beacons. *Animal Behaviour*, **71**, 109–116.

Hoefler, C. D., Taylor, M. and Jakob, E. M. (2002). Chemosensory response to prey in *Phidippus audax* (Araneae, Salticidae) and *Pardosa milvina* (Araneae, Lycosidae). *Journal of Arachnology*, **30**, 155–158.

Hollis, K. L. (1982). Pavlovian conditioning of signal-centered action patterns and autonomic behavior: a biological analysis of function. *Advances in the Study of Behavior*, **12**, 1–64.

Hoyer, S. C., Eckart, A., Herrel, A., *et al.* (2008). Octopamine in male aggression of *Drosophila*. *Current Biology*, **18**, 159–167.

Huseynov, E. F., Cross, F. R. and Jackson, R. R. (2005). Natural diet and prey-choice behaviour of *Aelurillus muganicus* (Araneae: Salticidae), a myrmecophagic jumping spider from Azerbaijan. *Journal of Zoology*, **267**, 159–165.

Huseynov, E. F., Jackson, R. R. and Cross, F. R. (2008). The meaning of predatory specialization as illustrated by *Aelurillus m-nigrum*, an ant-eating jumping spider (Araneae: Salticidae) from Azerbaijan. *Behavioural Processes*, **77**, 389–399.

Jackson, R. R. (1979). Nests of *Phidippus johnsoni* (Araneae, Salticidae): characteristics, pattern of occupation, and function. *Journal of Arachnology*, **7**, 47–58.

Jackson, R. R. (2002). Trial-and-error derivation of aggressive-mimicry signals by *Brettus* and *Cyrba*, spartaeine jumping spiders (Araneae: Salticidae) from Israel, Kenya, and Sri Lanka. *New Zealand Journal of Zoology*, **29**, 95–117.

Jackson, R. R. and Blest, A. D. (1982). The distances at which a primitive jumping spider, *Portia fimbriata*, makes visual discriminations. *Journal of Experimental Biology*, **97**, 441–445.

Jackson, R. R. and Carter, C. M. (2001). Geographic variation in reliance on trial-and-error signal derivation by *Portia labiata*, an araneophagic jumping spider from the Philippines. *Journal of Insect Behavior*, **14**, 799–827.

Jackson, R. R. and Li, D. Q. (1998). Prey preferences and visual discrimination ability of *Cyrba algerina*, an araneophagic jumping spider (Araneae: Salticidae) with primitive retinae. *Israel Journal of Zoology*, **44**, 227–242.

Jackson, R. R. and Li, D. Q. (2001). Prey-capture techniques and prey preferences of *Zenodorus durvillei*, *Z. metallescens* and *Z. orbiculatus*, tropical ant-eating jumping spiders (Araneae: Salticidae) from Australia. *New Zealand Journal of Zoology*, **28**, 299–341.

Jackson, R. R. and Li, D. Q. (2004). One-encounter search-image formation by araneophagic spiders. *Animal Cognition*, **7**, 247–254.

Jackson, R. R. and Wilcox, R. S. (1993a). Spider flexibly chooses aggressive mimicry signals for different prey by trial and error. *Behaviour*, **127**, 21–36.

Jackson, R. R. and Wilcox, R. S. (1993b). Observations in nature of detouring behaviour by *Portia fimbriata*, a web-building araneophagic jumping spider (Araneae, Salticidae) from Queensland. *Journal of Zoology*, **230**, 135–139.

Jackson, R. R., Carter, C. M. and Tarsitano, M. S. (2001). Trial-and-error solving of a confinement problem by a jumping spider, *Portia fimbriata*. *Behaviour*, **138**, 1215–1234.

Jackson, R. R., Clark, R. J. and Harland, D. P. (2002a). Behavioural and cognitive influences of kairomones on an araneophagic jumping spider. *Behaviour*, **139**, 749–775.

Jackson, R. R., Li, D., Fijn, N. and Barrion, A. (1998). Predator-prey interactions between aggressive-mimic jumping spiders (Salticidae) and araneophagic spitting spiders (Scytodidae) from the Philippines. *Journal of Insect Behavior*, **11**, 319–342.

Jackson, R. R., Pollard, S. D. and Cerveira, A. M. (2002b). Opportunistic use of cognitive smokescreens by araneophagic jumping spiders. *Animal Cognition*, **5**, 147–157.

Jackson, R. R., Pollard, S. D., Li, D. and Fijn, N. (2002c). Interpopulation variation in the risk-related decisions of *Portia labiata*, an araneophagic jumping spider (Araneae, Salticidae), during predatory sequences with spitting spiders. *Animal Cognition*, **5**, 215–223.

Jackson, R. R., Walker, M. W., Pollard, S. D. and Cross, F. R. (2006). Influence of seeing a female on the male-male interactions of a jumping spider, *Hypoblemum albovittatum*. *Journal of Ethology*, **24**, 231–238.

Jakob, E. M. (1991). Costs and benefits of group living for pholcid spiders: losing food, saving silk. *Animal Behaviour*, **41**, 711–722.

Jakob, E. M. (1994). Contests over prey by group-living pholcids (*Holocnemus pluchei*). *Journal of Arachnology*, **22**, 39–45.

Jakob, E. M. (2004). Individual decisions and group dynamics: why pholcid spiders join and leave groups. *Animal Behaviour*, **68**, 9–20.

Jakob, E. M., Skow, C. D., Haberman, M. P. and Plourde, A. (2007). Jumping spiders associate food with color in a T maze. *Journal of Arachnology*, **35**, 487–492.

Japyassu, H. F. and Caires, R. A. (2008). Hunting tactics in a cobweb spider (Araneae-Theridiidae) and the evolution of behavioral plasticity. *Journal of Insect Behavior*, **21**, 258–284.

Japyassu, H. F. and Viera, C. (2002). Predatory plasticity in *Nephilengys cruentata* (Araneae: Tetragnathidae): relevance for phylogeny reconstruction. *Behaviour*, **139**, 529–544.

Johnson, J. C. (2005). Cohabitation of juvenile females with mature males promotes sexual cannibalism in fishing spiders. *Behavioral Ecology*, **16**, 269–273.

Johnson, O., Becnel, J. and Nichols, C. D. (2009). Serotonin 5-HT$_2$ and 5-HT$_{1A}$-like receptors differentially modulate aggressive behaviors in *Drosophila melanogaster*. *Neuroscience*, **158**, 1292–1300.

Kasumovic, M., Elias, D. O., Punzalan, D., Mason, A. C. and Andrade M. C. B. (2009). Experience affects the outcome of agonistic contests without affecting the selective advantage of size. *Animal Behaviour*, **77**, 1533–1538.

Kawecki, T. J. (2010). Evolutionary ecology of learning: insights from fruit flies. *Population Ecology*, **52**, 15–25.

Koh, T. H. and Li, D. Q. (2003). State-dependent prey type preferences of a kleptoparasitic spider *Argyrodes flavescens* (Araneae: Theridiidae). *Journal of Zoology*, **260**, 227–233.

Kreiter, N. and Wise, D. H. (1996). Age-related changes in movement patterns in the fishing spider, *Dolomedes triton* (Araneae, Pisauridae). *Journal of Arachnology*, **24**, 24–33.

LeGuelte, L. (1969). Learning in spiders. *American Zoologist*, **9**, 145–152.

Li, D. Q. (2000). Prey preferences of *Phaeacius malayensis*, a spartaeine jumping spider (Araneae: Salticidae) from Singapore. *Canadian Journal of Zoology*, **78**, 2218–2226.

Li, D. and Jackson, R. R. (2003). A predator's preference for egg-carrying prey: a novel cost of parental care. *Behavioral Ecology and Sociobiology*, **55**, 129–136.

Li, D. and Lee, W. S. (2004). Predator-induced plasticity in web-building behaviour. *Animal Behaviour*, **67**, 309–318.

Li, D. Q., Jackson, R. R. and Barrion, A. (1997). Prey preferences of *Portia labiata*, *P. africana*, and *P. schultzi*, araneophagic jumping spiders (Araneae: Salticidae) from the Philippines, Sri Lanka, Kenya, and Uganda. *New Zealand Journal of Zoology*, **24**, 333–349.

Li, D. Q., Jackson, R. R. and Harland, D. P. (1999). Prey-capture techniques and prey preferences of *Aelurillus aeruginosus*, *A. cognatus*, and *A. kochi*, ant-eating jumping spiders (Araneae: Salticidae) from Israel. *Israel Journal of Zoology*, **45**, 341–359.

Lubin, Y., Ellner, S. and Kotzman, M. (1993). Web relocation and habitat selection in a desert widow spider. *Ecology*, **74**, 1915–1928.

Moller, P. and Görner, P. (1994). Homing by path integration in the spider *Agelena labyrinthica* Clerck. *Journal of Comparative Physiology, A*, **174**, 221–229.

Möller, R. (2002). Insects could exploit UV–green contrast for landmark navigation. *Journal of Theoretical Biology*, **214**, 619–631.

Mooney, K. A. and Haloin, J. R. (2006). Nest site fidelity of *Paraphidippus aurantia* (Salticidae). *Journal of Arachnology*, **34**, 241–243.

Morse, D. H. (1988). Cues associated with patch-choice decisions by foraging crab spiders *Misumena vatia*. *Behaviour*, **107**, 297–313.

Morse, D. H. (1991). Location of successful strikes on prey by juvenile crab spiders *Misumena vatia* (Araneae, Thomisidae). *Journal of Arachnology*, **27**, 171–175.

Morse, D. H. (1993). Choosing hunting sites with little information: patch-choice responses of crab spiders to distant cues. *Behavioral Ecology*, **4**, 61–65.

Morse, D. H. (1999). Choice of hunting site as a consequence of experience in late-instar crab spiders. *Oecologia*, **120**, 252–257.

Morse, D. H. (2000a). The effect of experience on the hunting success of newly emerged spiderlings. *Animal Behaviour*, 2000, **60**, 827–835.

Morse, D. H. (2000b). The role of experience in determining patch-use by adult crab spiders. *Behaviour*, **137**, 265–278.

Morse, D. H. (2000c). Flower choice by naive young crab spiders and the effect of subsequent experience. *Animal Behaviour*, **59**, 943–951.

Morse, D. H. (2007). *Predator Upon a Flower: Life History and Fitness in a Crab Spider*. Cambridge, MA: Harvard University Press.

Morse, D. H. and Fritz, R. S. (1982). Experimental and observational studies of patch-choice at different scales by the crab spider *Misumena vatia*. *Ecology*, **63**, 172–182.

Müller, M. and Wehner, R. (1988). Path integration in desert ants, *Cataglyphis fortis*. *Proceedings of the National Academy of Sciences of the USA*, **85**, 5287–5390.

Nakamura, T. and Yamashita, S. (2000). Learning and discrimination of colored papers in jumping spiders (Araneae, Salticidae). *Journal of Comparative Physiology, A*, **186**, 897–901.

Nakata, K. (2007). Prey detection without successful capture affects spider's orb-web behaviour. *Naturwissenschaften*, **94**, 853–857.

Nakata, K. and Ushimaru, A. (1999). Feeding experience affects web relocation and investment in web threads in an orb-web spider, *Cyclosa argenteoalba*. *Animal Behaviour*, **57**, 1251–1255.

Nakata, K., Ushimaru, A. and Watanabe, T. (2003). Using past experience in web relocation decisions enhances the foraging efficiency of the spider *Cyclosa argenteoalba*. *Journal of Insect Behavior*, **16**, 371–380.

Nørgaard, T. (2005). Nocturnal navigation in *Leucorchestris arenicola* (Araneae, Sparassidae). *Journal of Arachnology*, **33**, 533–540.

Nørgaard, T., Henschel, J. R. and Wehner, R. (2007). Use of local cues in the night-time navigation of the wandering desert spider *Leucorchestris arenicola* (Araneae, Sparassidae). *Journal of Comparative Physiology, A – Neuroethology, Sensory, Neural, and Behavioral Physiology*, **193**, 217–222.

Nørgaard, T., Nilsson, D.-E., Henschel, J. R., Garm, A., and Wehner, R. (2008). Vision in the nocturnal wandering spider *Leucorchestris arenicola* (Araneae: Sparassidae). *Journal of Experimental Biology*, **211**, 816–823.

Ortega-Escobar, J. (2006). Role of the anterior lateral eyes of the wolf spider *Lycosa tarentula* (Araneae, Lycosidae) during path integration. *Journal of Arachnology*, **34**, 51–61.

Patt, J. M. and Pfannenstiel, R. S. (2008). Odor-based recognition of nectar in cursorial spiders. *Entomologia Experimentalis et Applicata*, **127**, 64–71.

Peakall, D. B. (1971). Conservation of web proteins in the spider *Araneus diadematus*. *Journal of Experimental Zoology*, **176**, 257–264.

Pearce, J. M. and Bouton, M. E. (2001). Theories of associative learning in animals. *Annual Review of Psychology*, **52**, 111–139.

Peckham, G. W. and Peckham, E. G. (1887). Some observations on the mental powers of spiders. *Journal of Morphology*, **1**, 383–419.

Persons, M. H. and Rypstra, A. L. (2000). Preference for chemical cues associated with recent prey in the wolf spider *Hogna helluo* (Araneae: Lycosidae). *Ethology*, **106**, 27–35.

Persons, M. H. and Rypstra, A. L. (2001). Wolf spiders show graded antipredator behavior in the presence of chemical cues from different sized predators. *Journal of Chemical Ecology*, **27**, 2493–2504.

Persons, M. H. and Uetz, G. W. (1996a). The influence of sensory information on patch residence time in wolf spiders (Araneae: Lycosidae). *Animal Behaviour*, **51**, 1285–1293.

Persons, M. H. and Uetz, G. W. (1996b). Wolf spiders vary patch residence time in the presence of chemical cues from prey (Araneae, Lycosidae). *Journal of Arachnology*, **24**, 76–79.

Persons, M. H. and Uetz, G. W. (1997). Foraging patch residence time decisions in wolf spiders: is perceiving prey as important as eating prey? *Ecoscience*, **4**, 1–5.

Persons, M. H. and Uetz, G. W. (1998). Presampling sensory information and prey density assessment by wolf spiders (Araneae, Lycosidae). *Behavioral Ecology*, **9**, 360–366.

Persons, M. H., Walker, S. E., Rypstra, A. L. and Marshall, S. D. (2001). Wolf-spider predator avoidance tactics and survival in the presence of diet-associated predator cues (Araneae: Lycosidae). *Animal Behaviour*, **61**, 43–51.

Pourié, G. and Trabalon, M. (2001). Plasticity of agonistic behaviour in relation to diet and contact signals in experimentally group-living *Tegenaria atrica*. *Chemoecology*, **11**, 175–181.

Pruitt, J. N. and Riechert, S. E. (2009). Frequency-dependent success of cheaters during foraging bouts might limit their spread within colonies of a socially polymorphic spider. *Evolution*, **63**, 2966–2973.

Pruitt, J. N., Riechert, S. E. and Jones, T. C. (2008). Behavioural syndromes and their fitness consequences in a socially polymorphic spider, *Anelosimus studiosus*. *Animal Behaviour*, **76**, 871–879.

Punzo, F. (1980). Neurochemical changes associated with learning in *Schistocerca americana* (Orthoptera: Acrididae). *Journal of the Kansas Entomological Society*, **53**, 787–796.

Punzo, F. (1983). Localization of brain-function and neurochemical correlates of learning in the mud crab, *Eurypanopeus depressus* (Decapoda). *Comparative Biochemistry and Physiology, A*, **75**, 299–305.

Punzo, F. (1988a). Learning and localization of brain-function in the tarantula spider, *Aphonopelma chalcodes* (Orthognatha, Theraphosidae). *Comparative Biochemistry and Physiology, A – Physiology*, **89**, 465–470.

Punzo, F. (1988b). Physiological amino-acids in the central nervous-system of the tarantulas, *Aphonopelma chalcodes* and *Dugesiella echina* (Orthognatha, Theraphosidae). *Comparative Biochemistry and Physiology, C – Pharmacology, Toxicology, and Endocrinology*, **90**, 381–383.

Punzo, F. (1997). Leg autotomy and avoidance behavior in response to a predator in the wolf spider, *Schizocosa avida* (Araneae, Lycosidae). *Journal of Arachnology*, **25**, 202–205.

Punzo, F. (2002a). Food imprinting and subsequent prey preference in the lynx spider, *Oxyopes salticus* (Araneae: Oxyopidae). *Behavioural Processes*, **58**, 177–181.

Punzo, F. (2002b). Early experience and prey preference in the lynx spider, *Oxyopes salticus* Hentz (Araneae: Oxyopidae). *Journal of the New York Entomology Society*, **110**, 255–259.

Punzo, F. and Alvarez, J. (2002). Effects of early contact with maternal parent on locomotor activity and exploratory behavior in spiderlings of *Hogna carolinensis* (Araneae: Lycosidae). *Journal of Insect Behavior*, **15**, 455–465.

Punzo, F. and Ludwig, L. (2002). Contact with maternal parent and siblings affects hunting behavior, learning, and central nervous system development in spiderlings of *Hogna carolinensis* (Araneae: Lycosidae). *Animal Cognition*, **5**, 63–70.

Punzo, F. and Preshkar, C. (2002). Environmental, chemical cues associated with prey and subsequent prey preference in the wolf spider *Hogna carolinensis* Hentz (Araneae, Lycosidae). *Journal of Environmental Biology*, **23**, 341–345.

Punzo, F. and Punzo, T. (2001). Monoamines in the brain of tarantulas (*Aphonopelma hentzi*) (Araneae, Theraphosidae): differences associated with male agonistic interactions. *Journal of Arachnology*, **29**, 388–395.

Reyes-Alcubilla, C., Ruiz, M. A. and Ortega-Escobar, J. (2009). Homing in the wolf spider *Lycosa tarantula* (Araneae, Lycosidae): the role of active locomotion and visual landmarks. *Naturwissenschaften*, **96**, 485–494.

Riechert, S. E. (1985). Decisions in multiple goal contexts: habitat selection of the spider, *Agelenopsis aperta* (Gertsch). *Zeitschrift Tierpsychologie*, **70**, 53–69.

Rodríguez, R. L. and Gamboa, E. (2000). Memory of captured prey in three web spiders (Araneae: Araneidae, Linyphiidae, Tetragnathidae). *Animal Cognition*, **3**, 91–97.

Rypstra, A. L., Schmidt, J. M., Reif, B. D., DeVito J. and Persons, M. H. (2007). Tradeoffs involved in site selection and foraging in a wolf spider: effects of substrate structure and predation risk. *Oikos*, **166**, 853–863.

Salomon, M. (2007). Western black widow spiders express state-dependent web-building strategies tailored to the presence of neighbours. *Animal Behaviour*, **73**, 865–875.

Sandoval, C. P. (1994). Plasticity in web design in the spider *Parawixia bistriata*: a response to variable prey type. *Functional Ecology*, **8**, 701–707.

Scholtz, G. and Edgecombe, G. D. (2006). The evolution of arthropod heads: reconciling morphological, developmental and palaeontological evidence. *Development Genes and Evolution*, **216**, 395–415.

Seah, W. K. and Li, D. (2001). Stabilimenta attract unwelcome predators to orb webs. *Proceedings of the Royal Society of London, B*, **31**, 309–318.

Sebrier, M. A. and Krafft, B. (1993). Influence of prior experience on prey consumption behaviour in the spider *Zygiella x-notata*. *Ethology, Ecology, and Evolution*, **5**, 541–547.

Seyfarth, E.-A. and Barth, F. G. (1972). Compound slit sense organs on the spider leg: mechanoreceptors involved in kinesthetic orientation. *Journal of Comparative Physiology*, **78**, 176–191.

Seyfarth, E.-A., Hergenröder, R., Ebbes, H. and Barth, F. G. (1982). Idiothetic orientation of a wandering spider: compensation of detours and estimates of goal distance. *Behavioral Ecology and Sociobiology*, **11**, 139–148.

Shettleworth, S. J. (1998). *Cognition, Evolution, and Behavior*. New York: Oxford University Press.

Shettleworth, S. J., (2001). Animal cognition and animal behaviour. *Animal Behaviour*, **61**, 277–286.

Shettleworth, S. J. (2009). The evolution of comparative cognition: is the snark still a boojum? *Behavioural Processes*, **80**, 210–217.

Skow, C. D. (2007). Jumping spiders and aposematic prey: the role of contextual cues during avoidance learning. Ph.D. thesis, University of Massachusetts at Amherst.

Skow, C. D. and Jakob, E. M. (2006). Jumping spiders attend to context during learned avoidance of aposematic prey. *Behavioral Ecology*, **17**, 34–40.

Smith, H. M. (2009). The costs of moving for a diurnally cryptic spider. *Journal of Arachnology*, **37**, 84–91.

Strausfeld, N. J. (2009). Brain organization and the origin of insects: an assessment. *Proceedings of the Royal Society, B – Biological Sciences*, **276**, 1929–1937.

Strausfeld, N. J. and Barth, F. G. (1993). Two visual systems in one brain: neuropils serving the secondary eyes of the spider *Cupiennius salei*. *Journal of Comparative Neurology*, **328**, 43–62.

Strausfeld, N. J., Hansen, L., Li, Y. S., Gomez, R. S. and Ito, K. (1998). Evolution, discovery, and interpretations of arthropod mushroom bodies. *Learning and Memory*, **5**, 11–37.

Strausfeld, N. J., Strausfeld, C. M., Loesel, R., Rowell, D. and Stowe, S. (2006). Arthropod phylogeny: onychophoran brain organization suggests an archaic relationship with a chelicerate stem lineage. *Proceedings of the Royal Society of London, B*, **273**, 1857–1866.

Strausfeld, N. J., Weltzien, P. and Barth, F. G. (1993). Two visual systems in one brain: neuropils serving the principal eyes of the spider *Cupiennius salei*. *Journal of Comparative Neurology*, **328**, 63–75.

Su, K. F. Y. and Li, D. (2006). Female-biased predation risk and its differential effect on the male and female courtship behaviour of jumping spiders. *Animal Behaviour*, **71**, 531–537.

Tarsitano, M. S. (2006). Route selection by a jumping spider (*Portia labiata*) during the locomotory phase of a detour. *Animal Behaviour*, **72**, 1437–1442.

Tarsitano, M. S., and Andrew, R. (1999). Scanning and route selection in the jumping spider *Portia labiata*. *Animal Behaviour*, **58**, 255–265.

Tarsitano, M. S., and Jackson, R. R. (1994). Jumping spiders make predatory detours requiring movement away from prey. *Behaviour*, **131**, 65–73.

Tarsitano, M. S., and Jackson, R. R. (1997). Araneophagic jumping spiders discriminate between detour routes that do and do not lead to prey. *Animal Behaviour*, **53**, 257–266.

Tarsitano, M. S., Jackson, R. R. and Kircher, W. H. (2000). Signals and signal choices made by the araneophagic jumping spider *Portia fimbriata* while hunting the orb-weaving web spiders *Zygiella x-notata* and *Zosis geniculatus*. *Ethology*, **106**, 595–615.

Taylor, P. W. and Elwood, R. W. (2003). The mismeasure of animal contests. *Animal Behaviour*, **65**, 1195–1202.

Taylor, P. W. and Jackson, R. R. (2003). Interacting effects of size and prior injury in jumping spider conflicts. *Animal Behaviour*, **65**, 787–794.

Theodoratus, D. H. and Bowers, M. D. (1999). Effects of sequestered iridoid glycosides on prey choice of the prairie wolf spider, *Lycosa carolinensis*. *Journal of Chemical Ecology*, **25**, 283–295.

Tinbergen, N. and Kruyt, W. (1938). On the orientation of the digger wasp *Philanthus triangulum* Fabr. III. Selective learning of landmarks. In *The Animal in its World* (ed. N. Tinbergen). Cambridge, MA: Harvard University Press, pp. 146–196.

Toft, S. (1997). Acquired food aversion of a wolf spider to three cereal aphids: intra- and interspecific effects. *Entomophaga*, **42**, 63–69.

Toft, S. (1999). Prey choice and spider fitness. *Journal of Arachnology*, **27**, 301–307.

Uetz, G. W. and Hieber, C. S. (1997). Colonial web-building spiders: balancing the costs and benefits of group-living. In *Evolution of Social Behavior in Insects and Arachnids* (ed. J. C. Choe and B. J. Crespi). Cambridge, UK: Cambridge University Press.

Uetz, G. W. and Norton, S. (2007). Preference for male traits in female wolf spiders varies with the choice of available males, female age and reproductive state. *Behavioral Ecology and Sociobiology*, **61**, 631–641.

VanderSal, N. D., and Hebets, E. A. (2007). Cross-modal effects on learning: a seismic stimulus improve color discrimination learning in a jumping spider. *Journal of Experimental Biology*, **210**, 3689–3695.

Venner, S., Bel-Venner, M.-C., Pasquet, A., and Leborgne, R. (2003). Body-mass-dependent cost of web-building behavior in an orb-weaving spider, *Zygiella x-notata*. *Naturwissenschaften*, **90**, 269–272.

Venner, S., Pasquet, A. and Leborgne, R. (2000). Web-building behaviour in the orb-weaving spider *Zygiella x-notata*: influence of experience. *Animal Behaviour*, **59**, 603–611.

Vollrath, F. (1987). Foraging, growth and reproductive success. In *Ecophysiology of Spiders* (ed. W. Nentwig). Berlin: Springer, pp. 357–370.

Vollrath, F. and Houston, A. (1986). Previous experience and site-tenacity in the orb spider *Nephila* (Araneae, Araneidae). *Oecologia*, **70**, 305–308.

Wehner, R., and Srinivasan, M. V. (2003). Path integration in insects. In *The Neurobiology of Spatial Behaviour* (ed. K. J. Jeffery). Oxford, UK: Oxford University Press, pp. 9–30.

Wells, M. S. (1988). Effects of body size and resource value on fighting behavior in a jumping spider. *Animal Behaviour*, **36**, 321–326.

Whitehouse, M. E. A. (1997). Experience influences male-male contests in the spider *Argyrodes antipodiana* (Theridiidae: Araneae). *Animal Behaviour*, **53**, 913–926.

Wilder, S. M. and Rypstra, A. L. (2008a). Diet quality affects mating behaviour and egg production in a wolf spider. *Animal Behaviour*, **76**, 439–445.

Wilder, S. M. and Rypstra, A. L. (2008b). Prior encounters with the opposite sex affect male and female mating behavior in a wolf spider (Araneae, Lycosidae). *Behavioral Ecology and Sociobiology*, **62**, 1813–1820.

Wullschleger, B. and Nentwig, W. (2002). Influence of venom availability on a spider's prey-choice behaviour. *Functional Ecology*, **16**, 802–807.

Zevenbergen, J. M., Schneider, N. K. and Blackledge, T. A. (2008). Fine dining or fortress? Functional shifts in spider web architecture by the western black widow *Latrodectus hesperus*. *Animal Behaviour*, **76**, 823–829.

Kleptoparasitic spiders of the subfamily Argyrodinae: a special case of behavioural plasticity

MARY WHITEHOUSE

Throughout this book we have seen numerous examples of the flexible nature of spider behaviour. This includes flexibility in silk and web production and design; foraging, anti-predatory and deceptive behaviour; and sociality and courtship behaviour. We have also seen how behavioural plasticity and learning enhances the flexibility of these different behaviours. In this chapter we will look at a subfamily of spiders, Argyrodinae (Theridiidae), to see how all these forms of flexibility contribute to the success of this group. Argyrodinae are by no means the most successful group of spiders, nor are they likely to be the most intelligent (if it were possible to measure such a thing in spiders, that award would undoubtedly go to individuals in the *Portia* genus) but they are an interesting group of spiders that illustrate many of the concepts discussed in the book, and they also show some unusual takes on common themes.

10.1 Introduction

The subfamily Argyrodinae, which contains over 200 species, is well known for its association with the webs of other spiders, and the range of foraging techniques this group uses to exploit other spiders. For example, there are species that glean insects off the edge of the web (e.g. Hénaut, 2000, Kullmann, 1959), eat the silk from the web (e.g. Cangialosi, 1991, Grostal and Walter, 1997, Kerr and Quenga, 2004, Miyashita *et al.*, 2004), steal food bundles caught and wrapped by the host spider (e.g. Hénaut *et al.*, 2005, Legendre, 1960, Miyashita, 2001, Vollrath, 1979a), feed with the host (Baba *et al.*, 2007, Vollrath, 1984, Whitehouse, 1997a), attack the host while it is moulting (Cangialosi, 1990,

Spider Behaviour: Flexibility and Versatility, ed. Marie Elisabeth Herberstein. Published by Cambridge University Press. © Cambridge University Press 2011.

Tanaka, 1984, Whitehouse, 1986) and actively prey on the host or its young (Eberhard, 1979, Larcher and Wise, 1985, Smith Trail, 1980) by either by throwing a sticky thread (Eberhard, 1979, Whitehouse, 1987a) or by lunging at them (Whitehouse, 1986). Some species perform a range of the behaviours listed above while others specialise in only a few.

Not only is this subfamily flexible in its expression of foraging behaviours, but also in its social organisation. Within the family Theridiidae, Argyrodinae form a sister clade to social theridiids (Agnarsson, 2002, 2004; see Chapter 8) that form colonies in which individuals cooperate in prey capture, feed together on prey items and may have communal brood care (Buskirk, 1981, Krafft, 1979, Kullmann, 1972). These cooperative species are considered to have evolved from species showing subsocial maternal care. Argyrodinae show characteristics of subsocial maternal care: they only lay a few eggs (up to about 30 eggs per egg sac) and the female often stays with the egg sac until it has hatched or is close to hatching. There is even one species currently placed in the genus *Argyrodes*, *A. flavipes*, that is a communal social spider and does not exploit the webs of other spider species (Whitehouse and Jackson, 1998). Thus the Argyrodinae group contains species which range from a communal social spider and group-forming kleptoparasitic species to solitary araneophagic species. The common ancestry of Argyrodinae with social spiders may explain why the Argyrodinae have invaded and exploited the webs of other spiders using a range of behaviours. It also may have facilitated the formation of groups around the webs of their hosts.

The range of social organisation in Argyrodinae (from solitary to group living) also results in an array of approaches to courtship, mating and competition for food. In a solitary species, the most important aspect of mating and courtship is to locate a suitable mate. In a group-living species, locating a mate is less of a problem, while successfully courting a partner and competing against other suitors to secure a viable mating is crucial. Competition for mates may indicate why at least one group-living kleptoparasitic species, *Argyrodes antipodianus*, uses over 30 different vibratory displays during courtship (Whitehouse and Jackson, 1994). In this species there are also individual differences in the tactics used to compete for mates (Whitehouse, 1991), and individuals learn their relative fighting abilities (Whitehouse, 1997b).

Thus Argyrodinae show a breadth of behavioural flexibility in nearly all aspects of their lives. The previous chapters have discussed many of these behaviours in spiders in general. In this chapter, I will draw together the arguments from the other chapters to demonstrate how all these forms of flexibility contribute to the success of Argyrodinae. First, I will discuss the relationship between phylogeny and Argyrodinae foraging behaviours in order to understand how such a range of foraging behaviours could have evolved. Next, I will

focus on web building in Argyrodinae and discuss some of the concepts introduced in Chapter 3. This chapter will then concentrate on to the kleptoparasitic
behaviours themselves, examining adaptive trade-offs (as discussed in
Chapter 2) and the role of anti-predatory behaviour (as discussed in Chapter 4)
in shaping Argyrodinae kleptoparasitic behaviour, including the potential to
learn to improve foraging techniques. Chapter 9 presents a critique on the
difference between learning and behavioural plasticity. I will further examine
these concepts with respect to flexibility in kleptoparasitic behaviours, and
flexibility in araneophagic behaviour.

In the final two sections of this chapter I will look at the effect of social
grouping on the courtship and mating behaviour of Argyrodinae. In the first of
these I will discuss how group-living Argyrodinae have avoided some of the
obstacles to adaptive radiation experienced by social spiders, as discussed in
Chapter 8. In the last section I will use social grouping as a reference to discuss
the degree of complexity (as discussed in Chapter 7) in the courtship behaviour
of different species. This will elaborate the discussion on male–male competition presented in Chapters 7 and 9, and differences seen between individuals of
Argyrodinae.

An overriding theme of this chapter is that the shared origin of Argyrodinae
with social theridiids has provided Argyrodinae with the tools to exploit other
spider's webs; the interaction between the degree of sociality expressed by
different Argyrodinae species and their propensity to exploit other spider's
webs has generated the flexibility seen in all behaviours in the Argyrodinae.

10.2   Phylogeny and the flexibility of Argyrodinae foraging behaviours

To exploit the host, Argyrodinae use a mixture of seven key foraging
behaviours: (1) moving onto the host's web and consuming its silk; (2) gleaning
insects off the host's web that have been ignored by the host; (3) stealing food
bundles wrapped by the host; (4) feeding off a food bundle that the host is
feeding on; (5) attacking and consuming a host while it is vulnerable during
moulting; (6) attacking hosts or their offspring by lunging at them, and (7)
catching hosts by throwing a thread of silk with large glue droplets over the
host.

How these behaviours evolved and the relationships between them have
been difficult questions to answer, but are similar to questions on the phylogenetic relationship between different web-building behaviours, as discussed
in Chapter 3. The question that predominates research on Argyrodinae foraging
behaviour is 'how flexible are these foraging behaviours?' For example, do

different genera within Argyrodinae predominantly use one of these behaviours, while species in another genus use another, or do species within the same genera use several different techniques? Alternatively, are these behaviours so interchangeable that the same species will use different behaviours depending on circumstance? In order to address these questions we need to consider the phylogenetic relationships within the Argyrodinae.

The large subfamily Argyrodinae, which consists of over 200 species, has been difficult to categorise phylogenetically (Agnarsson, 2004, Whitehouse et al., 2002, M. Whitehouse, C. Lambkin et al., unpublished data). Argyrodes was first described as a genus by Simon in 1893. He considered Argyrodes to be distinct from two related genera, Rhomphaea and Ariamnes (Simon, 1893). When Exline and Levi (1962) reviewed the American species of Argyrodes they included Rhomphaea and Ariamnes in a single genus, Argyrodes. They recognised six species groups in this large genus: Argyrodes, Rhomphaea, Ariamnes, Cordillera, Cancellatus and Trigonum, which together appeared to form a monophyletic clade (Exline and Levi, 1962). Nevertheless, lumping such a diverse group of animals into a single genus was counterproductive in terms of clarity and understanding, and was never fully accepted (e.g. Whitehouse, 1987a). Consequently, Yoshida (2001) elevated Argyrodes to the subfamily level, Argyrodinae, leaving Argyrodes as a genus and resurrecting the genera Rhomphaea, Ariamnes and Spheropistha. This elevation was strongly supported by Agnarsson (2004) in his comprehensive review of the Theridiidae, where he placed the subfamily Argyrodinae within the clade of theridiid spiders that display subsocial maternal care and sociality. Agnarsson (2004) supported resurrecting Rhomphaea and Ariamnes as genera, and elevated the species group Trigonum to genus level, renaming it Neospintharus, and combined the Cancellatus and Cordillera species groups, naming this genus Faiditus.

Thus the current subfamily Argyrodinae contains six genera: Rhomphaea, Ariamnes, Argyrodes, Spheropistha, Neospintharus and Faiditus. The two main foraging methods in Argyrodinae are araneophagy (eating other spiders) and kleptoparasitism (taking food from other animals). How are these foraging behaviours distributed among the Argyrodinae genera?

Extensive research within Argyrodinae indicates that species in different genera tend to have similar foraging behaviours. Table 10.1 lists some of the currently known Argyrodinae. The table focuses on species about which something is known of their foraging behaviour. The table illustrates that spiders in the genera Rhomphaea and Ariamnes are araneophagic, and do not form groups around the webs of other spiders. Neospintharus is araneophagic, but it also gleans insects off the host's web. Faiditus and Argyrodes are largely kleptoparasitic, with

Table 10.1 *A list of Argyrodinae and their hosts and prey based on published reports*

As the table focuses on the foraging behaviours used by Argyrodinae with each host, not all hosts of Argyrodinae are shown here. The social status (facultatively aggregating, colonial or social) of host spiders is based on Whitehouse and Lubin, 2005. The potential group size of Argyrodinae is given as 1, 2 or many, as the number of Argyrodinae on a host's web is partially dependent on host web size (although most groups would contain less than 15 individuals). Nomenclature is based on Platnick (2010).

Genus	Species	Potential number in a group	Host's/prey's web	Host family	Locality	Host web-type	Argyrodinae foraging behaviour	References
Argyrodes	flavipes	Many	Own web	None	Australia	Argyrodinae's own web (tangle web)	Capture insects by wrapping them and feeding in a group, eat conspecifics, eat conspecific eggs	Whitehouse and Jackson, 1998
Argyrodes	antipodianus	Many	Eriophora pustulosa	Araneidae	New Zealand	Ecribellate vertical orb	Glean insects, eat silk, steal food bundles, feed with host, eat moulting host, attack spiderlings by lunging	Whitehouse, 1986, 1988, Whitehouse and Jackson, 1993
		Many	Nephila edulis	Nephilidae	Australia	Ecribellate vertical orb; facultatively aggregating	Glean insects, steal food bundles	Elgar, 1993
		Many	Nephila plumipes	Nephilidae	Australia	Ecribellate vertical orb; facultatively aggregating	Glean insects, eat silk, steal food bundles	Grostal and Walter, 1997

		Host	Family	Location	Web	Behavior	Reference
Argyrodes	Many	*Cyrtophora hirta*	Araneidae	Australia	Non-sticky horizontal orb with retreat + barrier web	?	Elgar et al., 1983
argentatus	Many	*Argiope appensa*	Araneidae	Guam	Ecribellate vertical orb	Glean insects, eat silk, steal food bundles, feed with the host, eat host	Kerr, 2005
	Many	*Cyrtophora moluccensis*	Araneidae	Guam	Non-sticky horizontal domed orb + barrier web; colonial	Glean insects, steal food bundles	Kerr and Quenga, 2004
	Many	*Argiope argentata*	Araneidae	Panama	Ecribellate vertical orb	Glean insects, eat silk, steal food bundles	Robinson and Olazarri, 1971
	Many	*Nephila pilipes*	Nephilidae	New Guinea	Ecribellate vertical orb	Glean insects, steal food bundles, feed with host	Robinson and Robinson, 1973
Argyrodes	Many	*Cyrtophora citricola*	Araneidae	Sardinia	Non-sticky horizontal orb + barrier web; colonial	Glean insects, steal food bundles, did not feed with host	Kullmann, 1959
argyrodes	Many	*Zygiella x-notata*	Araneidae	Sardinia	Ecribellate vertical orb; facultatively aggregating	Glean insects, eat silk, steal food bundles	Kullmann, 1959
	Many	*Argiope lobata*	Araneidae	Sardinia	Ecribellate vertical orb	Steal food bundles, feed with host	Wiehle, 1928

Table 10.1 (cont.)

Genus	Species	Potential number in a group	Host's/prey's web	Host family	Locality	Host web-type	Argyrodinae foraging behaviour	References
Argyrodes	argyrodes sub. gibbosus	Many	Cyrtophora citricola	Araneidae	Florida	Non-sticky horizontal orb + barrier web; colonial	Steal prey, eat eggs	Edwards, 2006
Argyrodes	bonadea	Many	Nephila clavata	Nephilidae	Japan	Ecribellate vertical orb + barrier web	Glean insects	Miyashita, 2001
Argyrodes		Many	Nephila pilipes	Nephilidae	Japan	Ecribellate vertical orb + barrier web	Glean insects	Miyashita, 2001
Argyrodes	elevatus	Many	Argiope argentata	Araneidae	Costa Rica	Ecribellate vertical orb	Glean insects, eat silk, steal food bundles, feed with host, eat host, eat spiderlings	Vinson, 1863, Vollrath, 1979a, Vollrath, 1979a, Vollrath, 1984
		Many	Nephila clavipes	Nephilidae	Costa Rica	Ecribellate vertical orb + barrier web; facultatively aggregating	Glean insects, steal food bundles, feed with host, eat eggs	Vollrath, 1979a
Argyrodes	fissifrons	Many	Psechrus argentatus	Psechridae	Australia	Cribellate sheet web + barrier web	Glean insects, eat other 'guest' Philoponella undulata (Uloboridae)	Elgar, 1994

Genus	Species	No.	Host species	Host family	Location	Web type	Behavior	Reference
Argyrodes	*fissifrons = kumandai*	?	*Agelena limbata*	Agelenidae	Japan	Non-sticky sheet web + barrier threads	Attack moulting host	Tanaka, 1984
		?	*Parasteatoda japonicum*	Theridiidae	Japan	Ecribellate tangle web	Attack host	Tanaka, 1984
		?	*Linyphia* sp.	Linyphiidae	Japan	Non-sticky sheet web + barrier threads	Attack host	Tanaka, 1984
		?	*Octonoba varians*	Uloboridae	Japan	Cribellate vertical orb	Attack host and eat eggs	Tanaka, 1984
Argyrodes	*flavescens*	Many	*Nephila clavata*	Nephilidae	Japan	Ecribellate vertical orb + barrier web	Glean insects, eat silk	Miyashita et al., 2004
		Many	*Nephila pilipes*	Nephilidae	Japan	Ecribellate vertical orb + barrier web	Glean insects, eat silk	Miyashita et al., 2004
		?	*Gasteracantha cancriformis*	Araneidae	Japan	Ecribellate vertical orb	Glean insects, eat silk	Miyashita et al., 2004
		?	*Leucauge blanda*	Tetragnathidae	Japan	Ecribellate vertical orb	Glean insects, eat silk	Miyashita et al., 2004
		?	*Nephila*	Nephilidae	Japan	Ecribellate vertical orb	Steal food bundles, feed with host	T. Miyashita, pers. comm.
Argyrodes	*incisifrons*	?	*Cyrtophora hirta*	Araneidae	Australia	Non-sticky horizontal orb with retreat + barrier web	Glean insects, steal food bundles, feed with host	Elgar et al., 1983
Argyrodes	*kumadai*	Many	*Cyrtophora moluccensis*	Araneidae	Japan	Non-sticky horizontal domed orb + barrier web; colonial	Glean insects, steal food bundles, feed with host	Baba et al., 2007

Table 10.1 (cont.)

Genus	Species	Potential number in a group	Host's/prey's web	Host family	Locality	Host web-type	Argyrodinae foraging behaviour	References
		1	Agelena silvatica	Agelenidae	Japan	Non-sticky horizontal sheet web + barrier web and a retreat	Glean insects	Baba et al., 2007
Argyrodes	malgaches, = zonatus	Many	Nephila madagascariensis	Nephiliidae	France	Ecribellate vertical orb	Glean insects, do not feed with host	Legendre, 1960
Argyrodes	miniaceus	Many	Nephila pilipes	Nephiliidae	New Guinea	Ecribellate vertical orb	Glean insects, steal food bundles, feed with host	Robinson and Robinson, 1973
Argyrodes	progiles, = projeles?	?	Stegodyphus sarasinorum	Eresidae	India	Cribellate tangle web; social spider		Bradoo, 1983
		?	Nephila clavata	Nephiliidae	India	Ecribellate vertical orb + barrier web		Bradoo, 1983
Argyrodes	sp.	?	Theridion evexum	Theridiidae	Costa Rica	Ecribellate tangle web	Eat eggs	Barrantes and Weng, 2007
Faiditus	caudatus	Many	Nephila clavipes	Nephiliidae	Panama	Ecribellate vertical orb + barrier web; facultatively aggregating	Glean insects, eat silk, eat spiders, eat eggs, eat spiderlings	Vollrath, 1976, Vollrath, 1987

		Many	Nephila clavipes	Nephilidae	Mexico	Ecribellate vertical orb + barrier web; facultatively aggregating	Glean insects, steal food bundles	Hénaut et al., 2005
Faiditus	globosus	Many	Nephila clavipes	Nephilidae	Mexico	Ecribellate vertical orb + barrier web; facultatively aggregating	Glean insects, steal food bundles, feed with host	Hénaut et al., 2005
		?	Gasteracantha cancriformis	Araneidae	Mexico	Ecribellate vertical orb	Glean insects, steal food bundles, feed with host	Hénaut, 2000
Faiditus	ulutans	Many	Anelosimus eximius	Theridiidae	Peru	Ecribellate tangle web; social spider	Glean insects, eat silk, steal food bundles, eat host	Cangialosi, 1990
Spheropistha	spp.	?	?		Japan	?	Glean insects	Yoshida, 2001
Spheropistha	melanosoma	?	Parasteatoda	Theridiidae	Japan	Ecribellate tangle web	Eat spiderlings	T. Miyashita, pers. comm.
Spheropistha	miyashita	?	Nephila, Eriophora	Nephilidae, Araneidae	Japan	Ecribellate vertical orb	Glean insects, eat silk	T. Miyashita, pers. comm.
Neospintharus	baboquivari	1?	Philoponella oweni	Uloboridae	USA?	Cribellate orb web; colonial	Eat eggs, eat host	Smith Trail, 1980
Neospintharus	trigonum	?	Linyphia triangularis	Linyphiidae	USA	Non-sticky dome-shaped sheet web+ barrier web	Attack host	Houser et al., 2005
		1	Own web		USA	Argyrodinae's own web (tangle web)	Capture insects	Cangialosi, 1997

Table 10.1 (cont.)

Genus	Species	Potential number in a group	Host's/prey's web	Host family	Locality	Host web-type	Argyrodinae foraging behaviour	References
		1	Frontinella communis	Linyphiidae	USA	Non-sticky bowl-shaped sheet web + barrier web	?	Cangialosi, 1997
		1	Pityohyphantes costatus	Linyphiidae	USA	Sheet web + barrier web and retreat	Eat host, chase host off web, capture insects	Cangialosi, 1997
		1	Neriene radiata	Linyphiidae	USA	Non-sticky dome-shaped sheet web + barrier web	Eat host, chase host off web, capture insects	Cangialosi, 1997
		1–2	Neriene radiata	Linyphiidae	USA	Non-sticky dome-shaped sheet web + barrier web	Capture insects on host web, attack male by biting and then wrap host, steal food bundles by dislodging host, scavenge dead hosts	Larcher and Wise, 1985
		1–2	Metepeira labyrinthea	Araneidae	USA	Ecribellate vertical incomplete orb web + barrier and retreat	Capture insects, attack host by biting, scavenge dead hosts	Larcher and Wise, 1985
Rhomphaea	fictilium	1	Philoponella oweni	Uloboridae	USA?	Cribellate orb web; colonial spider	Eat host	Smith Trail, 1980

No.	Predator genus	Predator species	Host	Host family	Country	Non-sticky	Behaviour	Reference
1			Frontinella communis	Linyphiidae	USA	Non-sticky bowl-shaped sheet web + barrier web	Eat host	Archer, 1946
1			Argiope trifasciata	Araneidae	?	Ecribellate vertical orb	Eat host	Horton, 1982
1	Rhomphaea	projiciens	Metazygia sp.	Araneidae	Costa Rica		Eat host	Eberhard, 1979
1	Rhomphaea	urquharti?	Achaearanea sp.	Theridiidae	New Zealand	Argyrodinae's own web and prey's web (ecribellate tangle web)	Attack by throwing sticky silk thread	Whitehouse, 1987a
1			Leucauge dromedaria	Tetragnathidae	New Zealand	Argyrodinae's own web	Attack by throwing sticky silk thread	Whitehouse, 1987a
1			Badumna longinqua	Desidae	New Zealand	Cribellate cob web	Eat host	Whitehouse, 1987a
1			Eriophora pustulosa	Araneidae	New Zealand	Ecribellate vertical orb	Attack by throwing sticky silk thread	Whitehouse, 1987a
1	Ariamnes	attenuatus	Ballooning spiders, mainly non-web-building species	Various	Colombia	Argyrodinae's own web – few strands	Attack by throwing sticky silk thread, catch insects using same technique	Eberhard, 1979
1	Ariamnes	colubrinus	Male spiders	Various	Australia	Argyrodinae's own web – few strands	Attack by throwing sticky silk thread, catch insects using same technique	Clyne, 1979
1			Male Sidymella rubrosignata	Thomisidae	Australia	Argyrodinae's own web – few strands	Attack by throwing sticky silk thread	Clyne, 1979

the occasional opportunistic attack on spiderlings or the host while moulting. While the behaviour of species in the *Spheropistha* genus has not been reported in the English literature, it has been reported in the Japanese literature (T. Miyashita, pers. comm.). Like *Faiditus* and *Argyrodes*, *Spheropistha* appears to be kleptoparasitic, although at least one species also attacks spiderlings (Miyashita, pers. comm.; Table 10.1). Thus kleptoparasitic and araneophagic behaviours are distributed in different genera.

A number of arguments have been put forward to explain the relationship between araneophagy and kleptoparasitism within Argyrodinae. Four pathways have been proposed by which kleptoparasitism and free-living araneophagy may have evolved (Whitehouse *et al.*, 2002). First, ecological pressures, rather than evolutionary history, may have dictated the species-specific behaviour, indicating that there is no relationship between phylogeny and behaviour (Model 1). Alternatively, araneophagy and kleptoparasitism may each have evolved once, in which case there are three possible models: free-living araneophagy may have evolved from kleptoparasitism (Model 2). Smith Trail (1980) argued that the kleptoparasitic skills of interpreting the host's vibrations could pre-adapt Argyrodinae for safely stalking and capturing the host itself. Alternatively, kleptoparasitism may have evolved from araneophagy (Model 3). Vollrath (1984) supported this model although he argued that Argyrodinae would initially invade other spiders' webs and chase out the owner, and then later adopt araneophagic behaviours that would pre-adapt them to kleptoparasitism. Finally, both kleptoparasitism and araneophagy may have evolved separately (Model 4). Whitehouse (1987a) proposed this argument based on differences in the araneophagic techniques of species from the predominantly araneophagic (*Rhomphaea* and *Ariamnes*) and kleptoparasitic (*Argyrodes*) genera. Spiders in the *Rhomphaea* and *Ariamnes* genera catch spiders by throwing a thread covered with large glue droplets over the prey spider (Eberhard, 1979, Whitehouse, 1987a). Spiders in the *Argyrodes* genus catch spiders by lunging at them with their front legs (Whitehouse, 1986).

The phylogenetic relationship between kleptoparasitic and araneophagic genera is unclear. Recent molecular and morphological phylogenies have produced conflicting results (Agnarsson, 2004, Arnedo *et al.*, 2004, Whitehouse *et al.*, 2002). Work produced using six American species (which was part of a larger study of Theridiidae) indicates that araneophagic genera are more derived, while kleptoparasitic genera are more basal, suggesting that araneophagy may have evolved from kleptoparasitism (Agnarsson, 2004). However, the work was based on morphological and behavioural characters. Work using five spiders of Argyrodinae also from the Americas (and also as part of a larger study) that used nuclear and michondrial DNA characters found that the two representatives of the araneophagic genera, *Rhomphaea* and *Ariamnes*, evolved on separate branches (Arnedo *et al.*, 2004). Microchondrial DNA characters on 24 species of Argyrodinae mainly from Australia also indicated that the araneophagic genera *Rhomphaea* and *Ariamnes* were not closely related, and that the American *Ariamnes* were quite distinct from the Australian *Ariamnes* (Whitehouse and Lambkin, unpublished data).

These results show that more phylogenetic work is needed to produce a consensus tree using species from all continents to resolve the relationship between genera. The current molecular data indicate inconsistency in the current morphological taxonomy, which may be confounded by rapid radiation within the subfamily. Argyrodinae seem to radiate rapidly on newly colonised landmasses (e.g. the radiation of *Ariamnes* in Hawaii; Gillespie and Rivera, 2007) and this could result in convergent evolution within the subfamily, which may explain the discrepancy in the position on the molecular phylogenetic tree of *Ariamnes*-like Argyrodinae from Australia and America.

The confusion between results in the phylogenetic studies suggests that the evolution of foraging behaviours in Argyrodinae may be flexible; possibly in much the same way as the evolution of web-building behaviour is in spiders in general (Chapter 3). Therefore, despite broad behavioural differences between kleptoparasitic and araneophagic genera, there is still a lot to establish about the evolution of foraging behaviours within Argyrodinae.

10.3   Argyrodinae and webs

As mentioned in Chapter 3, spider silk and spider webs vary considerably. The webs of some species (such as the Araneidae) contain silk with sticky glue droplets, while others (e.g. Uloboridae) achieve adhesion using very fine cribellate silk. Other webs have no specific stickiness and just rely on the web structure to knock down the prey (e.g. Agelenidae; see Chapter 3).

Spider webs vary greatly in size and in structure (e.g. tangle webs, vertical orb webs and horizontal sheet webs). Webs may be occupied by a solitary spider or there could be hundreds of spiders in a social spider colony. Webs can also vary between individuals of the same species, and within the same individual, depending on environmental constraints and hunger levels (Chapter 3).

For kleptoparasites such as the Argyrodinae, exploiting these different web types presents several problems: (1) the physical constraints due to the different silk types, (2) the need to interpret the vibrations from the different web shapes, and (3) the need to respond to the behaviour of one or multiple hosts. In addition the Argyrodinae need to adjust to the idiosyncrasies of each host species; such as whether they feed at the centre hub of the web or in a retreat; whether they suspend their food bundles at the hub or scatter them over the web; or whether they respond aggressively when they detect Argyrodinae on the web or ignore them. Given this diversity, can individual Argyrodinae adjust to a range of webs, or do different species specialise on a particular web type?

All Argyrodinae build some form of tangle web (sometimes called a space web). *Ariamnes* builds a flimsy web consisting of one main horizontal strand (supported by a few vertical strands) upon which it hunts spiders that have ventured onto the web (Eberhard, 1979). *Rhomphaea* builds a similar web and also catches spiders on this thread. However, it also invades other spiders' webs to capture the owner. It does not seem to build a web when venturing onto another spider's web (Whitehouse, 1987a). Kleptoparasitic Argyrodinae, such as those in the *Argyrodes* genus, build a small, scaffolding-like web attached to the web of their host (or even amongst the tangle web of their host). It uses this structure to make forays into the host's web and uses it as a scaffolding into which it hoists large food bundles cut out of the host's web (Robinson and Robinson, 1973, Whitehouse, 1986).

Faiditus ululans does a variation on scaffolding technique – it cuts holes through the tangled web of its host's (*Anelosimus eximius*) colony like tunnels. When *F. ululans* is chased by a host spider it swings though the tunnels on its own silk attached to the host's silk above (Cangialosi, 1991).

Thus the scaffolding web is a novel approach to web use not discussed in Chapter 3. Instead of using its web to catch prey directly, kleptoparasitic Argyrodinae build a scaffolding web to navigate around the sticky silk of the host web. The scaffolding web is also an anti-predatory device: *Argyrodes* can swing into it and into safety at any time it is detected and attacked by the host (Whitehouse, 1986). By attaching a scaffolding web to the host's web, kleptoparasitic Argyrodinae also reduce the impact of web variability between hosts on its foraging behaviour. This could increase the variety of webs that it can exploit.

Table 10.1 lists the main hosts and prey of Argyrodinae studied to date. Because Argyrodinae may use webs for shelter and may not feed in all the webs where it is found (Whitehouse, 1988) only the main hosts or hosts for which foraging behaviours have been described are included. Hosts exploited by kleptoparasitic Argyrodinae mainly build ecribellate or non-sticky webs. Some build sheet webs, but the majority build vertical orb webs. Conspicuous by their rarity are cribellate webs. The ability of *Argyrodes antipodianus* to kleptoparasitise the cribellate webs of *Badumna longinqua* (Desidae) was quite poor (Whitehouse, 1988). First, the kleptoparasite stuck to the silk and had difficulty removing itself (while it could walk through glue droplets on araneid webs). Second, it was more likely to be eaten, and finally it had a very low success rate at obtaining food (Whitehouse, 1988). Cribellate hosts of kleptoparasitic Argyrodinae are rare, but include the social spider *Phryganoporus candidus* (Desidae; = *Badumna candida*), which is a host to *Argyrodes alannae* and *A. rainbowi* in Australia

(Whitehouse, personal observation), and *Stegodypus sarasinorum* which is the host of *Argyrodes projeles* in India (Bradoo, 1983). Details on how these Argyrodinae obtain food from their cribellate hosts are not known.

Of the 15 *Argyrodes* and three *Faiditus* kleptoparasitic Argyrodinae in Table 10.1, only *Faiditus ululans* does not exploit at least one orb-web spider (Orbiculariae). Of these, ten exploit a *Nephila* species. The preference for orb-web spiders, especially *Nephila* (Miyashita, 2002) suggests that these webs may have characteristics particularly suited for kleptoparasitism (Hénaut *et al.*, 2005, Miyashita, 2002, Vollrath, 1987, Whitehouse *et al.*, 2002). *Nephila* build large, permanent webs that have a three-dimensional barrier web attached. Permanent webs are likely to be easier for Argyrodinae to locate than more transient webs. Permanence also reduces the need for Argyrodinae to remake and relocate their own scaffolding web. A vertical orb increases the effectiveness of a scaffolding web as a structure into which to swing to safety. *Nephila* also remain at the central hub of the web and do not build a retreat to the side. Stealing food from retreats is likely to be more risky than stealing food from the hub because scaffolding webs cannot be used so there is little means of escape should the kleptoparasite be detected by the host. The hub of the web is likely to be less risky for Argyrodinae than a retreat because Argyrodinae can connect their scaffolding web directly to the hub, making the hub easily accessible, and if Argyrodinae are attacked by the host, they can swing away to safety.

Nephila is also behaviourally ideal for kleptoparasitic Argyrodinae. They are big spiders that rarely go after small flies caught on their webs. These small flies are therefore available for Argyrodinae to glean. They are also slower than other species to respond to prey, so trapped prey is easier for an Argyrodinae to steal (Hénaut, 2000) and gives an Argyrodinae a better chance of escape if detected. *Nephila* also store their food bundles at the hub and feed at the hub (Hénaut, 2000, Robinson and Robinson, 1973), which makes them easier and less risky for an Argyrodinae to locate and exploit. Given the good fit of *Nephila* to the needs of Argyrodinae, work is required to test if *Argyrodes* and *Faiditus* evolved their kleptoparasitic behaviours to exploit *Nephila* webs specifically (and then later attacked other orb-web spiders) or whether they evolved their kleptoparasitic behaviours independently of the presence of *Nephila*. In addition, the preference by *Argyrodes* and *Faiditus* for orb-web spiders and *Nephila* in particular suggests some limitations on kleptoparasitism. So how flexible are kleptoparasitic behaviours?

10.4   Flexibility of kleptoparasitic behaviours

Before flexibility within kleptoparasitism can be discussed, the use of the term 'kleptoparasitism' needs to be addressed. There has been some debate as to whether Argyrodinae are kleptoparasites, which implies a cost to the host, or merely kleptobionts, indicating that they take food that is of no consequence to the host (Elgar, 1993, Vollrath, 1984). Supporters of the term kleptobiont argue that a direct fitness cost to the host is rarely measured and only inferred (Hénaut et al., 2005, Vollrath, 1984) and that some Argyrodinae only eat the silk and glean small insects off the host's web that the large host would not consume anyway (Legendre, 1960). However, even silk production is costly (Opell, 1998, Tanaka, 1989), a nutritious resource in itself (Sherman, 1994, Townley and Tillinghast, 1988) and many hosts take down their webs each day, eating the silk as they do so, thereby consuming both the silk and any small prey caught in the silk. So even if kleptoparasites consume only the silk, let alone eat small prey, they impose a cost to the host spiders that take down their web daily.

Even hosts that do not take down their webs diurnally, such as *Nephila* species, suffer a cost from Argyrodinae infestations (Grostal and Walter, 1997, Larcher and Wise, 1985, Rypstra, 1981). These studies have shown that hosts readily move when the concentration of kleptoparasites is too high. Because of the exploitative relationship between Argyrodinae and their hosts, it is reasonable to classify the foraging behaviours of Argyrodinae as kleptoparasitic or araneophagic, and then focus on how kleptoparasitism and araneophagy is expressed within this group.

Within the kleptoparasitic species there are further more fine-scale definitions. From his work in Panama, Vollrath identified specialist and generalist kleptoparasitic Argyrodinae (Vollrath, 1984). Vollrath found that *Argyrodes elevatus* used a range of foraging techniques but it was largely limited to *Nephila* webs. Alternatively, *Faiditus caudatus* exploits a range of hosts (Vollrath, 1984, although these are not identified) but its kleptoparasitic behaviour is largely limited to gleaning insects from around the edge of the host's web.

Vollrath suggested that specialist species use more complex behaviours that require a detailed 'understanding' of the host's web construction and the host's behaviour in order for the kleptoparasite to be successful without being eaten. Two behaviours that could be described as specialist behaviours are feeding with the host and stealing wrapped food bundles. *Argyrodes elevatus* attempts to steal food from its host *Nephila clavipes* only once it detects wrapping vibrations on the web (Vollrath, 1979b), indicating that it is finely tuned into the behaviour of its host.

Generalist kleptoparasites, by contrast, remain on the outer reaches of the host's web where they glean insects and eat silk. They do not require a detailed 'understanding' of the host's behaviour, and therefore may be able to exploit a greater range of hosts.

In Chapter 2, Nelson and Jackson caution against the use of diametrically opposed terms such as generalist and specialist feeders. In particular, they query whether the commonly held view that there is a trade-off between behavioural specialisation to capture prey and variety of prey types attacked: 'the jack of all trades is the master of none'. They argue that some spiders, such as *Portia fimbriata*, are able to develop specialist prey-capture techniques for a number of prey (Chapter 2, Jackson and Hallas, 1986, Jackson and Wilcox, 1990). Thus there may be no need for a trade-off and an individual Argyrodinae could use a specialist behaviour (such as feeding with the host) for a number of hosts. Cangialosi (1997) also does not agree with the term 'specialist kleptoparasite'. She argues that the Argyrodinae *Neospintharus trigonum* could be specialist of many species. For example, *N. trigonum* changes its foraging techniques depending on whether it is exploiting *Neriene radiata* or *Pityohyphantes costatus*; with *N. radiata* it is more likely to take over the host's web, possibly killing the host in the process, while with the larger *P. costatus*, whose web also has a retreat, it is more likely to kleptoparasitise the web.

Argyrodes kumadai of Japan is another good example of where this dichotomy may not be a useful approach. This spider uses a range of foraging techniques when kleptoparasitising *Cyrtophora moluccensis* that include stealing food bundles and feeding with the host (Baba *et al.*, 2007) and therefore it behaves as a specialist kleptoparasite. However, when it kleptoparasitises *Agelena silvatica*, it limits its foraging behaviours to that of a generalist by only gleaning insects off the host's web (Baba *et al.*, 2007). Thus *A. kumadai* maintains its flexibility in host choice by modifying the kleptoparasitic techniques it uses with its different hosts. Nevertheless, *A. kumadai* illustrates that while it may not be useful to describe Argyrodinae species as specialists and generalists, it may be useful to identify specific kleptoparasitic behaviours as more or less specialised, based on the degree to which Argyrodinae need to interact with the host in order for them to be successful.

Table 10.1 provides information on 15 species of *Argyrodes* and three species of *Faiditus*. Because the genus *Argyrodes* has only recently been split into *Argyrodes, Rhomphaea, Neospintharus, Ariamnes, Faiditus* and *Spheropistha* (Agnarsson, 2004, Yoshida, 2001), there may still be species within this genus that should be placed elsewhere. *Argyrodes fissifrons* appears to be a behavioural outlier in the *Argyrodes* as it attacks a range of other spiders and little is known about *Argyrodes* sp. In addition, *Argyrodes flavipes* is a social spider, and is also probably in the wrong genus. Therefore the following discussion on the kleptoparasitic Argyrodinae will not include these species.

Kleptoparasitic Argyrodinae use two behaviours – stealing wrapped food bundles and feeding with the host – that could be described as specialist behaviours. Of the 15 species of *Argyrodes* in Table 10.1, seven steal food bundles and feed with the host; of the three species of *Faiditus*, all steal food bundles and one feeds with the host. So at this stage there appears to be no indication that species using specialist and generalist kleptoparasitic behaviours are confined to separate genera.

Not surprisingly, most of the studies that have looked in detail at the foraging behaviours of kleptoparasitic Argyrodinae have focused on their interactions with orb-web spiders, especially *Nephila* (Table 10.1). Thus reports of Argyrodinae using specialist behaviours on non-orb-web spiders may be under-represented. Nevertheless, of the seven species reported to feed with the host, all feed with orb-web spiders, while of the nine species reported to steal the host's food bundles, all do so from orb webs except *Faiditus ululans*, which steals food bundles from the social spider *Anelosimus eximius* (Theridiidae; Cangialosi, 1990). So at least one species can use a specialist behaviour on a non-orb-web spider. *Neospintharus trigonum* also steals food bundles from the linyphiid *Neriene radiata*, but is does so by dislodging the host rather than stealthily removing it (Cangialosi, 1997). Of all the hosts or prey listed in Table 10.1, only five produce cribellate silk. In addition, *Faiditus subdolus* has been found on *Philoponella oweni* webs (Smith Trail, 1980), while *Argyrodes allanae* and *A. rainbowi* have been found on *Phryganoporus candidus* webs (Whitehouse, personal observation).

Because of limited information it is not possible to conclude if kleptoparasitic Argyrodinae that use specialised foraging behaviours are limited to only a few hosts (stenophagy) while those that use more generalised behaviours attack a greater range of hosts (europhagy). Indeed, as Chapter 2 pointed out, such linkages may not be useful. What we can say is that there is a strong bias among kleptoparasitic Argyrodinae to exploit only a few types of orb webs, and that to date, feeding with the host has only occurred on these webs; even to the extent that within one species, *Argyrodes kumadai*, feeding with the host was used with its orb-web host *Cyrtophora moluccensis*, but not with its sheet-web host *Agelena silvatica* (Baba *et al.*, 2007).

10.4.1   *Predation risk and flexibility of kleptoparasitic behaviours*

A reason why feeding with the host may be limited to a few orb-web spiders while other foraging behaviours are used with a wider range of hosts is because they vary in the extent to which they expose the Argyrodinae to the risk of predation by the host: the less dangerous the behaviour, the lower the risk of using it with several hosts without modification; the more dangerous the behaviour, the more likely that it will only be used with a limited number of suitable hosts.

Gleaning insects and feeding on the silk are probably the least dangerous foraging methods, as they only require stealth to avoid detection from the host. Stealing large food bundles is more complex as the Argyrodinae need to cut the food free without alerting the host. This has to be done carefully with the use of silk threads to replace the food bundles so that the loss of web tension does not alert the host to the theft. To do this, Argyrodinae attach the dragline silk to the host web, holding onto the silk connected to the food bundle while cutting it. Once cut, the Argyrodinae slowly let the dragline take the strain of the cut thread and attach the thread back onto the web, or else they just slowly release the thread, allowing the rest of the web take up the strain (Vollrath, 1979a, Whitehouse, 1986). The food bundles are then transferred from the host's web to the scaffolding web of Argyrodinae, where the host usually cannot locate it.

Feeding with the host is probably the most dangerous and difficult foraging behaviour any kleptoparasitic Argyrodinae uses, as well as the most effective in terms of the energy gained per time foraging (Whitehouse, 1997a). To feed with the host, the kleptoparasite must be undetected while feeding within a few millimetres of the mouthparts of a potential predator (Legendre, 1960, Robinson and Robinson, 1973). By feeding with the host, Argyrodinae are able to tap into much greater food reserves than they could otherwise obtain, and they can consume them very quickly. Animals will accept a high predation risk when the rate of food uptake is high (Berger-Tal *et al.*, 2010, Kotler and Blaustein, 1995) as part of a trade-off between food and safety (Brown, 1988), which may explain why Argyrodinae feed with the host despite the dangers (Whitehouse, 1997a).

Foraging behaviours with higher predation risks may also need to be more flexible in order to tailor that behaviour to a specific host, thereby reducing predation risk. Argyrodinae only feed with orb-web spider hosts. However, individuals in a species of Argyrodinae may not always have access to the same host species. The abundance of host species may vary between seasons and at different times of the year (Miyashita, 2002). Thus different hosts are often present for different generations of Argyrodinae who may need to modify their behaviour to suit their host (Baba *et al.*, 2007). Learning is more likely to develop if there is variation between generations but consistency within generations (Stephens, 1993). Thus it could be advantageous for a species of Argyrodinae using risky foraging techniques to be able to learn how to modify its behaviour to suit potentially different hosts.

But Argyrodinae have a very limited cognitive capacity. In Chapter 9, the neurobiological basis of learning is described. The part of the brain that is attracting the greatest interest with respect to learning and cognition is the protocerebrum, which is primarily a visual centre (Chapter 9). Unlike Salticidae, Argyrodinae have poor vision, and so have not needed to develop a ganglion in the protocerebrum to process visual information. If a ganglion developed for visual assessment is also used in cognition, then this may have further constrained the cognitive abilities of Argyrodinae.

Nevertheless there is evidence that some kleptoparasitic Argyrodinae are able to modify their behaviour, improving with experience their ability to exploit a particular host. Vollrath (1984) reports an experiment in which some *A. elevatus* that had been deprived of experience of a *Nephila* host's web as juveniles were provided with the opportunity to steal food bundles from a *Nephila* web. He describes a trend in which the likelihood of finding a food bundle and successfully stealing the food bundle improved with experience.

Argyrodes antipodianus in Australia has access to large orb-web spiders such as *Nephila* (which are about 100 times heavier than *A. antipodianus*). However, the same species in New Zealand is largely limited to the webs of the orb-web spider *Eriophora pustulosa*, which is considerably smaller (only about 10 times as heavy as *A. antipodianus*). Because *E. pustulosa* is more similar in size to *A. antipodianus* than *Nephila*, it is harder for *A. antipodianus* to move undetected around the smaller host's web, and feeding with *E. pustulosa* is more problematic. For example, while *A. antipodianus* can easily feed with *Nephila* from the same side of the web, it is difficult for *A. antipodianus* to feed on the same side of the web as *E. pustulosa* without being detected. *Eriophora pustulosa* usually feeds at the hub with its food bundle slightly poking through the plane of the web. The best position for *A. antipodianus* to feed with *E. pustulosa* is from the other side of the web, where the food bundle is exposed, and *A. antipodianus* has some protection should the host detect its presence.

To see if *A. antipodianus* needed to learn how to feed with *E. pustulosa*, *A. antipodianus* from New Zealand, which had never been exposed to orb webs, were tested on orb webs as adults and compared with *A. antipodianus* that were experienced with orb webs (Whitehouse, 1992, Whitehouse, unpublished data). Results showed that naive *A. antipodianus* were just as likely to move onto an orb web and towards the hub to feed as experienced individuals, but that experienced spiders were faster than naive spiders at reaching the hub, and experienced *A. antipodianus* were more likely to move to the other side of the orb web if they approached from the wrong side than naive individuals. Thus *A. antipodianus*, like other spiders discussed in Chapter 9, is able to improve its prey-capture technique with experience. Feeding on the same side of the web as *E. pustulosa* is a detouring error (see Chapter 9) that experienced *A. antipodianus* correct; however, it is not an error when it occurs on the webs of other larger potential hosts. *Argyrodes antipodianus* is thereby maintaining flexibility in its kleptoparasitic foraging behaviour in order to modify it to specific hosts.

This is also a clear example of where the distinction between foraging and anti-predatory defence is blurred, as discussed in Chapter 4. However, *A. antipodianus* give a new twist to flexibility in anti-predatory behaviour by the way it uses learning to adjust its behaviour to a specific predation threat.

There are many other examples where Argyrodinae modify their behaviour to tailor it to a particular host. For example, *A. elevatus* searches for food bundles only at the hub in *Nephila* webs, but in *Argiope* webs it does so both at the hub and in the orb web (Vollrath, 1979a). *Argyrodes argyrodes* gleans insects and steals food bundles from *Cyrtophora citricola* and *Zygiella x-notata*, but does not feed with them, while with *Argiope* it does not glean insects but does feed with the host (Kullmann, 1959). *Faiditus ululans* modifies its stealing strategy depending on the number of host spiders that respond to capture the prey (Cangialosi, 1991). *Argyrodes kumadai* uses a range of kleptoparasitic techniques with *Cyrtophora moluccensis*, but with *Agelena silvatica* it only gleans insects (Baba *et al.*, 2007). *Neospintharus trigonum* also changes its foraging techniques depending on whether it is exploiting *Neriene radiata* or *Pityohyphantes costatus* (Cangialosi, 1997). It would be interesting to know if learning plays a role in these behaviours as well.

In Chapter 2, Nelson and Jackson discuss ecotypic variation in the predatory behaviour of different populations of *Portia fimbriata*. The exploitation by *A. antipodianus* of *E. pustulosa* webs in New Zealand but not Australia may be an example of this. However, although *A. antipodianus* are not normally found on *E. pustulosa* webs in Australia, we do not know whether Australian *A. antipodianus* could learn to adapt to these webs if given the opportunity.

10.5   Flexibility of araneophagic behaviours

Argyrodinae that predominantly attack other spiders (araneophagy), are those in the *Neospintharus*, *Rhomphaea*, and *Ariamnes* genera. They seem to be less restrictive than the kleptoparasites in the type of spider they exploit, although reports are also more vague, as prey is described as 'ballooning spiders', 'web builders' or '*Linyphia, Araneus and Frontinella*' (Table 10.1). *Ariamnes* and *Rhomphaea* capture spiders by throwing a thread covered in large glue droplets over the prey. Some use small leg movements to create vibrations on the web to attract the spider prey towards them (Whitehouse, 1987a).

Spiders in the genus *Neospintharus* seem to be opportunistic araneophages (Cangialosi, 1997). For example, it seems that the relative size of *Neospintharus trigonum* to the host spider may influence whether it is a predator or a kleptoparasite of the host (Cangialosi, 1997, Larcher and Wise, 1985). *Neospintharus trigonum*'s method of catching prey consists of biting the prey and then wrapping it (Cangialosi, 1997), which is more similar to the technique used by kleptoparasitic species (see below) than the true araneophages.

Many predominantly kleptoparasitic species of *Faiditus* and *Argyrodes* attack spiders. The webs of some host species, such as *Crytophora moluccensis*, are used by both their young and by other non-kleptoparasitic spiders as frameworks from which to construct their own webs (Berry, 1987, Lubin, 1974, Proctor, 1992). This provides Argyrodinae kleptoparasitising these webs with the opportunity to attack non-host spiders such as the eggs and young of *C. moluccensis* (Lubin, 1974). Argyrodinae such as *Faiditus caudatus* also attack the eggs of other hosts such as *Nephila clavipes* (Vollrath, 1976). Some kleptoparasitic Argyrodinae such as *A. kumandai* and *A. antipodianus* feed on moulting hosts (Tanaka, 1984, Whitehouse, 1986). *Argyrodes kumandai* attacks its much larger host by biting its joints while it is moulting and vulnerable. As the host is unable to defend itself, *A. kumandai* begins to feed and thereby kills the host (Tanaka, 1984). Other kleptoparasitic Argyrodinae such as *F. ululans* attack small hosts (Cangialosi, 1990), while others (*A. antipodianus, A. elevatus, F. caudatus*) attack spiderlings (see Table 10.1).

The two kleptoparasitic species in which the araneophagic capture technique is well known are *Faiditus ululans* and *Argyrodes antipodianus*. They attack small spiders using a completely different method from that used by spiders in the *Ariamnes* and *Rhomphaea* genera: they lunge at their prey with their front two pairs of legs, and scoop the small spiders towards their mouthparts where they are bitten (Whitehouse, 1986, Whitehouse *et al.*, 2002).

Although both predominantly araneophagic and predominantly kleptoparasitic Argyrodinae use quite different prey capture methods to catch spiders (lunging and throwing silk), both will lure spiders towards themselves using aggressive mimicry. When catching small theridiids (*Achaearanea* sp.), *A. antipodianus* slightly 'shuffles' its tarsi on the web. This creates vibrations that appear to attract the theridiid to within lunging distance (Whitehouse, 1986). Likewise, *Rhomphaea* sp. from New Zealand uses small leg movements that appear to attract the prey to within striking distance of its sticky silk (Whitehouse, 1987a).

Both Chapter 4 and Chapter 6 discuss aggressive mimicry. Chapter 6 notes that among spiders, aggressive mimicry is most commonly used against web-building spiders. The vibratory deception used by Argyrodinae follows this pattern. In Chapter 4 aggressive mimicry vibrations are also argued to be anti-predatory, given that the spider being hunted could eat the hunting spider. While this is unlikely to be the case when kleptoparasitic Argyrodinae catch very small spiders, it could influence signals broadcast by araneophagic Argyrodinae when they target spiders similar in size to themselves. This possibility needs to be explored.

Argyrodes antipodianus only opportunistically attacks spiderlings, and this behaviour was observed under laboratory conditions. The frequency at which it attacks spiderlings as part of its normal foraging behaviour is unknown, but is assumed to be less frequent than its kleptoparasitic foraging behaviours. Additionally, whether *A. antipodianus* attacks spiderlings depends on whether spiderlings are present around the host's web. Thus some *A. antipodianus* may be exposed to this food source while others may not. This potential variability between generations but consistency within a generation suggests that this behaviour is a potential candidate for learning (Stephens, 1993). As *A. antipodianus* can adjust its 'feeding with the host' behaviour to accommodate different hosts, can it also improve its ability to feed on spiderlings to take advantage of when they are plentiful?

To see if *A. antipodianus* was able to improve its ability to catch spiderlings, the ability of inexperienced adult *A. antipodianus* to catch *Achaearanea* spiderlings was compared with that of experienced adult *A. antipodianus* and inexperienced juvenile *A. antipodianus*. Experienced adults were less likely to make mistakes (for example, lunge in the wrong direction) than inexperienced adults, and more successful at catching spiderlings, but they were no better than inexperienced juveniles (Whitehouse, 1992, Whitehouse, unpublished data). In Chapter 9, learning is defined as 'a sustained change in behavioural performance resulting from a change in the cognitive representation of relationships between cues'. However, from the limited data available, it seems that experience in catching spiderlings stops the deterioration of the ability of *A. antipodianus* to catch spiderlings rather than stimulates its development. As such, it is not strictly learning as described above, but it appears to be an example of 'use it or lose it' behavioural plasticity.

10.6   Sociality and foraging behaviours

Within the Theridiidae, the Argyrodinae form a clade with social spiders and spiders with subsocial maternal care (Agnarsson, 2004). This phylogenetic association may explain some of the foraging characteristics of Argyrodinae, while at the same time Argyrodinae may have avoided some of the constraints normally confronted by social spiders. Cooperative social spiders cooperate in prey capture, feed together on prey items and may have communal brood care (Buskirk, 1981, Kullmann, 1972; see Chapter 8 for a complete discussion on cooperative social spiders). Cooperative species are considered to have evolved from species showing subsocial maternal care, where one mother cares for her offspring but once the mother dies, the offspring stay together for some time, dispersing before maturing to the adult stage (Evans, 1998). The transition from subsocial to cooperative social groups involves a transition from an outbreeding system to one with regular inbreeding, which is thought to be driven by the high cost of dispersal. Cooperative social spiders are uncommon, with only 25 species in six different families, representing as many as 19 independent evolutionary transitions to sociality (Chapter 8). The level of inbreeding in these species seems to have seriously limited their chances of adaptive radiation, indicating that the development of sociality in spiders is an evolutionary dead end (see Chapter 8 for a discussion of this).

Argyrodinae seem to have avoided this fate. Like subsocial and social spiders, kleptoparasitic Argyrodinae produce few offspring per clutch, and form groups consisting of up to 45 spiders around the same *Nephila* web (Vollrath, 1984). However, unlike theridiid social spiders, Argyrodinae are not highly inbred. In contrast to the social spiders, dispersal costs seem low for Argyrodinae species as all life stages regularly move between host webs (Whitehouse and Jackson, 1993) reducing the likelihood of inbreeding and associated constraints. Thus there has been no restriction on species radiation in Argyrodinae, given that there are over 200 species of Argyrodinae.

Nevertheless, other factors associated with spider sociality may be relevant to Argyrodinae. In a recent approach to sociality, Whitehouse and Lubin (2005) emphasised that that social groups may have primarily a reproductive, protective or foraging function, depending on whether they enhance the reproductive, protective or foraging aspect of the animal's life (sociality may serve a mixture of these functions). By identifying which function influences a particular social behaviour we can determine how that social behaviour will change under different conditions, and which models are most pertinent. Using this approach with spiders, they argued that unlike eusocial insects where the groups are largely governed by the reproductive function of their groups, the group characteristics of social spiders are largely governed by the foraging function of the group.

The function of groups of kleptoparasitic Argyrodinae species is strictly foraging. Spiders are congregating around the host spiders to secure food, not to raise offspring. Thus models relating to the dynamics of foraging groups will be most relevant to Argyrodinae. For example, the cooperative hunting model (Packer and Ruttan, 1988) investigates the conditions in which cooperation, cheating or scavenging is expected in foraging groups. Packer and Ruttan (1988) argue that a population of pure cooperators could be an evolutionarily stable strategy (ESS) only if the typical prey is small enough to be monopolised by one hunter. If large animals are the usual prey, cheaters and scavengers could invade, as their strategy will yield larger individual benefits.

This model is very relevant to kleptoparasitic Argyrodinae because they have taken the concept of cheating, in a cooperative hunting sense, to an extreme. For example, when kleptoparasitic Argyrodinae feed with the host (who cannot monopolise its large prey) they cheat the host by both exploiting the prey-capture ability of the host and also its digestive enzymes, especially as the host is consuming a prey much larger than Argyrodinae could digest on its own (Cangialosi, 1990, 1991, Elgar 1993, Legendre, 1960, Smith Trail, 1980, Vollrath, 1976, 1984, Whitehouse, 1997a).

While foraging, kleptoparasitic Argyrodinae like *A. antipodianus* are flexible in the degree of tolerance they show towards conspecifics, which is also in agreement with predictions of the cooperative hunting model. According to the model, individuals will fight over a resource that can be controlled by one individual, but not fight for a resource that cannot be controlled (Packer and Ruttan, 1988). *Argyrodes antipodianus* will rest within a couple of centimetres of conspecifics on the scaffolding web when they are not feeding, thereby showing tolerance. But when feeding *A. antipodianus* will fight vigorously over a food bundle in the scaffolding web, and for control of the scaffolding thread attached to or near a food bundle upon which the host is feeding. Thus they will fight for a foraging resource they can control. However, once *A. antipodianus* is at the hub of the host's web, near the host and trying to feed on the host's food bundle, they will touch another feeding *A. antipodianus* but do not respond aggressively towards them (Whitehouse, 1997a). Thereby *A. antipodianus* show tolerance towards conspecifics when all are feeding on a resource they cannot dominate, in agreement with predictions based on the cooperative hunting model.

However, cooperative hunting dynamics are unlikely to be the main factor influencing Argyrodinae's tolerance of conspecifics when feeding with the host. To feed with the host, the Argyrodinae must be within a few millimetres of the mouthparts of the much larger host that would readily consume the Argyrodinae individual if it were caught. As any vibration would alert the host to the presence of the Argyrodinae, not responding to conspecifics at the hub enables *A. antipodianus* to reduce the risk of detection and therefore predation by the host (Whitehouse, 1997a). Thereby intraspecific tolerance is also an anti-predatory response.

The predisposition of Argyrodinae to tolerate conspecifics may have originated from its common origin with social and subsocial theridiids. The juveniles of spiders with maternal care form feeding groups. Thus these spiders are tolerant of other spiders sharing their web. Tolerance of sharing webs with other spiders would pre-adapt Argyrodinae to invade other spider's webs to steal food. It may also have pre-adapted them to avoid responding aggressively to the presence of other conspecifics when it is not expedient to do so.

In summary, flexibility with respect to the tolerance of *A. antipodianus* towards conspecifics appears to be influenced by a number of factors: (a) a genetic disposition of tolerance towards conspecifics, (b) cooperative hunting dynamics and the possibility of cheating or controlling a food resource, and (c) the opportunity to reduce predation risk in the trade-off between food and safety. If the findings for *A. antipodianus* are applicable to other kleptoparasitic Argyrodinae, then there are a number of factors maintaining the flexibility of tolerance towards conspecifics in Argyrodinae.

10.7   Competition for mates and mating behaviour

An intriguing question in the courtship and mating behaviour of animals is why are some courtships expressed as simple displays while others are complex? The expression of spider courtship and mating behaviour is discussed in Chapter 7 from the perspective of sexual selection. However, in order for sexual selection to have a strong influence, spiders need to have access to more than one mate. As Chapter 7 points out, the biggest selective constraint on mating in some solitary species can be finding a mate.

In social species where competition for mates is high, sexual selection should have a strong influence on the expression of courtship and mating behaviour. Although this effect may be dulled in social spiders with high inbreeding levels, group-living Argyrodinae are not constrained by inbreeding and therefore may experience strong sexual selection pressures.

Argyrodinae range from solitary to group-living species, thus these spiders represent a great opportunity to study the effect of sociality and access to mates on the evolution of courtship and mating behaviour. Solitary araneophagic Argyrodinae are likely to have less access to mates than group-forming kleptoparasitic Argyrodinae. Thus solitary Argyrodinae may have more simple courtship displays than kleptoparasitic Argyrodinae, as solitary males are not subject to the same level of competition from other males.

Factors that influence the complexity of the courtship and mating behaviour of spiders are often associated with female receptivity, female choice or even cryptic female choice (Aisenberg and Eberhard, 2009, Shamble *et al.*, 2009). These mechanisms require that the female has access to a number of suitors from which she can choose the sperm she will use. Thus female choice may be particularly relevant to the courtship behaviour of group-forming kleptoparasitic Argyrodinae, where access to suitors is high.

The courtship behaviour of *Argyrodes antipodianus* appears to fit the model of a complex courtship display by a group-living kleptoparasitic Argyrodinae. During courtship and mating, the displays are very variable, and the interaction can last up to eight hours. The courtship and mating sequence of *A. antipodianus* falls into three phases. Phase one starts when the male locates the female's web and finishes with the first mating. Vibratory displays in this phase are limited to the males shuddering in response to the female's silk. If the female is receptive, she taps the silk. Both sexes tap as they move towards each other and they mate for a few minutes (Whitehouse and Jackson, 1994). Females receive enough sperm from this mating to produce offspring. Phase two, which is very variable in length (up to 3 hours), is a period of quite intricate courtship vibratory displays where males and females performed up to 30 different forms of tapping, bouncing, pulling and shuddering, interspersed with relatively long mating bouts (6 s to 4 minutes) in no predictable order. In phase three, which usually lasts about half an hour, the male appears to be depositing a sperm plug. This phase is terminated by the female chasing the male away (Whitehouse, 1991, Whitehouse and Jackson, 1994).

The courtship behaviour of another *Argyrodes*, *A. zonatus*, has been briefly described (Legendre, 1960). In this spider the female seizes the cephalothoracic protrusions of the male with her pedipalps and performs elaborate vibratory courtship displays caused by plucking the silk with her legs. The courtship behaviour of the male is not described, although Legendre noted that many males court the female simultaneously. Although this description clearly indicates that the female put her mouthparts on the cephalothoracic protrusions of the male, it is difficult to say if the courtship was complex or simple.

Most of the complexity in the courtship display of *A. antipodianus* is seen in the second phase after the first mating (Whitehouse, 1991), which is surprising, given that the female can produce offspring after just the first mating (Whitehouse, personal observation). This indicates that cryptic female choice may be influencing the courtship complexity of *A. antipodianus*. Cryptic female choice occurs when females favour the use of one male's sperm over another after mating has occurred (Aisenberg and Eberhard, 2009). Aisenberg and Eberhard (2009) suggested that one of the strongest supports for the existence of cryptic female choice is courtship behaviour during sperm transfer, such as the complex courtship display by *A. antipodianus* in phase two.

Alternatively, the prolonged mating sequence may be part of a strategy to make the female unreceptive to subsequent suitors. In *Drosophila*, males produce a substance that reduces the female's propensity to re-mate (Bretman *et al.*, 2010). In the Argyrodinae, males are renowned for the strange protrusions at the front of the cephalothorax. These protuberances vary between genera: males in the genus *Argyrodes* possess two pronounced hairy protuberances, one behind the other; *Neospintharus* males also have two protuberances with hairs, but they are not so close to each other; *Faiditus* males have a hairy cavity below the eyes; *Rhomphaea* either have a single protuberance between the eyes or none at all, while *Ariamnes* have no protuberances.

Beneath these protuberances, at least in the *Argyrodes* genus, are clypeal glands (Legendre and Lobez, 1975), which produce a secretion that can been seen on the hairs of the protuberances (Whitehouse, 1987b). To mate, the females in the genus *Argyrodes* place their mouthparts between the male's protuberances (Legendre, 1960, Whitehouse and Jackson, 1994). As she moves her mouthparts over the protuberances, she is possibly consuming the secretion produced by the clypeal glands (Whitehouse and Jackson ,1994). Thus the courtship behaviour may be multimodal (as discussed in Chapter 7) consisting of vibratory and taste stimuli.

The role of the clypeal secretion is unclear. It may work as an anti-aphrodisiac, reducing female re-mating. By engaging in a long complicated courtship, the male may be enticing the female to feed on more of this secretion, while at the same time giving himself time to make more secretions while he is away from the female performing the courtship displays or to give himself time to make a sperm plug. Alternatively, the secretion may enhance cryptic female choice, where males are judged by the quality of the secretion, which may be a nuptial gift. The role of this substance would be an interesting avenue to explore.

The courtship behaviour of a solitary araneophage, *Rhomphaea urquharti* from New Zealand, has also been described (Whitehouse, 1987a). This solitary species, which has no protrusions, has a more simple courtship, consisting of up to 16 vibratory displays. During the initial phase the male scrapes his pedipalp over the female's epigynum before jumping away, which suggests a strong anti-predatory aspect to the courtship display. Towards the end of the sequence the pedipalp is inserted for longer and it starts to swell, suggesting sperm transfer. The courtship display of *R. urquharti* is most complex prior to copulation. This species, like many *Rhomphaea*, does not have cephalothoracic protruberances, and the female does not place her mouth on the male's cephalothorax, so clypeal secretions are unlikely to be affecting this courtship behaviour or female re-mating.

The comparison between *A. antipodianus* and *R. urquharti* fits into the prediction that group-forming kleptoparasitic Argyrodinae will have more complex courtship displays than solitary araneophagic Argyrodinae. However, these are only two species, and the comparison is confounded by the presence and absence of the cephalothoracic protruberances.

Faiditus ululans forms groups around the social spider *Anelosimus eximius* (Theridiidae). It is kleptoparasitic in that it will glean insects and steal food bundles from the host, but it does not feed with the host (Cangialosi, 1990). It will also feed on dead host spiders. The courtship behaviour of *F. ululans* is described as simplistic (Cangialosi, 1990) and seems to be similar to phase one of the courtship and mating behaviour of *A. antipodianus*. Thus the mating behaviour of this Argyrodinae does not support the idea that group-forming Argyrodinae have more complex courtship behaviours than solitary Argyrodinae. The mating position of *F. ululans* is not described, although it does have a hairy groove below the eyes that could contain pores for clypeal gland excretions. Males in this species seem to move quickly between females, mating with many females consecutively (Cangialosi, 1990). It is possible that males in this species are less likely to actively compete for mates (through prolonged courtship and male–male competition) but may try to dilute the presence of other males' sperm by mating often with as many females as possible. More work is needed to test this idea.

Thus the courtship behaviour of Argyrodinae, at least in some species, is flexible in terms of the number of displays used and their order. The courtship behaviour is also variable between species, as is manifested in the range of cephalothoracic protuberances in Argyrodinae. Whether the complexity of the courtship display can be predicted based on the social organisation of the Argyrodinae, the form of the cephalothoracic protuberances, the presence of clypeal glands, or all of the above, requires further investigation.

10.7.1   Male–male interactions

One factor that strongly influences the courtship behaviour of *A. antip- odianus* is the fact that more than one male can be courting the same female. If two males try to court a female at the same time, they often fight for access to the female (see Chapter 7 for a review of factors influencing male–male competition in spiders). Classical game theory models supported arguments that males use contests to assess the fighting ability of their opponent (e.g. Enquist and Leimar, 1983). More recent developments in game theory have acknowledged that animals may assess themselves more than their opponents (Arnott and Elwood, 2009, Taylor and Elwood, 2003). Despite these developments, the influence of experience on combat tactics has received little work (see Chapter 7 for a discussion of this).

In *A. antipodianus*, males move through a series of escalations, which climax with grappling and biting, when fighting for access to females (Whitehouse, 1991). In these fights the males' experience of winning or losing previous fights strongly influences the outcome of the fight (Whitehouse, 1997b). This was demonstrated in an experiment in which pairs of male spiders were matched for size. The pairs were then split up, with one of the pair trained to lose contests (experiencing many training fights with large opponents) while the other was trained to win contests (experiencing many training fights with small opponents). When the trained spiders were tested against their partners, the male that had been trained to win contests was more likely to win the fight against the male of the same size who had only experienced losing contests (Whitehouse, 1997b). These findings demonstrate that *A. antipodianus*' assessment of its fighting ability is flexible, and that it can learn to be a winner or loser.

This result suggests that *A. antipodianus* is more likely to assess its own like-lihood of winning a contest, rather than assess the ability of its opponent to win a contest. This argument is supported by the fact that inaugural fights between large male *A. antipodianus* matched for size are more likely to escalate than fights between small males matched for size. It seems that *A. antipodianus* is modifying its self-assessment of its ability to win fights after experiencing a number of wins or loses (Whitehouse, 1997b).

How *A. antipodianus* assesses itself is unclear. The training may have influenced the contests by altering the spider's perception of its own fighting ability within the population, possibly by following a Bayesian strategy (Iwasa *et al.*, 1981, Valone and Brown, 1989), or by developing a rule of thumb (Bouskila and Blumstein, 1992). To follow a Bayesian strategy, a spider would adjust the estimation of its fighting ability by raising it after a win, and lowering it after a loss. If the spider were altering the perception of itself, a competitor would need to apply more effort and escalate the contest to a higher level to convince a trained winner to lose, but less effort to convince a trained loser to lose.

Alternatively, experience may have affected the outcome of the contests presented here through the development of a rule of thumb (Bouskila and Blumstein, 1992). For example, experience may alter how much effort a spider will put into a fight. This strategy requires no assessment of the opponent's fighting abilities, nor of the animal's own fighting abilities. The rule of thumb is: if I am prepared to escalate further than my opponent, I win, and will increase the energy I put into the next contest. If my opponent escalates further than me, I lose, and I will reduce the energy I put into the next contest. Thus the level of escalation is predetermined before each contest, even though it is based on the results of previous contests.

Thus *A. antipodianus*' ability to learn to be winners or losers is not as flexible as it first appears. While males can learn to modify their fighting behaviour and therefore are flexible in the amount of effort they use in a fight, they are unlikely to be directly assessing their opponents fighting abilities.

10.7.2   *Differences between individuals*

Another interesting aspect of the mating and courtship behaviour of *A. antipodianus* is that when males fight for a female, the loser of the contest does not leave, but stays near the courting and mating pair. During phase two of the courtship/mating sequence (after the first mating) the second male also tries to court and mate with the female. He will try to disrupt the mating pair by orientating towards them and then drumming or shuddering. The first male may respond to the presence of the second male by chasing him away, but this can be hazardous as the second male can circle back to the female and mate with her while his opponent is out searching for him. Alternatively, the first male may focus on the female by performing courtship displays while moving towards her (apparently ignoring the second male). This can lead to both the first and second male courting the female simultaneously (Whitehouse, 1991).

There seem to be individual differences in the likelihood that a first male will either chase the second male or ignore him (Whitehouse, 1991, Whitehouse, personal observation). In a small study which looked in detail at only a few groups of two courting males and one female, some first males did not tolerate the presence of the second male courting the female, and chased the second male whenever it was detected. In other interactions, the first male appeared to ignore the second male and continued to court the female, rarely attacking the second male.

Could these differences indicate a basic form of animal personality? Animal personality, or behavioural syndrome, is when individuals within a species show different responses to the same stimuli, but these differences are consistent in different contexts (Dingemanse *et al.*, 2010, Sih *et al.*, 2004). For example, a male that is aggressive when fighting another male may also be aggressive when trying to mate with a female. Behavioural syndromes actually indicate a reduction in flexibility in an animal's ability to respond to different situations, but an increase in flexibility in the types of responses to the same stimuli within a species.

Different *A. antipodianus* males appear to differ in their aggressiveness to the same stimuli. For example, large males with no fighting experience are more likely to escalate higher in their first male/male contest than small males (Whitehouse, 1997b). If these individual differences translate to the differences in courtship and mating behaviours between males, then this could indicate the development of a behavioural syndrome. This is an avenue of research that needs further investigation.

10.8   Conclusions and outlook

In this chapter the approaches to spider flexibility developed in the preceding chapters have been applied to the subfamily Argyrodinae. Argyrodinae are not the most successful group of spiders, nor the most intelligent, but their origins have enabled them to develop diverse approaches to web use; foraging behaviour, anti-predatory behaviour, deceptive behaviour, social behaviour, courtship and mating behaviour.

Argyrodinae owe their success to their common ancestry with the social theridiids, which has meant that they have the tools (such as tolerance of other spiders on the same web) to exploit other spider's webs. The form of the exploitation is related to the relative sizes of the Argyrodinae and the host: when the host is a lot larger than the Argyrodinae, the Argyrodinae steal from the host; when the host is the same size as the Argyrodinae, the Argyrodinae are likely to attack the host.

The interaction between the degree of tolerance expressed by different Argyrodinae species, and their propensity to exploit other spider's webs, has generated the flexibility seen in all behaviours in the Argyrodinae. For example, small Argyrodinae needed safe ways to exploit the webs of large hosts that are also potential predators. To do this they construct their own web attached to the host web. This scaffolding web has enabled a few Argyrodinae to exploit cribellate webs (on which they can get stuck), as well as ecribellate tangle webs, sheet webs and orb webs. Orb webs, and especially *Nephila* webs, are the preferred host webs of kleptoparasitic Argyrodinae, and here they use specialised and lucrative but dangerous foraging techniques, such as feeding with the host. Kleptoparasitic Argyrodinae are more tolerant of each other when feeding on the web next to the host than when moving stolen food bundles onto the support web. The ability of Argyrodinae to vary their tolerance may have been influenced by cooperative hunting dynamics, which indicate that Argyrodinae would fight for the controllable food source on the support web, but tolerate conspecifics on the uncontrollable food source at the hub. The genetic disposition towards tolerance would also enhance tolerance at the hub as fighting there would increase predation risk from the host at the hub.

The varying degrees of sociality in Argyrodinae may also influence courtship and mating behaviour. It would be interesting to do a comparative experiment testing if social Argyrodinae, in which competition for mates is strong, have more complex courtship displays than solitary Argyrodinae, which may have more problems finding a mate.

The protocerebrum of spiders is thought to be the centre of vision, learning and cognition. As Argyrodinae have very limited vision, the development of this area is likely to be limited in comparison with visual spiders such as salticids. Thus Argyrodinae need to apply their learning capacity very strategically. For example, there is no evidence that kleptoparasitic Argyrodinae recognise each other individually, but they can modify their response to contests for mates based on their past experience in fights, and they show individual differences in the strategies used to compete for mates and secure matings. In addition, Argyrodinae are able to modify their kleptoparasitic repertoire to suit the host they are exploiting, and they can modify the specialised foraging technique 'feeding with the host' to improve its effectiveness with different hosts. They even have the behavioural plasticity to enhance their exploitation of transient food sources (spiderlings) when these are abundant.

Species in the subfamily Argyrodinae use flexibility strategically in all aspects of their behaviour, even though they are not the most cognisant spiders. Thus they demonstrate that spiders should not be dismissed as mere automatons, and that in spiders the interaction between phylogenetic constraints and environmental opportunities can produce very dynamic responses.

Acknowledgements

I would like to thank Christine Lambkin, Sharon Downes, Tadashi Miyashita and especially Marie Herberstein for comments on the manuscript. I would also like to thank Robert Jackson for getting me interested in spiders and *Argyrodes* in the first place!

References

Agnarsson, I. (2002). Sharing a web: on the relation of sociality and kleptoparasitism in theridiid spiders (Theridiidae, Araneae). *Journal of Arachnology*, **30**, 181–188.

Agnarsson, I. (2004). Morphological phylogeny of cobweb spiders and their relatives (Araneae, Araneoidea, Theridiidae). *Zoological Journal of the Linnean Society*, **141**, 447–626.

Aisenberg, A. and Eberhard, W. G. (2009). Female cooperation in plug formation in a spider: effects of male copulatory courtship. *Behavioral Ecology*, **20**, 1236–1241.

Archer, A. F. (1946). The Theridiidae or comb-footed spiders of Alabama. *Alabama Museum of Natural History*, **22**, 1–67.

Arnedo, M. A., Coddington, J., Agnarsson, I. and Gillespie, R. G. (2004). From a comb to a tree: phylogenetic relationships of the comb-footed spiders (Araneae, Theridiidae) inferred from nuclear and mitochondrial genes. *Molecular Phylogenetics and Evolution*, **31**, 225–245.

Arnott, G. and Elwood, R. W. (2009). Assessment of fighting ability in animal contests. *Animal Behaviour*, **77**, 991–1004.

Baba, Y. G., Walters, R. J. and Miyashita, T. (2007). Host-dependent differences in prey acquisition between populations of a kleptoparasitic spider *Argyrodes kumadai* (Araneae: Theridiidae). *Ecological Entomology*, **32**, 38–44.

Barrantes, G. and Weng, J. L. (2007). Natural history, courtship, feeding behaviour and parasites of Theridion evexum (Araneae: Theridiidae). *Bulletin of the British Arachnological Society*, **14**, 61–65.

Berger-Tal, O., Mukherjee, S., Kotler, B. P. and Brown, J. S. (2010). Complex state-dependent games between owls and gerbils. *Ecology Letters*, **13**, 302–310.

Berry, J. W. (1987). Notes on the life history and behavior of the communal spider *Cyrtophora moluccensis* (Doleschall) (Araneae, Araneidae) in Yap, Caroline Islands. *Journal of Arachnology*, **15**, 309.

Bradoo, B. L. (1983). A new record of commensalism between *Argyrodes progiles* Tikader (Araneae: Theridiidae) and *Stegodyphus sarasinorum* Karsch. *Current Science*, **52**, 217–218.

Bouskila, A. and Blumstein, D. T. (1992). Rules of thumb for predation hazard assessment: predictions form a dynamic model. *American Naturalist*, **139**, 162–176.

Bretman, A., Lawniczak, M. K. N., Boone, J. and Chapman, T. (2010). A mating plug protein reduces early female remating in *Drosophila melanogaster*. *Journal of Insect Physiology*, **56**, 107–113.

Brown, J. S. (1988). Patch use as an indicator of habitat preference, predation risk, and competition. *Behavioral Ecology and Sociobiology*, **22**, 37–47.

Buskirk, R. E. (1981). Sociality in the Arachnida. In *Social Insects* (ed. H. R. Hermann). London: Academic Press, pp. 281–367.

Cangialosi, K. R. (1990). Life cycle and behaviour of the kleptoparasitic spider, *Argyrodes ululans* (Araneae, Theridiidae). *Journal of Arachnology*, **18**, 347–358.

Cangialosi, K. R. (1991). Attack strategies of a spider kleptoparasite: effects of prey availability and host colony size. *Animal Behaviour*, **41**, 639–647.

Cangialosi, K. R. (1997). Foraging versatility and the influence of host availability in *Argyrodes trigonum* (Araneae, Theridiidae). *Journal of Arachnology*, **25**, 182–193.

Clyne, D. (1979). *The Garden Jungle*. Sydney, Australia: Collins.

Dingemanse, N. J., Kazem, A. J. N., Réale, D. and Wright, J. (2010). Behavioural reaction norms: animal personality meets individual plasticity. *Trends in Ecology and Evolution*, **25**, 81–89.

Eberhard, W. G. (1979). *Argyrodes attenuatus* (Theridiidae): a web that is not a share. *Psyche*, **86**, 407–413.

Edwards, G. B. (2006). *Cyrtophora citricola* (Araneae: Araneidae), a colonial tentweb orbweaver established in Florida. *Florida Department of Agriculture and Consumer Services Entomology Circular*, **411**(Mar/Apr), 1–4.

Elgar, M. A. (1993). Interspecific associations involving spiders: kleptoparasitism, mimicry and mutualism. *Memoirs of the Queensland Museum*, **33**, 411–430.

Elgar, M. A. (1994). Experimental evidence of a mutualistic association between two web-building spiders. *Journal of Animal Ecology*, **63**, 880–886.

Elgar, M. A., Pope, B. and Williamson, I. (1983). Observations on the spatial distribution and natural history of *Cyrtophora hirta* (L. Koch) (Araneae: Araneidae) in Queensland, Australia. *Bulletin of the British Arachnological Society*, **6**, 83–87.

Enquist, M. and Leimar, O. (1983). Evolution of fighting behaviour: decision rules and assessment of relative strength. *Journal of Theoretical Biology*, **102**, 387–410.

Evans, T. A. (1998). Factors influencing the evolution of social behaviour in Australian crab spiders (Araneae: Thomisidae). *Biological Journal of the Linnean Society*, **63**, 205–219.

Exline, H. and Levi, H. W. (1962). American spiders of the genus *Argyrodes* (Araneae, Theridiidae). *Bulletin of the Museum of Comparative Zoology*, **127**, 75–202.

Gillespie, R. G. and Rivera, M. A. J. (2007). Free-living spiders of the genus *Ariamnes* (Araneae, Theridiidae) in Hawaii. *Journal of Arachnology*, **35**, 11–37.

Grostal, P. and Walter, D. E. (1997). Kleptoparasites or commensals? Effects of *Argyrodes antipodianus* (Araneae: Theridiidae) on *Nephila plumipes* (Araneae: Tetragnathidae). *Oecologia*, **11**, 570–574.

Hénaut, Y. (2000). Host selection by a kleptoparasitic spider. *Journal of Natural History*, **34**, 747–753.

Hénaut, Y., Delme, J., Legal, L. and Williams, T. (2005). Host selection by a kleptobiotic spider. *Naturwissenschaften*, **92**, 95–99.

Horton, C. C. (1982). Predators of two orb-web spiders (Araneae, Araneidae). *Journal of Arachnology*, **11**, 47.

Houser, J. D., Jennings, D. T. and Jakob, E. M. (2005). Predation by *Argyrodes trigonum* on *Linyphia triangularis*, an invasive sheet-web weaver in coastal Maine. *Journal of Arachnology*, **33**, 193–195.

Iwasa, Y., Higashi, M. and Yamamura, N. (1981). Prey distribution as a factor determining the choice of optimal foraging strategy. *American Naturalist*, **117**, 710–723.

Jackson, R. R. and Hallas, S. E. A. (1986). Comparative biology of *Portia africana, P. albimana, P. fimbriata, P. labiata, P. shultzi*. *New Zealand Journal of Zoology*, **13**, 423–489.

Jackson, R. R. and Wilcox, R. S. (1990). Aggressive mimicry, prey-specific predatory behavior and predator-recognition in the predator-prey interactions of *Portia fimbriata* and *Euryattus* sp., jumping spiders from Queensland. *Behavioral Ecology and Sociobiology*, **26**, 111–119.

Kerr, A. M. (2005). Behavior of web-invading spiders *Argyrodes argentatus* (Theridiidae) in *Argiope appensa* (Araneidae) host webs in Guam. *Journal of Arachnology*, **33**, 1–6.

Kerr, A. M., and Quenga, A. S. (2004). Population variation of web-invading spiders (Theridiidae: *Argyrodes* spp.) on host webs in Guam, Mariana Islands, Micronesia. *Journal of Natural History*, **38**, 671–680.

Kotler, B. P. and Blaustein, L. (1995). Titrating food and safety in a heterogeneous environment: when are the risky and safe patches of equal value? *Oikos*, **74**, 251–258.

Krafft, B. (1979). Organisation et évolution des sociétés d'araignées. *Journal de Psychologie*, **1**, 23–51.

Kullmann, E. J. (1959). Beobachtungen und Betrachtungen zum Verhalten der Theridiide *Conopistha argyrodes* Walckenaer (Araneae). *Mitteilungen aus dem Museum fuer Naturkunde in Berlin*, **35**, 275–292.

Kullmann, E. J. (1972). Evolution of social behaviour in spiders. *American Zoologist*, **12**, 419–426.

Larcher, S. F. and Wise, D. H. (1985). Experimental studies of the interactions between a web-invading spider and two host species. *Journal of Arachnology*, **13**, 43–59.

Legendre, R. (1960). Quelques remarques sur le comportement des *Argyrodes* malgaches. *Annalées des Sciences Naturelles Zoologie*, **12**, 507–512.

Legendre, R. and Lopez, A. (1975). Ultrastructure de la glande clypéale des mâles d'araignées appartenant au genre *Argyrodes* (Theridiidae). *Comptes Rendues de l'Académie des Sciences, Paris*, **281**, 1101–1103.

Lubin, Y. D. (1974). Adaptive advantages and the evolution of colony formation in *Cyrtophora* (Araneae: Araneidae). *Zoological Journal of the Linnean Society*, **34**, 321–339.

Miyashita, T. (2001). Competition for a limited space in kleptoparasitic *Argyrodes* spiders revealed by field experiments. *Population Ecology*, **43**, 97–103.

Miyashita, T. (2002). Population dynamics of two species of kleptoparasitic spiders under different host availabilities. *Journal of Arachnology*, **30**, 31–38.

Miyashita, T., Maezono, Y. and Shimazaki, A. (2004). Silk feeding as an alternative foraging tactic in a kleptoparasitic spider under seasonally changing environments. *Journal of Zoology*, **262**, 225–229.

Opell, B. D. (1998). Economics of spider orb-webs: the benefits of producing adhesive capture thread and of recycling silk. *Functional Ecology*, **12**, 613–624.

Packer, C. and Ruttan, L. (1988). The evolution of cooperative hunting. *American Naturalist*, **132**, 159–198.

Platnick, N. I. (2010). *The World Spider Catalog*, version 11.0. American Museum of Natural History. Online at http://research.amnh.org/iz/spiders/catalog/

Proctor, H. (1992). Cohabitation of six species of spiders in webs of *Cyrtophora moluccensis* (Araneae, Araneidae) in Moorea, French Polynesia. *Journal of Arachnology*, **20**, 144–145.

Robinson, M. H. and Olazarri, J. (1971). Units of behavior and complex sequences in the predatory behavior of *Argiope argentata* (Fabricius) (Araneae: Araneidae). *Smithsonian Contributions to Zoology*, **65**, 1–36.

Robinson, M. H. and Robinson, B. (1973). Ecology and behavior of the giant wood spider *Nephila maculata* (Fabricius) in New Guinea. *Smithsonian Contributions to Zoology*, **149**, 1–76.

Rypstra, A. L. (1981). The effect of kleptoparasitism on prey consumption and web relocation in a Peruvian population of the spider *Nephila clavipes*. *Oikos*, **37**, 179–182.

Shamble, P. S., Wilgers, D. J., Swoboda, K. A. and Hebets, E. A. (2009). Courtship effort is a better predictor of mating success than ornamentation for male wolf spiders. *Behavioral Ecology*, **20**, 1242–1251.

Sherman, P. M. (1994). The orb-web: an energetic and behavioural estimator of a spider's dynamic foraging and reproductive strategies. *Animal Behaviour*, **48**, 19–34.

Sih, A., Bell, A. and Johnson, J. C. (2004). Behavioral syndromes: an ecological and evolutionary overview. *Trends in Ecology and Evolution*, **19**, 372–378.

Simon, E. (1893). *Histoire Naturelle des Araignées*. Paris: Librairie Encyclopédique de Roret.

Smith Trail, D. (1980). Predation by *Argyrodes* (Theridiidae) on solitary and communal spiders. *Psyche*, **87**, 349–355.

Stephens, D. W. (1993). *Learning and Behavioural Ecology: Incomplete Information and Environmental Predictability*. New York: Chapman and Hall.

Tanaka, K. (1984). Rate of predation by a kleptoparasitic spider, *Argyrodes fissifrons*, upon a large host spider *Agelena limbata*. *Journal of Arachnology*, **12**, 363–367.

Tanaka, K. (1989). Energetic cost of web construction and its effect on web relocation in the web-building spider *Agelena limbata*. *Oecologia*, **81**, 459–464.

Taylor, P. W. and Elwood, R. W. (2003). The mismeasure of animal contests. *Animal Behaviour*, **65**, 1195–1202.

Townley, M. A. and Tillinghast, E. K. (1988). Orb web recycling in *Araneus cavaticus* (Araneae, Araneidae) with an emphasis on the adhesive spiral component, gabamide. *Journal of Arachnology*, **16**, 303–319.

Valone, T. S. and Brown, J. S. (1989). Measuring patch assessment abilities of desert granivores. *Ecology*, **70**, 1800–1810.

Vinson, A. (1863). *Aranéides des îles de la Réunion, Maurice et Madagascar*. Paris: Rovel.

Vollrath, F. (1976). Konkurrenzvermeidung bei tropischen kleptoparasitischen Haubennetzspinnen der Gattung *Argyrodes* (Arachnida: Araneae: Theridiidae). *Entomologica Germanica*, **3**, 104–108.

Vollrath, F. (1979a). Behaviour of the kleptoparasitic spider *Argyrodes elevatus* (Araneae, Theridiidae). *Animal Behaviour*, **27**, 515–521.

Vollrath, F. (1979b). Vibrations: their signal and function for a spider kleptoparasite. *Science*, **205**, 1149–1150.

Vollrath, F. (1984). Kleptobiotic interactions in invertebrates. In *Producers and Scavengers: Strategies of Exploitation and Parasitism* (ed. C. J. Barnard). London: Croom Helm, pp. 61–94.

Vollrath, F. (1987). Kleptobiosis in spiders. In *Ecophysiology of Spiders* (ed. W. Nentwig). Heidelberg, Germany: Springer Verlag, pp. 61–94.

Whitehouse, M. E. A. (1986). The foraging behaviours of *Argyrodes antipodiana* (Araneae, Theridiidae), a kleptoparasitic spider from New Zealand. *New Zealand Journal of Zoology*, **13**, 151–168.

Whitehouse, M. E. A. (1987a). Spider eat spider: the predatory behaviour of *Rhomphaea* sp. indet. from New Zealand. *Journal of Arachnology*, **15**, 355–362.

Whitehouse, M. E. A. (1987b). The external structural detail of the protrusions on the cephalothorax of male *Argyrodes antipodiana*. *Bulletin of the British Arachnological Society*, **7**, 142–144.

Whitehouse, M. E. A. (1988). Factors influencing specificity and choice of host in *Argyrodes antipodiana* (Theridiidae). *Journal of Arachnology*, **16**, 349–355.

Whitehouse, M. E. A. (1991). To mate or fight? Male-male competition and alternative mating strategies in *Argyrodes antipodiana* (Theridiidae, Araneae). *Behavioural Processes*, **23**, 163–172.

Whitehouse, M. E. A. (1992). Behavioural plasticity in the New Zealand spider *Argyrodes antipodiana*. Ph.D. thesis, University of Canterbury, New Zealand.

Whitehouse, M. E. A. (1997a). The benefits of stealing from a predator: foraging rates, predation risk, and intraspecific aggression in the kleptoparasitic spider *Argyrodes antipodiana*. *Behavioral Ecology*, **8**, 665–667.

Whitehouse, M. E. A. (1997b). Experience influences male-male contests in the spider *Argyrodes antipodiana* (Theridiidae: Araneae). *Animal Behaviour*, **53**, 913–923.

Whitehouse, M. E. A. and Jackson, R. R. (1993). Group structure and time budgets of *Argyrodes antipodiana* (Araneae, Theridiidae), a kleptoparasitic spider from New Zealand. *New Zealand Journal of Zoology*, **20**, 201–206.

Whitehouse, M. E. A. and Jackson, R. R. (1994). Intraspecific interactions of *Argyrodes antipodiana* (Araneae: Theridiidae), a kleptoparasitic spider from New Zealand. *New Zealand Journal of Zoology*, **21**, 253–268.

Whitehouse, M. E. A. and Jackson, R. R. (1998). Predatory behaviour and parental care in *Argyrodes flavipes*, a social spider from Queensland. *Journal of Zoology*, **244**, 95–105.

Whitehouse, M. E. A. and Lubin, Y. D. (2005). The functions of societies and the evolution of group living: spider societies as a test case. *Biological Reviews*, **80**, 1–15.

Whitehouse, M. E. A., Agnarsson, I., Miyashita, T., *et al.* (2002). *Argyrodes*: phylogeny, sociality and interspecific interactions: – a report on the *Argyrodes* symposium, Badplaas, 2001. *Journal of Arachnology*, **30**, 238–245.

Wiehle, H. (1928). Beiträge zur Biologie der Araneen. *Zeitschrift für Morphologie und Ökologie der Tiere*, **11**, 115–151.

Yoshida, H. (2001). The genus *Rhomphaea* (Araneae: Theridiidae) from Japan, with notes on the subfamily Argyrodinae. *Acta Arachnologica*, **50**, 183–192.

Index

Printed in the United States
By Bookmasters